1998
YEAR BOOK OF
GERIATRICS AND GERONTOLOGY®

Statement of Purpose

The Year Book Service

The Year Book series was devised in 1901 by practicing health professionals who observed that the literature of medicine and related disciplines had become so voluminous that no one individual could read and place in perspective every potential advance in a major specialty. In the final decade of the 20th century, this recognition is more acutely true than it was in 1901.

More than merely a series of books, Year Book volumes are the tangible results of a unique service designed to accomplish the following:

- to *survey* a wide range of journals of proven value
- to *select* from those journals papers representing significant advances and statements of important clinical principles
- to provide *abstracts* of those articles that are readable, convenient summaries of their key points
- to provide *commentary* about those articles to place them in perspective

These publications grow out of a unique process that calls on the talents of outstanding authorities in clinical and fundamental disciplines, trained literature specialists, and professional writers, all supported by the resources of Mosby, the world's preeminent publisher for the health professions.

The Literature Base

Mosby and its editors survey more than 1,000 journals published worldwide, covering the full range of the health professions. On an annual basis, the publisher examines usage patterns and polls its expert authorities to add new journals to the literature base and to delete journals that are no longer useful as potential Year Book sources.

The Literature Survey

The publisher's team of literature specialists, all of whom are trained and experienced health professionals, examines every original, peer-reviewed article in each journal issue. More than 250,000 articles per year are scanned systematically, including title, text, illustrations, tables, and references. Each scan is compared, article by article, to the search strategies that the publisher has developed in consultation with the 270 outside experts who form the pool of Year Book editors. A given article may be reviewed by any number of editors, from one to a dozen or more, regardless of the discipline for which the paper was originally published. In turn, each editor who receives the article reviews it to determine whether the article should be included in the Year Book. This decision is based on the article's inherent quality, its probable usefulness to readers of that Year Book, and the editor's goal to represent a balanced picture of a given field in each volume of the Year Book. In addition, the editor indicates when to include figures and tables from the article to help the YEAR BOOK reader better understand the information.

Of the quarter million articles scanned each year, only 5% are selected for detailed analysis within the YEAR BOOK series, thereby assuring readers of the high value of every selection.

The Abstract

The publisher's abstracting staff is headed by a seasoned medical professional and includes individuals with training in the life sciences, medicine, and other areas, plus extensive experience in writing for the health professions and related industries. Each selected article is assigned to a specific writer on this abstracting staff. The abstracter, guided in many cases by notations supplied by the expert editor, writes a structured, condensed summary designed so that the reader can rapidly acquire the essential information contained in the article.

The Commentary

The YEAR BOOK editorial boards, sometimes assisted by guest commentators, write comments that place each article in perspective for the reader. This provides the reader with the equivalent of a personal consultation with a leading international authority—an opportunity to better understand the value of the article and to benefit from the authority's thought processes in assessing the article.

Additional Editorial Features

The editorial boards of each YEAR BOOK organize the abstracts and comments to provide a logical and satisfying sequence of information. To enhance the organization, editors also provide introductions to sections or individual chapters, comments linking a number of abstracts, citations to additional literature, and other features.

The published YEAR BOOK contains enhanced bibliographic citations for each selected article, including extended listings of multiple authors and identification of author affiliations. Each YEAR BOOK contains a Table of Contents specific to that year's volume. From year to year, the Table of Contents for a given YEAR BOOK will vary depending on developments within the field.

Every YEAR BOOK contains a list of the journals from which papers have been selected. This list represents a subset of the more than 1,000 journals surveyed by the publisher and occasionally reflects a particularly pertinent article from a journal that is not surveyed on a routine basis.

Finally, each volume contains a comprehensive subject index and an index to authors of each selected paper.

The 1998 Year Book Series

Year Book of Allergy, Asthma, and Clinical Immunology: Drs. Rosenwasser, Borish, Gelfand, Leung, Nelson, and Szefler

Year Book of Anesthesiology and Pain Management®: Drs. Tinker, Abram, Chestnut, Roizen, Rothenberg, and Wood

Year Book of Cardiology®: Drs. Schlant, Collins, Gersh, Graham, Kaplan, and Waldo

Year Book of Chiropractic®: Dr. Lawrence

Year Book of Critical Care Medicine®: Drs. Parrillo, Balk, Calvin, Franklin, and Shapiro

Year Book of Dentistry®: Drs. Meskin, Berry, Jeffcoat, Leinfelder, Roser, Summitt, and Zakariasen

Year Book of Dermatologic Surgery®: Drs. Greenway, Papadopoulos, Whitaker, and Barrett

Year Book of Dermatology®: Dr. Thiers

Year Book of Diagnostic Radiology®: Drs. Osborn, Groskin, Dalinka, Maynard, Pentecost, Rebner, Ros, Smirniotopoulos, and Young

Year Book of Drug Therapy®: Drs. Lasagna and Weintraub

Year Book of Emergency Medicine®: Drs. Wagner, Dronen, Davidson, King, Niemann, and Roberts

Year Book of Endocrinology®: Drs. Bagdade, Braverman, Horton, Kannan, Landsberg, Molitch, Morley, Nathan, Odell, Poehlman, Rogol, and Ryan

Year Book of Family Practice®: Drs. Berg, Bowman, Davidson, Dexter, and Scherger

Year Book of Gastroenterology®: Drs. Aliperti and Fleshman

Year Book of Geriatrics and Gerontology®: Drs. Beck, Burton, Ostwald, Rabins, Reuben, Roth, Shapiro, and Whitehouse

Year Book of Hand Surgery®: Drs. Amadio and Hentz

Year Book of Hematology®: Drs. Spivak, Bell, Ness, Quesenberry, Wiernik, and Horowitz

Year Book of Infectious Diseases: Drs. Keusch, Barza, Bennish, Poutsiaka, Skolnik, and Snydman

Year Book of Medicine®: Drs. Klahr, Cline, McCallum, Frishman, Utiger, Malawista, Mandell, and Jett

Year Book of Neonatal and Perinatal Medicine®: Drs. Fanaroff, Maisels, and Stevenson

Year Book of Nephrology, Hypertension, and Mineral Metabolism: Drs. Schwab, Bennett, Emmett, Hostetter, Kumar, and Toto

Year Book of Neurology and Neurosurgery®: Drs. Bradley and Gibbs

Year Book of Nuclear Medicine®: Drs. Gottschalk, Blaufox, Neumann, Strauss, and Zubal

Year Book of Obstetrics, Gynecology, and Women's Health: Drs. Mishell, Herbst, and Kirschbaum

Year Book of Occupational and Environmental Medicine®: Drs. Emmett, Frank, Gochfeld, and Hessl

Year Book of Oncology®: Drs. Ozols, Eisenberg, Glatstein, Loehrer, Tallman, and Wiersma

Year Book of Ophthalmology®: Drs. Wilson, Augsburger, Cohen, Eagle, Grossman, Laibson, Maguire, Nelson, Penne, Rapuano, Sergott, Spaeth, Tipperman, Ms. Gosfield, and Ms. Salmon

Year Book of Orthopedics®: Drs. Morrey, Beauchamp, Currier, Tolo, Trigg, Swiontkowski

Year Book of Otolaryngology–Head and Neck Surgery®: Drs. Paparella and Holt

Year Book of Pathology and Laboratory Medicine®: Drs. Raab, Cohen, Olson, Sirgi, and Stanley

Year Book of Pediatrics®: Dr. Stockman

Year Book of Plastic, Reconstructive, and Aesthetic Surgery®: Drs. Miller, Bartlett, Garner, McKinney, Ruberg, Salisbury, and Smith

Year Book of Psychiatry and Applied Mental Health®: Drs. Talbott, Ballanger, Frances, Lydiard, Meltzer, Schowalter, and Tasman

Year Book of Pulmonary Disease®: Drs. Jett, Maurer, Ryu, Strollo, and Wenzel

Year Book of Rheumatology®: Drs. Panush, Hadler, LeRoy, Liang, Reichlin, Simon, and Weinblatt

Year Book of Sports Medicine®: Drs. Shephard, Drinkwater, Eichner, Torg, Alexander, and Mr. George

Year Book of Surgery®: Drs. Copeland, Bland, Deitch, Eberlein, Howard, Luce, Seeger, Souba, and Sugarbaker

Year Book of Thoracic and Cardiovascular Surgery®: Drs. Ginsberg, Wechsler, and Williams

Year Book of Urology®: Drs. Andriole and Coplen

Year Book of Vascular Surgery®: Dr. Porter

1998
The Year Book of GERIATRICS AND GERONTOLOGY®

Editor
John R. Burton, M.D.
Professor of Medicine, The Johns Hopkins University School of Medicine; Director, Division of Geriatric Medicine, Johns Hopkins Bayview Medical Center; Clinical Director, Division of Geriatric Medicine and Gerontology, The Johns Hopkins University, Baltimore, Maryland

Mosby

St. Louis Baltimore Boston Carlsbad Naples New York Philadelphia Portland London
Madrid Mexico City Singapore Sydney Tokyo Toronto Wiesbaden

Mosby
Dedicated to Publishing Excellence

A Times Mirror Company

Managing Editor: Gina G. Byrd
Developmental Editor: Kelly J. Poirier
Manuscript Editor: Stephanie M. Geels
Production Assistant: Laura Bayless
Manager, Literature Services: Idelle L. Winer
Illustrations and Permissions Specialist: Steve Ramay

1998 EDITION

Printed in the United States of America
Composition by Reed Technology and Information Services, Inc.
Printing/binding by Maple-Vail

Editorial Office:
Mosby, Inc.
11830 Westline Industrial Drive
St. Louis, MO 63146

Customer Service:
customer.support@mosby.com
www.mosby.com/Mosby/CustomerSupport/index.html

International Standard Serial Number: 0894-2757
International Standard Book Number: 0-8151-9631-8

Associate Editors

John C. Beck, M.D.
Professor of Medicine Emeritus, University of California, Los Angeles, California

Sharon K. Ostwald, Ph.D., R.N., C.S.
Theodore J. and Mary E. Trumble Professor; Director, Center on Aging, University of Texas—Houston School of Nursing, Houston, Texas

Peter V. Rabins, M.D., M.P.H.
Professor of Psychiatry, The Johns Hopkins University School of Medicine, Baltimore, Maryland

David B. Reuben, M.D.
Associate Professor of Medicine; Chief, Division of Geriatrics; Director, Multicampus Division of Geriatric Medicine and Gerontology, University of California, Los Angeles, California

Jesse Roth, M.D.
Raymond and Anna Lublin Professor of Medicine; Director, Division of Geriatric Medicine and Gerontology, The Johns Hopkins University School of Medicine, Baltimore, Maryland

Jay R. Shapiro, M.D.
Professor of Medicine, Division of Geriatric Medicine and Gerontology, The Johns Hopkins University School of Medicine; Program Director, General Clinical Research Center, Johns Hopkins Bayview Medical Center, Baltimore, Maryland

Peter J. Whitehouse, M.D., Ph.D.
Director, Alzheimer Center, University Hospitals of Cleveland; Professor of Neurology and Chief, Division of Behavioral and Geriatric Neurology, Case Western Reserve University, Cleveland, Ohio

Table of Contents

Journals Represented

Mosby and its editors survey more than 1,000 journals for its abstract and commentary publications. From these journals, the editors select the articles to be abstracted. Journals represented in this YEAR BOOK are listed below.

Age and Ageing
American Journal of Alzheimer's Disease
American Journal of Cardiology
American Journal of Clinical Nutrition
American Journal of Epidemiology
American Journal of Geriatric Psychiatry
American Journal of Human Genetics
American Journal of Hypertension
American Journal of Medicine
American Journal of Obstetrics and Gynecology
American Journal of Pathology
American Journal of Physiology
American Journal of Psychiatry
American Journal of Public Health
American Journal of Respiratory and Critical Care Medicine
American Journal of Surgery
Annals of Internal Medicine
Annals of Neurology
Archives of Dermatology
Archives of Family Medicine
Archives of Neurology
Archives of Ophthalmology
Archives of Physical Medicine and Rehabilitation
British Journal of General Practice
British Journal of Psychiatry
British Medical Journal
Canadian Journal of Neurological Sciences
Cancer Research
Cell
Circulation
Clinical Nurse Specialist
Clinical Pharmacology and Therapeutics
Endocrinology
European Urology
General Hospital Psychiatry
Geriatric Nursing
Gerontologist
Heart
Hepatology
Infection Control and Hospital Epidemiology
International Journal of Eating Disorders
International Journal of Geriatric Psychiatry
Journal for Healthcare Quality
Journal of Bone and Joint Surgery (American Volume)
Journal of Bone and Mineral Research
Journal of Clinical Endocrinology and Metabolism
Journal of Clinical Epidemiology

Journal of Clinical Investigation
Journal of General Internal Medicine
Journal of Gerontological Nursing
Journal of Gerontology
Journal of Infectious Diseases
Journal of Internal Medicine
Journal of Medical Genetics
Journal of Neurology, Neurosurgery and Psychiatry
Journal of Neuropathology and Experimental Neurology
Journal of Neuroscience Nursing
Journal of Neurosurgery
Journal of PeriAnesthesia Nursing
Journal of Pharmacology and Experimental Therapeutics
Journal of the American College of Surgeons
Journal of the American Geriatrics Society
Journal of the American Medical Association
Journal of the Neurological Sciences
Lancet
Maturitas
Mechanisms of Ageing and Development
Medical Care
Medical Journal of Australia
Nature
Nature Genetics
Nature Medicine
Neurology
New England Journal of Medicine
Oncology Nursing Forum
Ophthalmology
Physical Therapy
Proceedings of the National Academy of Sciences
Psychiatric Services
Psychological Medicine
Research in Nursing and Health
Scandinavian Journal of Urology and Nephrology
Science
Stroke
Urologic Nursing

Standard Abbreviations

The following terms are abbreviated in this edition: acquired immunodeficiency syndrome (AIDS), cardiopulmonary resuscitation (CPR), central nervous system (CNS), cerebrospinal fluid (CSF), computed tomography (CT), deoxyribonucleic acid (DNA), electrocardiography (ECG), health maintenance organization (HMO), human immunodeficiency virus (HIV), intensive care unit (ICU), intramuscular (IM), intravenous (IV), magnetic resonance (MR) imaging (MRI), and ribonucleic acid (RNA).

Note

The Year Book of Geriatrics and Gerontology® is a literature survey service providing abstracts of articles published in the professional literature. Every effort is made to assure the accuracy of the information presented in these pages. Neither the editors nor the publisher of the YEAR BOOK OF GERIATRICS AND GERONTOLOGY® can be responsible for errors in the original materials. The editors' comments are their own opinions. Mention of specific products within this publication does not constitute endorsement.

To facilitate the use of the YEAR BOOK OF GERIATRICS AND GERONTOLOGY® as a reference tool, all illustrations and tables included in this publication are now identified as they appear in the original article. This change is meant to help the reader recognize that any illustration or table appearing in the YEAR BOOK OF GERIATRICS AND GERONTOLOGY® may be only one of many in the original article. For this reason, figure and table numbers will often appear to be out of sequence within the YEAR BOOK OF GERIATRICS AND GERONTOLOGY®.

Introduction

I am particularly pleased with the 1998 edition of the YEAR BOOK OF GERIATRICS AND GERONTOLOGY. By having the opportunity to read all of the abstracts and editorial comments, I have learned tremendously. I believe this YEAR BOOK will provide a very useful and balanced review for clinicians and gerontologists interested in the health care of the elderly and the aging process itself.

The same experienced editorial group in place from last year has continued for the 1998 YEAR BOOK. All have selected articles that will be very valuable for many to review. Each associate editor has shared his experiences and insights in the creation of the comments.

I am deeply grateful to all of the associate editors who reviewed literally thousands of articles from well over one thousand journals. Many of these journals are well-recognized, mainstream journals. Others represent those less likely to be seen by clinicans, yet containing valuable new information. The selected papers were published between November 1996 and the end of October 1997. All associate editors have selected figures and tables that will stand out in review of the YEAR BOOK and, I believe, will increase tremendously the value of the abstract.

This volume simply could not be produced without the tremendous dedication of the administrative assistants of each associate editor. Without their continued surveillance of the many articles that are reviewed, and the careful editing of the abstracts and comments, the timely publication of this 1998 YEAR BOOK simply could not occur. I would like to thank those individuals for their dedication and commitment: Lorraine Sherwood (Beck), Pam Hill (Roth), Kathleen Kuser (Shapiro), Kate Jakobsen (Rabins), Faith Reidenbach (Whitehouse), Stephanie Ngo (Reuben), and Dianne Kirven (Oswald).

I would especially like to thank Sharon Kuta, my administrative assistant, who has had the responsibility of assembling the entire YEAR BOOK. She works 12 months a year on this project, and, without her organization and dedication to the multiple versions of the text, we simply would not be able to produce it.

I and the associate editors are grateful to the staff of Mosby, Inc. for their continued commitment to produce a high-quality book. This has been a particularly difficult year, with the relocation of the offices of the YEAR BOOK from Chicago to St. Louis, and many worked above and beyond the call of duty to get this edition out on time. We are especially grateful to Kelly Poirier who, again this year, has been the developmental editor. Her equanimity and dedication, both of which she displayed in great quantity over the months, are deeply appreciated.

This year, I'd like to bring the attention of the readers to the fact that 96 different journals emanating from 32 countries have participated in the publishing of papers collected under the rubric "global theme issues on aging." Interested readers may thumb through journals in their own libraries and find a variety of articles that cover broadly the field of geriatic medicine and gerontology and provide truly a world perspective on aging.

I truly hope that you will find the 1998 YEAR BOOK OF GERIATRICS AND GERONTOLOGY a very valuable and easy-to-read review.

John R. Burton, M.D.

1 Clinical Geriatrics

Introduction

The knowledge used to provide evidence-based care for older persons continues to increase at a rapid pace. For purposes of this chapter, these advances can be categorized into five groups: (1) prevention, (2) clinical epidemiology, (3) geriatric syndromes, (4) diseases affecting organ systems, and (5) health care delivery.

Within "prevention," research has helped clarify the link between total cholesterol and death due to coronary heart disease, and several studies have helped define the indications and management of oral anticoagulation. Careful observational epidemiological studies have identified cancer risks associated with calcium channel blocker use and bone mineral density. The list of adverse effects of smoking and beneficial effects of estrogen continues to be extended. Among the geriatric syndromes, major advances in osteoporosis research have identified further benefits from hormonal, bisphosphonate, and vitamin D therapy.

Important advances have been made in several disease systems. In cardiology, research has been directed at evaluating new methods, through both pharmacology and clinical care, aimed at reducing the complications of congestive heart failure. Of note are major studies evaluating losartan and carvedilol. Clinical aspects of community-acquired pneumonia and bacterial endocarditis in older persons have been clarified in case series. The benefit of treating subclinical hypothyroidism has been studied in a small randomized clinical trial. The value of exercise programs to reduce symptoms of knee osteoarthritis has been studied in a large clinical trial.

Finally, several health care delivery studies are beginning to unravel some of the differences in care for older persons that is provided by managed care as compared with that provided by fee-for-service Medicare. Within the managed care environment, an innovative group clinic was able to reduce utilization below that of traditional managed care of older persons.

As the reader will soon discover, the choice of 1998 YEAR BOOK OF GERATRICS AND GERONTOLOGY selections indicates a field that continues to burgeon.

David B. Reuben, M.D.

Prevention

Clarifying the Direct Relation Between Total Cholesterol Levels and Death From Coronary Heart Disease in Older Persons

Corti M-C, Guralnik JM, Salive ME, et al (Natl Inst on Aging, Bethesda, Md; US Food and Drug Administration, Rockville, Md; Natl Inst for Research and Care of the Elderly, Fiesole, Italy; et al)

Ann Intern Med 126:753–760, 1997 1–1

Introduction.—There is debate over whether the total cholesterol level can predict coronary heart disease in older adults and whether cholesterol reduction is useful in primary prevention of coronary heart disease in this age group. Total cholesterol may have a different relationship to coronary heart disease in older vs. younger adults, or other factors—such as frailty and concomitant diseases—may intervene in the relationship between risk factor and outcome. Data from the Established Populations for Epidemiologic Study in the Elderly were used to assess the direct role of total cholesterol as a risk factor for coronary heart disease mortality in elderly people.

Methods.—The analysis included prospective data on a community-based cohort of 4,066 men and women, all at least age 65 at baseline. The mean age was 79; 5% of the cohort was African-American. In 1988, the subjects underwent interviews and blood sampling. They were followed up for mortality through 1992. Total cholesterol was evaluated as a predictor of mortality before and after adjustment for coronary heart disease risk factors and measures of frailty.

Results.—Two hundred fifty-two patients died of coronary heart disease events during follow-up. On unadjusted analyses, coronary heart disease mortality was highest for patients with the lowest total cholesterol levels (i.e., 160 mg/dL or less) and lowest for those with the highest total cholesterol levels (240 mg/dL or higher). Subsequent analyses adjusted for known risk factors for coronary heart disease and indicators of poor health, such as chronic diseases, low serum iron, and low serum albumin. Also, 44 patients who died of coronary heart disease within the first year of follow-up were excluded. These analyses showed that high total cholesterol levels were associated with a high risk of death from coronary heart disease. As total cholesterol level declined, so did the risk of coronary heart disease mortality (Figure).

Conclusion.—Elevated total cholesterol levels carry an increased risk of death from coronary heart disease in older adults. Factors related to comorbidity and frailty account for the apparent "adverse effects" of low cholesterol values in this age group reported in previous studies. The elderly should not be excluded from cholesterol screening studies, although judgment must be used in interpreting the results. The only way to tell whether cholesterol screening and lipid-reducing therapy are of benefit in the elderly is through randomized, controlled trials.

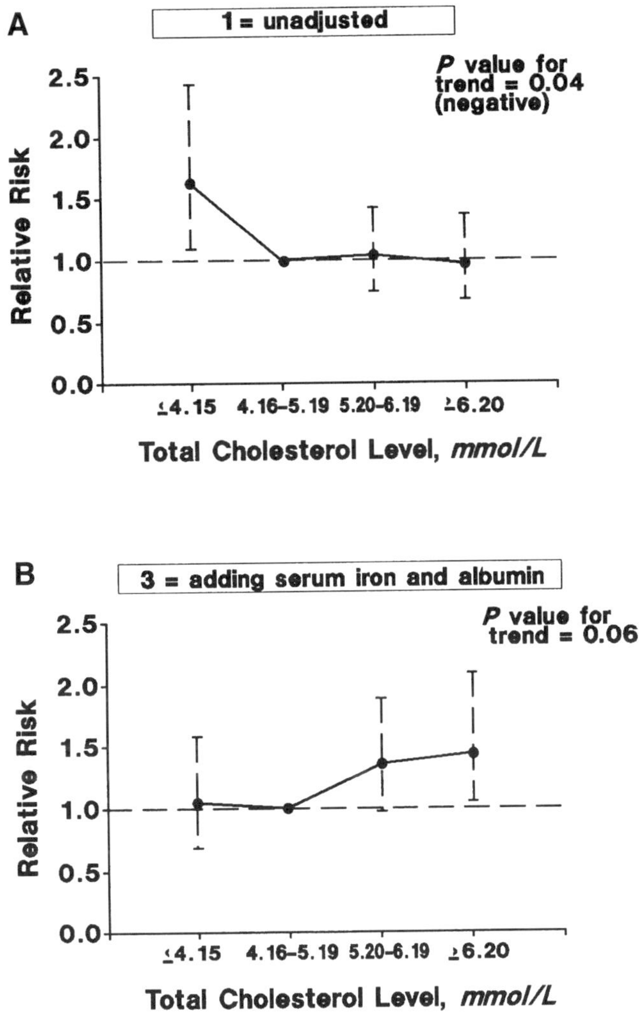

FIGURE.—Relative risks for death from coronary heart disease (*CHD*) according to total cholesterol level before and after stepwise inclusion of adjustment variables and exclusion of first-year events. Relative risks are from 4 separate community-stratified proportional-hazard models. A, model 1 is adjusted for high-density lipoprotein cholesterol levels only and includes all events. C, model 2 is adjusted for age, sex, and risk factors for coronary heart disease and includes all events. B, model 3 is adjusted for age, sex, risk factors for coronary heart disease and serum iron and albumin levels and includes all events. D, model 4 is adjusted for age, sex, risk factors for coronary heart disease and serum iron and albumin levels and excludes first-year events. Risk factors for coronary heart disease include high-density lipoprotein cholesterol level; isolated systolic hypertension; diastolic hypertension; alcohol consumption; smoking; and history of high blood pressure, diabetes, heart attack, and stroke. (Courtesy of Corti M-C, Guralnik JM, Salive ME, et al: Clarifying the direct relation between total cholesterol levels and death from coronary heart disease in older persons. *Ann Intern Med* 126:753–760, 1997.)

(*Continued*)

FIGURE (cont.)

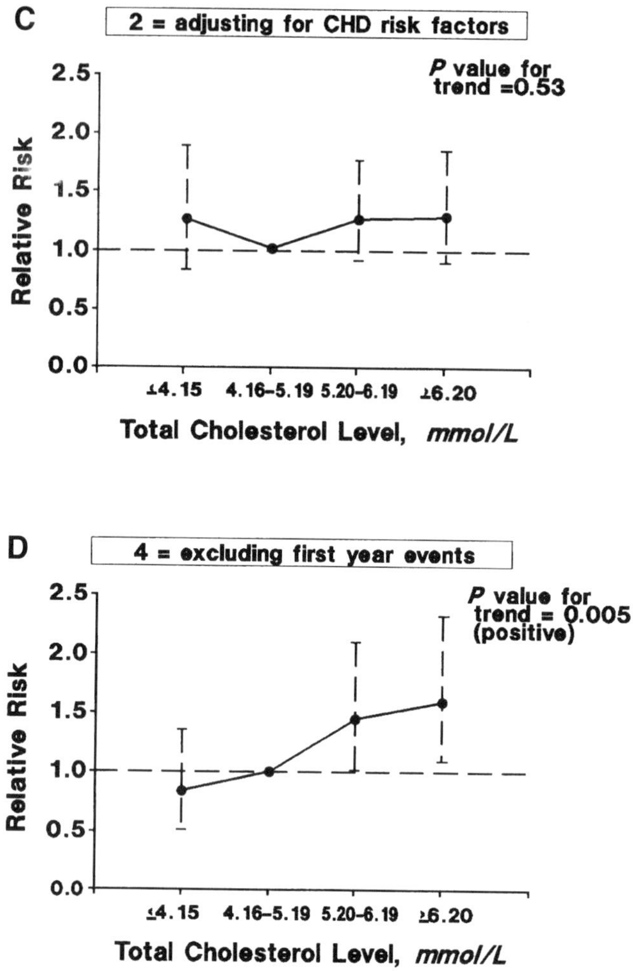

► The question of the importance of increased serum cholesterol levels in coronary artery disease remains unanswered. Several studies have demonstrated "J-shaped" curves with increased mortality associated with low cholesterol levels, and others have shown no relationship at all. This analysis of the Established Populations for Epidemiologic Studies in the Elderly examined the role of comorbidity and frailty as confounders that might explain previous findings.

Consistent with other studies, crude coronary heart disease mortality rates were highest in the lowest serum total cholesterol category. However, after adjustment for coronary heart disease risk factors, the inverse relationship disappeared. When further adjustment was made for serum markers of poor health (low iron and albumin), the direction of the relationship reversed.

Moreover, when coronary heart disease events during the first year of follow-up were excluded, both borderline and elevated total cholesterol levels were associated with significant risk for death from coronary heart disease. This research strongly suggests that the apparent "J-shaped" curve of the relationship between serum cholesterol and coronary artery mortality reflects 2 populations: the frail for whom hypocholesterolemia is an indication of poor health and those who are healthy and have the same cholesterol-to-coronary-disease relationship that has been demonstrated for middle-aged adults.

D.B. Reuben, M.D.

Serum Lipids and Incidence of Coronary Heart Disease: Findings From the Systolic Hypertension in the Elderly Program (SHEP)

Frost PH, for the Systolic Hypertension in the Elderly Research Group (Univ of California, San Francisco; et al)

Circulation 94:2381–2388, 1996 1–2

Objective.—The risk of coronary heart disease (CHD) in middle-aged individuals is directly related to total and LDL cholesterol level and inversely related to HDL cholesterol level. There is less information about CHD risk factors in individuals over age 60 even though most CHD incidents occur in men over 60 and women over 70. Findings of the Systolic Hypertension in the Elderly Program, a randomized, placebo-controlled, double-blind, multicenter clinical trial, show that CHD is associated with serum total cholesterol, non-HDL cholesterol, and LDL cholesterol levels in men and women.

Methods.—Blood pressure values, cholesterol levels, and triglyceride levels were measured in 4,736 individuals (14% black, 43% men) at least ≥60 with elevated blood pressure. Patients were randomly assigned to therapy or placebo groups. Outcomes were decreases in occurrence of fatal and nonfatal stroke and monitoring of major CHD incidents.

Results.—Mean systolic and diastolic blood pressures were 170 and 77 mm Hg, respectively; mean total cholesterol, HDL cholesterol, and non-HDL cholesterol levels were 236 mg/dL, 54 mg/dL, and 182 mg/dL, respectively; fasting triglyceride values were 144 mg/dL. Patients were followed up for an average of 4.5 years. Patients had 245 nonfatal myocardial infarctions or fatal CHD during the study. Multivariate analysis established a relation between myocardial infarction and CHD events and total cholesterol, LDL and non-HDL cholesterol levels, cholesterol measures to HDL ratios, and triglycerides.

Conclusion.—HDL was not a risk factor for CHD. Non-HDL cholesterol appears to be a CHD risk factor indicator in older individuals. Controlling non-HDL cholesterol levels could reduce the incidence of CHD by 23% to 30%. The patients in this study were healthy volunteers and therefore may not be representative of the older population. Whether reducing the risk factors will result in a clinical benefit to this cohort is not known.

► This is an important paper because of its convincing evidence of a relation between serum lipids and CHD in an older population, confirming much more limited studies than have been previously reported.[1–7] The multicenter SHEP study of systolic hypertension involved a large heterogeneous group of individuals of men and women age 60 or older who had extensive baseline measurements and systematic recording of both cardiovascular and noncardiovascular events. The large sample size and its racial heterogeneity are clearly advantageous over the previous studies that have been reported, but it must be emphasized that this study cannot be construed as population based because the selection criteria included established isolated systolic hypertension (in itself a risk factor) and a healthy older cohort interested in general health maintenance. The results, I believe, clearly support the inference that serum lipids are CHD risk factors in older American men and women and raises the intriguing issue of whether this risk reduction will be followed by clinical benefit. Clearly the SHEP study showed clinical benefit of blood pressure reduction, and other studies have shown substantial reduction in CHD mortality rate with smoking cessation. It would thus be attractive to support the view that reduction in lipid risk factors would lead to additional benefit. This finding is at least in part supported by the Scandinavian Simvastatin Survival Study,[8] which enrolled participants age 50 to 70 at baseline and monitored them for a mean of 5.4 years with clear benefit. However, the intriguing question of whether primary CHD prevention in adults older than 65 would lead to benefit remains unanswered.

J.C. Beck, M.D.

References

1. Barrett-Conner E, Suarez L, Khaw K, et al: Ischemic heart disease risk factors after age 50. *J Chron Dis* 37:903–908, 1984.
2. Castelli WP, Wilson WF, Levy D, et al: Cardiovascular risk factors in the elderly. *Am J Cardiol* 63:12H–19H, 1989.
3. Benfante R, Reed D: Is elevated serum cholesterol level a risk factor for coronary heart disease in the elderly? *JAMA* 263:393–396, 1990.
4. Rubin SM, Sidney S, Black DM, et al: High blood cholesterol in elderly men and the excess risk for coronary heart disease. *Ann Intern Med* 113:916–920, 1990.
5. Shipley MJ, Pocock SJ, Marmot MG: Does plasma cholesterol concentration predict mortality from coronary heart disease in elderly people? 18 year follow up in the Whitehall Study. *BMJ* 303:89–92, 1991.
6. Stamler J, Dyer AR, Shekelle RB, et al: Relationship of baseline major risk factors to coronary and all-cause mortality, and to longevity: Findings from long-term follow-up of Chicago cohorts. *Cardiology* 82:191–222, 1993.
7. Kannel WB, Larson M: Long-term epidemiologic prediction of coronary disease: The Framingham experience. *Cardiology* 82:137–152, 1993.
8. Scandinavian Simvastatin Survival Study Group: Randomized trial of cholesterol lowering in 4444 patients with coronary heart disease: The Scandinavian Simvastatin Survival Study (4S). *Lancet* 344:1383–1389, 1994.

Cost Effectiveness of Simvastatin Treatment to Lower Cholesterol Levels in Patients With Coronary Heart Disease

Johannesson M, for the Scandanavian Simvastatin Survival Study Group (Stockholm School of Economics, et al)

N Engl J Med 336:332–336, 1997 1–3

Objective.—The Scandinavian Simvastatin Survival Study showed that simvastatin brought about a 30% reduction in overall mortality in patients with coronary heart disease that was caused solely by a 42% reduction in mortality from coronary causes. Whether broad use of cholesterol-lowering drugs is merited depends on the cost effectiveness of such treatment. Estimates of the cost effectiveness of simvastatin in relation to age, sex, and baseline cholesterol values in patients with coronary heart disease were presented.

Methods.—Costs per year of life gained were estimated for 2,242 men and 2,410 women age 35–70, taking simvastatin to reduce cholesterol levels ranging from 213 to 309 mg/dL and who had a history of angina pectoris or acute myocardial infarction. Costs included intervention plus the direct and indirect costs associated with morbidity resulting from coronary disease.

Results.—The direct costs of intervention per year of life gained after 5 years of treatment ranged from $11,400 for men and $27,400 for women, age 35, with a pretreatment cholesterol level of 213 mg/dL, to $3,800 for men and $6,200 for women, age 70, with a pretreatment cholesterol level of 309 mg/dL. Seventy-year-old men and women with a pretreatment cholesterol level of 213 incurred direct costs of $6,200 and $13,300, respectively. When both direct and indirect costs were included, there was a net saving for every year of life gained for 35-year-old men and women at all pretreatment cholesterol levels. Intervention costs for men and women age 70 remained unchanged at all pretreatment cholesterol levels. These estimated cost-effectiveness ratios were within the range considered cost effective in other studies. Goldman et al. found higher cost-effectiveness ratios for women younger than 55 with cholesterol levels less than 250 mg/dL.

Conclusion.—Simvastatin therapy is effective and cost effective in reducing overall mortality and mortality from coronary events in patients with coronary heart disease. Cost estimate data were based on actual significant reductions in coronary events and overall mortality in a randomized clinical study. These estimates cannot be applied to primary intervention because patients in this study had coronary heart disease and were, therefore, at high risk for coronary events. Cerebrovascular events were reduced in this study by 30%.

▶ This is the third report of the Scandanavian Simvastatin Survival Study (4S) that deals with the cost effectiveness of the trial and sheds important light on this critical issue.[1, 2] This analysis addresses the cost effectiveness of lowering cholesterol levels with simvastatin in relation to the age, sex, and cholesterol levels of patients with coronary heart disease in a very large prospective study. The estimated cost-effectiveness ratios were well within the range that has been considered cost effective in other studies.[3-6] The use of simvastatin is cost effective in both men and women at the ages and cholesterol levels studied and reported in the article. It is important to emphasize that the 4S study was directed at persons who already had symptoms of coronary artery disease, and, thus, the data do not apply to primary prevention in which the absolute risks of coronary heart disease are much lower.

The paper confirms the American observations by Goldman, et al[6] and is probably more accurate because the study abstracted here was a prospective one and excluded the possible beneficial effects on cerebrovascular events. In the 4S study, cerebrovascular events were reduced by 30% and, thus, the cost-effectiveness ratio might have been even higher.

J.C. Beck, M.D.

References

1. Pedersen TR, Kjekshus J, Berg K, et al: Cholesterol lowering and the use of health care resources: Results of the Scandinavian Simvastatin Survival Study. *Circulation* 93:1796–1802, 1996.
2. Jönsson B, Johannesson M, Kjekshus J, et al: Cost-effectiveness of cholesterol lowering: Results from the Scandinavian Simvastatin Survival Study (4S). *Eur Heart J* 17:1001–1007, 1996.
3. Tosteson AN, Rosenthal DI, Melton LJ III, et al: Cost-effectiveness of screening perimenopausal white women for osteoporosis: Bone densitometry and hormone replacement therapy. *Ann Intern Med* 113:594–603, 1990.
4. Littenberg B, Garber AM, Sox HC Jr: Screening for hypertension. *Ann Intern Med* 112:192–202, 1990.
5. Hay JW, Wittels EH, Gotton AM Jr: An economic evaluation of lovastatin for cholesterol lowering and coronary artery disease reduction. *Am J Cardiol* 57:789–796, 1991.
6. Goldman L, Weinstein MC, Goldman PA, et al: Cost-effectiveness of HMG-CoA reductase inhibition for primary and secondary prevention of coronary heart disease. *JAMA* 265:1145–1151, 1991.

The Duration of Oral Anticoagulant Therapy After a Second Episode of Venous Thromboembolism

Schulman S, and the Duration of Anticoagulation Trial Study Group (Karolinska Hosp, Stockholm; et al)

N Engl J Med 336:393–398, 1997 1–4

Introduction.—Two recent multicenter trials have shown that extending the duration of oral anticoagulant therapy after a first episode of venous thromboembolism can reduce the rate of recurrence. Because the optimal duration of prophylactic oral anticoagulation after a second episode has not been determined, a multicenter trial was designed to compare the benefits of treatment for 6 months with indefinite treatment.

Methods.—During the 3-year enrollment period, 227 patients were randomly assigned to the 2 treatment groups. Eligible patients were at least 15-years-old and had a second episode of acute pulmonary embolism or deep-vein thrombosis in the leg, the iliac veins, or both. Initial treatment consisted of heparin for at least 5 days; oral anticoagulation with warfarin sodium or dicumarol was usually started at the same time as heparin therapy. The target chosen for the international normalized ratio was 2.0 to 2.85. Patients in the 6-month group discontinued oral anticoagulant therapy without tapering at their 6-month evaluation. Principal end points of the study were major hemorrhage, recurrent venous thromboembolism, and death.

Results.—There were 26 recurrences of venous thromboembolism during the 48 months of follow-up. Only 3 recurrences (2.6%) were in the indefinite therapy group, compared with 23 in the 6-month group (20.7%). No recurrence took place during anticoagulation therapy (the 3 patients in the indefinite therapy group had prematurely discontinued therapy). When compared with therapy of indefinite duration, the relative risk of recurrence in the group assigned to 6 months of oral anticoagulation therapy was 8.0 (Fig 1). Thirteen major hemorrhages occurred, 3 in the 6-month group (2.7%) and 10 in the indefinite treatment group (8.6%). The relative risk of major hemorrhage in the 6-month group was 0.3.

Discussion.—The risk of major hemorrhagic complications has been a deterrent to the long-term use of oral anticoagulant therapy after a second episode of venous thromboembolism. There was a trend toward an in-

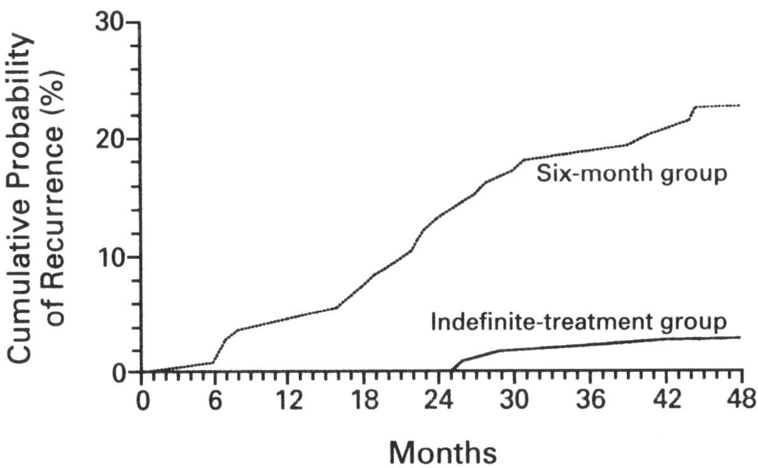

FIGURE 1.—Cumulative probability of recurrent venous thromboembolism in patients with a second episode, according to the duration of assigned anticoagulant therapy. (Reprinted by permission of *The New England Journal of Medicine*, from Schulman S, and the Duration of Anticoagulation Trial Study Group: The duration of oral anticoagulant therapy after a second episode of venous thromboembolism. *N Engl J Med* 336:393–398, 1997. Copyright 1997, Massachusetts Medical Society. All rights reserved.)

creased risk of major hemorrhage with indefinite duration of therapy, but this was offset by a much lower rate of recurrent thromboembolism.

► The acute and long-term treatment of thromboembolic disease continues to be in evolution. New regimens for the treatment of acute disease, including those that can be administered at home,[1] have been developed and studies are beginning to define the optimal duration of therapy for an initial episode.[2] In this randomized trial, the question was how long to maintain anticoagulation in patients who had a second episode of venous thromboembolism. In one arm of the study, patients were treated for 6 months and in the other arm, they were treated indefinitely. After 4 years of follow-up, 21% of those who had received only 6 months of treatment had recurrence compared with only 3% of those receiving therapy indefinitely. However, there were more major hemorrhages in the indefinite-treatment group. The study does not exclude the possiblity that subgroups exist for whom treatment does not need to be continued indefinitely or that prolonged (beyond 6 months) but not lifelong treatment may be effective. Nevertheless, until evidence to the contrary is provided, the prudent approach to treating recurrent thromboembolic disease is lifelong anticoagulation therapy.

D.B. Reuben, M.D.

References

1. The Columbus Investigators: Low-molecular weight heparin in the treatment of patients with venous thromboembolism. *N Engl J Med* 337:657–662, 1997.
2. Schulman S, Rhedin A-S, Linmarker P, et al: A comparison of six weeks with six months of oral anticoagulant therapy after a first episode of venous thromboembolism. *N Engl J Med* 332:1661–1665, 1995.

Correction of Excessive Anticoagulation With Low-dose Oral Vitamin K_1

Weibert RT, Le DT, Kayser SR, et al (Univ of California, San Diego; Univ of California, San Francisco)
Ann Intern Med 125:959–962, 1997 1–5

Background.—Many patients taking warfarin have excessive anticoagulation, with an international normalized ratio (INR) of greater than 5.0, which carries an increased risk of hemorrhage. Vitamin K_1 (phytonadione) was once well accepted as an effective treatment for reducing excessive anticoagulation. However, this treatment appears to have been neglected in recent years. The authors review their experience with the use of vitamin K_1 to correct excessive anticoagulation.

Methods.—The review included 81 patients experiencing anticoagulation with episodes of excessive anticoagulation and having an INR greater than 5.0. None had significant bleeding complications. All patients were managed with a single 2.5 mg oral dose of vitamin K_1 and withholding of 1 or 2 doses of warfarin. Twenty-four to 48 hours later, the INR was measured and the warfarin dose adjusted accordingly. All INRs were

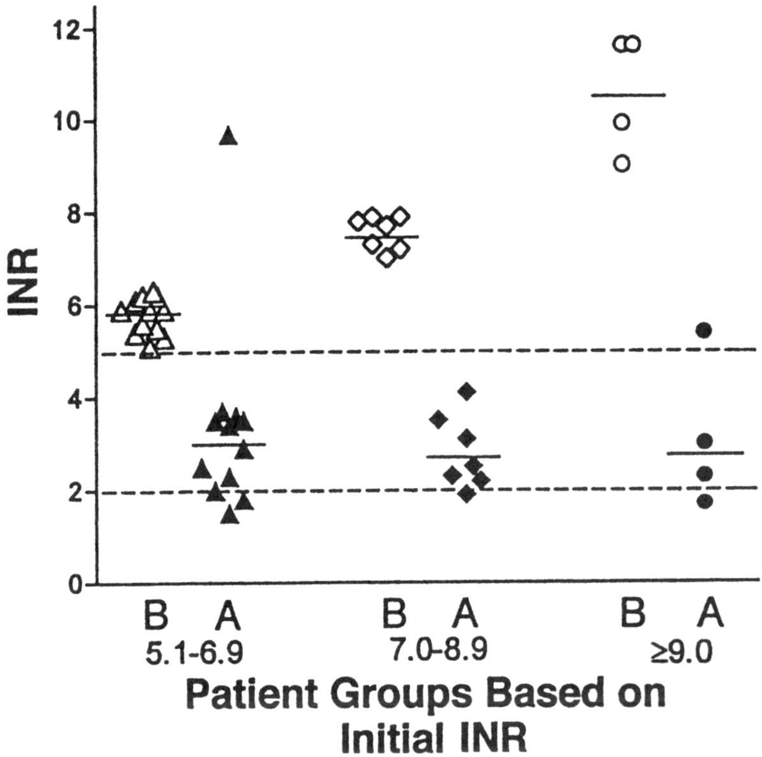

FIGURE 2.—The effect on the international normalized ratio (INR) 48 hours after patients received 2.5 mg of oral vitamin K_1 and had 2 doses of warfarin withheld. Data are grouped according to the initial INR for each patient. Open symbols (*B columns*) are INRs before patients received vitamin K_1; closed symbols (*A columns*) are INRs 48 hours after patients received vitamin K_1. The dashed lines delineate the target range for correcting excessive anticoagulation (an INR between 2.0 and 5.0). The solid lines delineate geometric mean INRs. (Courtesy of Weibert RT, Le DT, Kayser SR, et al: Correction of excessive anticoagulation with low-dose oral vitamin K_1. *Ann Intern Med* 125:959–962, 1997.)

measured using a portable capillary fingerstick monitor or automated photo-optical coagulometer.

Results.—In 96% of patients, giving oral vitamin K_1 successfully reduced the INR to less than 5.0 (Fig 2). In no case did the treatment cause resistance to subsequent anticoagulation. There were no cases of clinical thromboembolism.

Conclusions.—This experience shows the effectiveness of oral vitamin K_1 (combined with withholding 1 or 2 doses of warfarin) for patients with excessive anticoagulation. This is a reliable, safe, and inexpensive approach for patients who are not having a serious bleeding episode and whose INR is between 5.0 and 10.0. The authors hope that their experience will help to overcome the current reluctance to use vitamin K_1 for this indication.

► With the recognition that oral anticoagulation with warfarin is effective in reducing strokes in individuals with non-rheumatic atrial fibrillation, its use is increasing among older persons. Despite its effectiveness, oral anticoagulation is associated with the risk of bleeding, particularly when the INR exceeds 5.0. Unfortunately, even with the most meticulous monitoring, some patients' INR levels will periodically exceed the therapeutic range. In this case series, the authors evaluated the effect of giving 2.5 mg of oral vitamin K_1 on the INRs of patients who initially had INRs exceeding 5.0. It appears that giving 1 dose of Vitamin K and withholding 1 or 2 doses of warfarin is enough to bring the vast majority of patients back into a therapeutic range. When prescribing warfarin, it might be advisable to also prescribe Vitamin K for patients to have on hand should they become excessively over anticoagulated.

D.B. Reuben, M.D.

Does Multiple Risk Factor Reduction Explain the Reduction in Fall Rate in the Yale FICSIT Trial?

Tinetti ME, McAvay G, Claus E (Yale Univ, New Haven, Conn)
Am J Epidemiol 144:389–399, 1996 1–6

Background.—The risk of falls in older persons increases with the number of impairments in different areas. It follows that the risk of falls may be reduced by ameliorating as many of the impairments as possible. However, having many impairments may reduce the patient compensatory abilities. Compensatory abilities may be restored by means of a multiple risk factor abatement approach. In the Yale Frailty and Injuries Cooperative Studies of Intervention Techniques (FICSIT) trial, the rate of falls was significantly reduced among elderly individuals assigned to a multiple risk factor abatement intervention trial. This study assessed the relationship between changes in the studied risk factors and the occurrence of falls.

Methods.—The analysis included 301 community-dwelling older adults. Of those, 153 were assigned to a multifactorial targeted intervention (TI) and 148 to a social visit (SV) control group. The number of falls during a 6-month period was significantly reduced in the TI group. The 2 groups were compared for changes in risk factors related to falling.

Results.—Subjects assigned to the TI group showed significantly more improvement in several risk areas than those in the SV group, including postural blood pressure change, step length use of 4 or more medications, and unsafe tub and toilet transfers. There was also a borderline-significant change in balance favoring the TI group. As assessed by a composite risk factor score, 42% of subjects in the TI group were in the highest tertile for risk-factor reduction, compared to 22% of the SV group. For the T1 group, the rate of falls per person per year decreased to 0.83 among subjects with the least risk reduction, 0.62 in those with intermediate risk reduction, and 0.26 for those with the greatest risk reduction. Regardless of group assignment, fall rates were similar for patients who achieved the greatest and lowest risk reductions.

Conclusions.—Interventions to reduce multiple risk factors for falling among the elderly are feasible, assessable, and effective. Interventions designed to ameliorate postural blood pressure change, balance and transfers, and gait seem particularly effective; medication review should probably be included as well. The findings suggest that it is feasible and more appropriate to design a specific intervention protocol for the individual than to offer a standard protocol.

► Most problems in older adults, whether they be geriatric syndromes or a variety of chronic diseases, are the result of the accumulated effect of multiple risk factors. This is beautifully demonstrated in the article by Mary Tinetti and her colleques, which expands on the findings reported in the YEAR BOOK 2 years ago when the main findings of the study were reported in *The New England Journal of Medicine.*[1] The geriatric syndrome—falling—is an excellent model to address the components of the process of an intervention that leads to a favorable outcome. A multiple risk factor abatement strategy is often considered inappropriate because the problem to date with most of these studies has been the difficulty in determining which component or components were responsible for the treatment effect. This paper demonstrates that mechanisms of response can be addressed by analytic methodologies in multiple risk factor intervention studies. As had previously been reported,[1] the multiple risk factor reduction strategy of the Yale FICSIT Trial resulted in a significant reduction in fall rates among community-living older individuals. This present analysis demonstrates that the intervention resulted in a reduced presence or severity of at least 5 of the 8 targeted risk factors and that reductions in several of these risk factors were, in turn, associated with a reduction in the occurrence of falling. The important risk factors in this study were postural blood pressure change, balance, transfers, gait, and medications, because much of the improvement in postural blood pressure drop was related to medication review and adjustment. The important message from this analysis is that it is appropriate to tailor intervention protocols to individuals rather than to tailor individuals to a standardized protocol as is the more usual practice.

J.C. Beck, M.D.

Reference

1. Tinetti ME, Baker DI, McAvay G, et al: A multifactorial intervention to reduce the risk of falling among elderly people living in the community. *N Engl J Med* 331:821–827, 1994.

Effectiveness of Water Exercise on Postural Mobility in the Well Elderly: An Experimental Study on Balance Enhancement

Simmons V, Hansen PD (Northern Arizona Univ, Flagstaff; Univ of Puget Sound, Tacoma, Wash)

J Gerontol 51A:M233–M238, 1996 1–7

Introduction.—Falls are a common health problem in the elderly. Due to a fear of falling, older people tend to restrict their activity, which, in turn, may cause a decrease in functional mobility. This study was based on the hypothesis that older persons fear to make movement errors, restrict activity, and lose skill in postural tasks. It then applied training principles discovered through motor skill acquisition research. Because it was hypothesized that postural capabilities would improve by having the elderly exercise in a risk-free environment, water was chosen for the experiment.

Methods.—Fifty-two independently living elderly volunteers (age 80 ± 5.8 years) were randomly assigned into 1 of 4 groups: (1) land sitters, (2) water sitters, (3) land exercisers, and (4) water exercisers. For a period of 5 weeks, each group met twice per week for 45 minutes to perform exercises. Prior to the experiment and at the end of each week, the distance each individual could reach (functional reach) was measured.

Results.—At the beginning of the sessions, there were no significant differences in the functional reach of the groups. However, after 5 weeks, the functional reach was 13.4 ± 1.6 inches for the water exercisers, 11.3 ± 1.5 inches for the land exercisers, 9.6 ± 0.71 inches for the water sitters, and 9.3 ± 0.71 inches for the land sitters. The water exercisers had a large functional reach improvement for the first 2 weeks, a slower rate between the second and fourth weeks, and a larger improvement in weeks 4 and 5. While the land exercisers had a large improvement between the start and the end of the first week, they demonstrated slower improvement between the second week and the end of the test. The water and land sitters showed little improvement over the course of the study. After 10 months, 80% of the water exercisers were still exercising in the pool, while none of the land exercisers continued their program. There were no orthopedic injuries in the water exerciser group, while there was one broken hip and one fractured wrist in the land exerciser group.

Conclusion.—The production of movement errors in a water environment or the initiation of a novel exercise program on land enhanced the postural capabilities of elderly people. A wider range of movement without an increase in the risk of injury due to a fall was experienced by the participants in the water exercise program. They were able to reach farther at the end of the study, and were more compliant following the study.

▶ A variety of exercise programs have been designed to prevent falls and promote health in older persons, and many of these have been formally evaluated in clinical trials. Water exercises have become increasingly popular and may be safer because of the physical properties of water (e.g., buoyancy).

In this small trial, the effect of water exercise was compared to land exercise, using an identical protocol of 45-minute, twice-per-week exercises on functional reach. Two control groups were also used, one in water, the other on land. Both sets of exercisers improved over the 5 weeks, but the water exercisers improved the most. At 5 weeks, the difference between water exercisers and land exercisers was statistically significant. At 10–12 months after the last session of the study, 80% of the water exercisers were still exercising in the pool. Although the sample size of this study was small and the end point—functional reach—was not a clinical outcome, the study's findings are provocative and should stimulate further research on the benefits of water-based exercise programs.

D.B. Reuben, M.D.

Vitamin E Supplementation and In Vivo Immune Response in Healthy Elderly Subjects: A Randomized Controlled Trial

Meydani SN, Meydani M, Blumberg JB, et al (Tufts Univ, Boston; Dana Farber Cancer Inst, Boston; Veterans Affairs Med Ctr, Boston; et al)

JAMA 277:1380–1386, 1997 1–8

Background.—The humoral and cell-mediated immune responses both change with aging. One contributing factor is the aging-related increase in prostaglandin E_2 (PGE_2) production. Studies in mice have suggested that a high level of vitamin E supplementation can reduce PGE_2 production. Various levels of vitamin E supplementation were studied for their effects on measures of cell-mediated immunity in elderly people.

Methods.—The randomized, double-blind, placebo-controlled trial included 88 healthy adults age 65 or older. They were assigned to receive 8 months of treatment with vitamin E at a dose of 60, 200, or 800 mg/day or placebo. The indicators of cell-mediated immunity were selected for their clinical relevance: delayed-type hypersensitivity skin response (DTH); antibody responses to hepatitis B, tetanus and diphtheria, and pneumococcal vaccines; and autoantibodies to DNA and thyroglobulin.

Results.—By 4 months, some indicators of cell-mediated immunity were significantly improved in subjects taking vitamin E. For subjects in the 200 mg/day group, DTH increased by 65% and antibody titer to hepatitis B increased sixfold, compared with 17% and threefold, respectively, in the placebo group; 41% and threefold in the 60 mg/day group; and 49% and 2.5-fold in the 800 mg/day group. Antibody titer to tetanus vaccine also increased significantly in the subjects taking 200 mg/day of vitamin E. Antibody response to hepatitis B and DTH were greater for subjects with a serum α-tocopherol concentration of greater than 48.4 μmol/L. Other markers of cell-mediated immunity—antibody titer to diphtheria, immunoglobulin levels, levels of T and B cells, and autoantibody levels—were unaffected by vitamin E supplementation.

Conclusion.—High-level supplementation with vitamin E appears to enhance T-cell mediated immune function in healthy elderly people. The doses given in this study had no adverse effects. The findings suggest that an increased intake of vitamin E may be recommended for elderly people.

► As a result of age-related waning of immune function, older persons are more likely to incur infectious and neoplastic diseases. To date, there has been little evidence that this decline in immune function is preventable or reversible. In this randomized clinical trial of supplementation with vitamin E in 3 doses vs. placebo, all 3 doses resulted in augmented delayed-type hypersensitivity skin responses.

Although vitamin E had no effect on immunoglobulin levels, those receiving the higher doses of vitamin E (200 or 800 mg/day) had higher antibody titers to hepatitis B vaccine, an indication of improved T-cell–dependent function. All subjects had increased IgG antibody levels against pneumococcal vaccine, but those receiving 200 mg had the largest responses. Although these findings are very encouraging, it remains to be determined whether these increases in cell-mediated immunity as a result of vitamin E supplementation are associated with reductions in clinical events such as infections and tumors.

D.B. Reuben, M.D.

Vitamin E and Vitamin C Supplement Use and Risk of All-Cause and Coronary Heart Disease Mortality in Older Persons: The Established Populations for Epidemiologic Studies of the Elderly

Losonczy KG, Harris TB, Havlik RJ (Natl Inst on Aging, Bethesda, Md)

Am J Clin Nutr 64:190–196, 1996 1–9

Objective.—Free radical damage is a major component in the development of coronary heart disease. Vitamins C and E have been shown to reduce free radical damage. Studies of the relationship between vitamin C and cardiovascular disease have produced mixed results, and no studies have examined concurrent use of vitamins C and E. Results of a study of the protective effect against all-cause mortality, coronary heart disease mortality, cancer mortality, and other causes of mortality in an elder population by concurrent use of vitamins E and C were presented.

Methods.—Interviewers gathered information on use of vitamins C and E and other medications from 11,178 participants, age 67–105, in the Established Populations for Epidemiologic Studies for the Elderly from 1984 to 1993. Participants were reinterviewed every 3 years. All-cause mortality was the outcome measure.

Results.—By the end of the study period, there were 1,101 deaths from coronary heart disease, 761 deaths from cancer, and 1,719 deaths from other events. The relative risk (RR) of all-cause mortality for vitamin E users was 0.66 compared with nonuser participants; for mortality from coronary heart disease, it was 0.53; and for mortality from cancer, it was 0.41. Users of vitamins E and C had an RR of all-cause mortality of 0.58, compared with vitamin E users. Whereas vitamin E used alone reduced the risk of death by 20%, vitamin C use alone did not decrease mortality. Compared with nonusers, vitamin E and C users had a decreased risk of coronary heart disease mortality (RR = 0.42), whereas users of vitamin E only had an RR of 0.64. Information about dietary intake of vitamin E, fat, fiber, fruits, and vegetables, and vitamin supplement dosage and duration were not collected; nor were health habits or access to health care. Individuals with coronary disease were excluded from the study.

Conclusion.—Although vitamin E was shown to decrease the risk of mortality, vitamin C did not appear to add any extra benefit; these results agree with those of the Health Professionals Follow-Up Study. The reduced risk for cancer seen in vitamin E users may reflect a reduction in free radical damage to DNA and/or beneficial effects to the immune system.

▶ An increasing body of evidence suggests that antioxidant vitamins, especially vitamin E, reduce the risk of certain diseases. Studies of the association of vitamin C with cardiovascular disease, on the other hand, have been extremely conflicting. This article is the first study that examines the effect of concurrent vitamin E and vitamin C supplementation, although in the past it has been suggested that their actions may be synergistic. The study represents a secondary analysis of the Established Populations for Epidemiological Studies of the Elderly (EPESE), thus involving a study population of 11,178 subjects. The study tests the hypothesis that ingestion of vitamin E supplements has a protective effect against all-cause mortality, coronary heart disease mortality, cancer mortality and other remaining causes of mortality in an elderly population and that use of vitamin E with C supplements may enhance this protective effect.

There are a number of limitations to the database used for this secondary analysis. Among them are the following: (1) there was no information regarding the dietary intake of either vitamin; (2) there were no general dietary data available and, thus, one could not exclude the possibility that individuals taking vitamin E and C supplementation might not also have had other dietary habits that might lower the risk of mortality, such as lower fat intake and higher fiber intake; and (3) the dose of the supplementation for either vitamin was unknown, as was the duration of the supplementation. Finally, it is possible that in the EPESE subjects in this particular analysis, there might have been other confounding factors influencing the results, such as better health habits or better access to health care. Once more, the analysis gives no insight into mechanisms by which this benefit is brought about, and one can only conclude that prospective studies addressing mechanisms as well as the independent and combined effects of supplementation, controlling for some of the above factors, are sorely needed.

J.C. Beck, M.D.

Folic Acid Fortification of the Food Supply: Potential Benefits and Risks for the Elderly Population

Tucker KL, Mahnken B, Wilson PWF, et al (Tufts Univ, Boston; Natl Heart, Lung, and Blood Inst, Bethesda, Md)

JAMA 276:1879–1885, 1996 1–10

Objective.—Although the Food and Drug Administration (FDA) recommendation of 140 μg of folic acid supplementation per 100 g of cereal-grain product has been approved, some contend that higher levels are needed to provide adequate protection against neural tube defects. Others have expressed concern about the masking effects of higher folic acid doses on vitamin B_{12} deficiency. Increased folate intake has been shown to benefit the elderly, who have a 29% prevalence of hyperhomocysteinemia, by reducing homocysteine and, therefore, heart attacks and strokes. Results of a study of the potential benefits and risks of folic acid supplementation in the elderly were presented.

Methods.—Free homocysteine, vitamin B_{12}, and folate levels were determined in 747 participants, age 67–96, in the Framingham Heart Study. Participants completed a food questionnaire. Projected risk levels of disease and levels of homocysteine, folate, and vitamin B_{12} were compared statistically.

Results.—Projections indicate that fortifying the food supply with folic acid at the proposed level of 140 μg per 100 g of cereal-grain product would reduce the percentage of elderly persons with folate intake of less than 400 μg/day from 66% to 49%. At fortification levels of 280 μg, 350 μg, and 700 μg, percentages would be reduced to 32%, 26%, and 11%, respectively. Homocysteine levels decline with improved folate status. At fortification levels of 140 μg/day, the estimated risk of carotid artery stenosis was reduced by 3%, and the risk of coronary artery disease was reduced by 5%. Most individuals with low vitamin B_{12} levels also had low folate intake. Whereas the FDA cost-benefit ratio estimate of 140 μg of folate supplementation ranged from 1:24 to 1:29, and the California Birth Defects Monitoring Program cost-benefit ratio on prevalence of pernicious anemia at 350 μg of folate supplementation was 1:6.1, these estimates did not consider the cost saving resulting from a decreased incidence of homocysteine-related cardiovascular disease which, in this study, is calculated to be 25%.

Conclusion.—The benefits of folate fortification on reduction of homocysteine levels and, therefore, of heart disease outweigh the risks. The addition of cobalamin to folic acid supplementation would be beneficial. The relationship between folate and vitamin B_{12} deficiency—and, therefore, the cost effectiveness of treating all forms of vitamin B_{12} deficiency—could not be established in this study. This relationship needs to be identified in future studies.

► Previous volumes of this YEAR BOOK have dealt with the relationship between folate intake and homocysteine levels and the relationship between homocysteine levels and cardiovascular disease. This article, using the Framingham Heart Study database, examines the possible beneficial impact of several levels of folic acid intake on the risk of cardiovascular disease. It was instigated by the FDA proposal that, over the next several years, flour be fortified with folic acid in a concentration of 140 μg per 100 g of cereal-grain product. The potential risk of high folic intake is the masking of a B_{12} deficiency, and although there is at the moment a great deal of controversy about whether this actually occurs and whether the neurologic consequences of B_{12} deficiency are more severe in individuals with high folic intake, the potential risk remains in the absence of adequate data.

This secondary analysis suggests that the benefits of folic acid fortification on heart disease risk, through projected decreases in homocysteine levels, should greatly outweigh the possible risks of the FDA-mandated level of cereal-grain product fortification. Higher levels of folic acid fortification need to be approached with caution until the following are known: (1) the clinical course of various forms of vitamin B_{12} deficiency in older persons; (2) the measurement of the potential adverse effect of high folic intake on this clinical course; and (3) the most cost-effective approaches to identifying all forms of vitamin B_{12} deficiency.

J.C. Beck, M.D.

Clinical Epidemiology

A Prospective Study of Triglyceride Level, Low-Density Lipoprotein Particle Diameter, and Risk of Myocardial Infarction

Stampfer MJ, Krauss RM, Ma J, et al (Brigham and Women's Hosp, Boston; Harvard Med School, Boston; Lawrence Berkeley Natl Lab, Berkeley, Calif)

JAMA 276:882–888, 1996 1–11

Objective.—Although high triglyceride levels are associated with increased risk of myocardial infarction, results of studies of the relationship between triglyceride levels and coronary disease have been mixed. Triglyceride levels and the risk of coronary disease have been correlated with both low high-density lipoprotein cholesterol (HDL-C) and with a high low-density lipoprotein cholesterol (LDL-C)/HDL-C ratio. Because the smaller size of LDL particles may render them more prone to oxidation, low LDL diameter may be an independent risk factor for myocardial infarction. Because there are no prospective data available for evaluation, baseline blood samples from the Physicians' Health Study were prospectively analyzed to assess the impact of HDL-C subfractions and various apolipoproteins in the prediction of the risk of myocardial infarction.

Methods.—The randomized, double-blind, placebo-controlled, nested case-control 2 × 2 factorial trial of aspirin and β-carotene examined primarily nonfasting blood samples from 14,916 United States men age 40–84. The outcome measure was reported myocardial infarctions occurring during the 7-year follow-up period. Data on coronary risk factors were compared statistically.

Results.—The diameters of LDL particles of patients with myocardial infarction were significantly smaller than the diameters of age- and smoking-matched case controls (25.6 vs. 25.9 nm). Patients with myocardial infarction had significantly higher triglyceride levels than case controls (168 vs. 132 mg/dL). Low-density lipoprotein particle diameter was significantly and inversely related to triglyceride level ($r = 0.71$) and significantly and directly correlated with HDL-C level ($r = 0.60$). After controlling for additional risk factors, only triglyceride level significantly and independently predicted increased risk of myocardial infarction.

Conclusion.—Although elevated triglyceride levels increase the risk of coronary disease, their precise role has not been clarified, and study results have been mixed. The association between LDL particle diameter and risk of myocardial infarction loses significance after adjustment for triglyceride level. There was a very low cardiovascular mortality rate (15%) in the Physicians' Health Study compared with that of the general population of United States men of similar age.

▶ This article puts to rest the debate as to whether triglyceride levels are independent risk factors for myocardial infarction. It also addresses whether the question of low diameter LDL-C also acts as a risk factor independent of the triglycerides. The trial involved the Physicians' Health Study of 14,916 males, age 40–84, during a 7-year follow-up. The findings indicate that nonfasting triglyceride levels (as the majority of the blood samples were nonfasting) appear to be a strong and independent predictor of future risk of myocardial infarction, particularly when the total cholesterol level is also elevated. The role of the LDL particle diameter as an independent risk factor for myocardial infarction disappears after adjustment for triglyceride levels in this very large sample.

Unfortunately, this article gives no further insight as to the mechanisms by which this risk is translated into increased atherogenesis. In addition, the cardiovascular mortality rate in this large study was only 15% that of the general population of white United States males of comparable age. This raises the issue of whether the findings are broadly generalizable. The authors argue for their generalizability from the practical point of view that plasma triglyceride levels might aid in identifying high-risk individuals in whom a much more vigorous risk reduction intervention could be initiated. Clearly, this notion needs to be addressed in another study.

J.C. Beck, M.D.

Calcium-Channel Blockade and Incidence of Cancer in Aged Populations

Pahor M, Guralnik JM, Ferrucci L, et al (Catholic Univ, Rome; Natl Inst on Aging, Bethesda, Md; Istituto Nazionale Ricerca e Cura per Gli Anziani, Florence, Italy; et al)

Lancet 348:493–497, 1996 1–12

Background.—Although their effectiveness in treating hypertension and coronary heart disease is well known, calcium channel blockers also affect other organ systems to varying degrees. Now evidence suggests that calcium channel blockers can interfere with apoptosis, which helps destroy cancer cells. This study evaluated whether patients taking these drugs were at increased risk for developing cancer.

Methods.—As of 1992, the study included 5,052 participants, 65 or older, who had been interviewed in 1988 and who, at that time, had not been diagnosed with cancer. Medical histories contained information about daily doses of all medications and possible confounding factors, such as age and blood pressure. Comparisons were made between patients taking calcium channel blockers and those who were not. Separate comparisons were completed for patients taking verapamil, nifedipine, and diltiazem.

Findings.—Use of calcium channel blockers was associated with a significantly increased likelihood of having coronary heart disease, heart failure, hypertension, stroke, or diabetes; of being disabled; of having a lower systolic blood pressure; of being admitted to a hospital; and of having cancer. Even after other factors, such as smoking status, age, male gender, black race, and alcohol consumption, were factored out, patients taking calcium channel blockers were still at a significantly higher risk of developing cancer (1.72 hazard ratio). As the dose of calcium channel blocker increased, so did the risk of cancer. The risk was significantly increased for cancers of the uterus and adnexa and of the lymphatic and hemopoietic organs. The risk was increased (but not to statistical significance) for stomach, colon, rectum, breast, prostate, and urinary tract cancers, and it was close to 1:1 for liver, gallbladder, pancreas, and skin cancers. Lung cancer risk was reduced, but not significantly so. As for individual calcium channel blockers, patients taking verapamil were at the greatest risk of cancer ($P = 0.0002$), followed by those taking nifedipine ($P = 0.031$) and diltiazem ($P > 0.1$).

Conclusions.—Even after adjusting for possible confounding variables, the use of calcium channel blockers was associated with a greatly increased risk of cancer. Almost all organs were at increased cancer risk, which indicates a similar pathologic mechanism. These results should not prompt the withdrawal of calcium channel blockers; rather, they should be used as a springboard for further research into the noncardiovascular effects of these drugs.

► Calcium channel blockers are among the most frequently used agents for treatment of hypertension. They are effective in lowering blood pressure and appear to be the best single agents for treating African American men with this disorder. However, the short- and long-term side effects of this class of antihypertensive drugs are being increasingly recognized. Among the side effects that have been reported are constipation, gastrointestinal bleeding, and increased mortality after myocardial infarction.

In this study using the Established Populations for Epidemiologic Studies of the Elderly (EPESE), the investigators demonstrated an increase in the incidence of cancer among users of calcium channel blockers. In addition, the relationship between calcium channel blocker use and cancer was evident for many individual primary tumors. Lung cancer, was a notable exception. The relationship was stronger with higher daily doses of the drugs but was not equivalent across different specific agents. Verapamil had twice the hazard ratio of diltiazem.

The authors are correct to downplay the clinical implications of the study. It would be premature to change clinical regimens based on these findings. Nevertheless, it is wise to keep this association in mind and to be vigilant in maintaining cancer screening according to current guidelines for older persons who are receiving calcium channel blockers.

D.B. Reuben, M.D.

Bone Mineral Density and Risk of Breast Cancer in Older Women

Cauley JA, for the Study of Osteoporotic Fractures Research Group (Univ of Pittsburgh, Pa; et al)

JAMA 276:1404–1408, 1996 1–13

Introduction.—There is a positive correlation between bone mineral density (BMD) and early menarche, length of reproductive life, and parity in women. It is well known that there is a strong relation between menopausal loss of ovarian estrogens and rapid bone loss. Some investigations indicate an increased risk of breast cancer in women taking endogenous estrogen after menopause. A large number of nonblack women age 65 or older underwent BMD evaluation to determine if there is an increased risk of breast cancer in women with higher levels of BMD, and thus higher exposure to estrogen.

Methods.—A total of 9,704 women were recruited from 4 clinical centers over a 2-year period. At baseline, women underwent history and physical evaluation and analysis of radius and calcaneus BMD with dual-energy radiograph absorptiometry. Two years after baseline, these women underwent dual-energy radiograph absortiometry evaluation of the proximal femur and lumbar spine. Information about breast cancer was elicited through a questionnaire at 1 year and at a mean follow-up of 3.2 years later.

Results.—Of 6,854 women with complete information available at last follow-up, 97 had breast cancer. Women with breast cancer had a significantly higher BMD and a higher body mass index and mean body weight compared with women without breast cancer. The relative risk of breast cancer was 30% to 50% higher for each standard deviation increase in BMD. A direct relation was noted between age-adjusted BMD and risk of breast cancer. Women with low BMD had the lowest age-adjusted incidence rate of breast cancer. Compared with women with the lowest BMD, women with the highest BMD had a 2.0–2.5 times higher risk of breast cancer.

Conclusion.—There was a two-fold increased risk of subsequent breast cancer in women with the highest BMD of the radius, hip or spine. Findings suggest that the balance of risks and the benefits of hormone replacement therapy be thoroughly evaluated in each woman regarding BMD, osteoporosis, and breast cancer.

▶ Although evidence is mounting in support of the beneficial effects of estrogen on BMD, coronary heart disease, and skin changes associated with aging, exposure to estrogen has its dark side. The best-supported finding is the relation between exogenous estrogen and endometrial cancer. Some studies also have indicated an increased risk of breast cancer among women who have taken estrogen replacement therapy. In this analysis of the Study of Osteoporotic Fractures cohort, the authors demonstrated that increased BMD of the radius, hip, or spine is associated with increased risk of subsequent breast cancer. Because this association could be the result of estrogen replacement therapy, the authors excluded these cases from the analysis. Accordingly, they have linked breast cancer to a measure, albeit indirect, of endogenous estrogen. As efforts to increase bone density through estrogen replacement therapy increase, one would suspect that the risk of breast cancer will also increase. However, other methods of increasing BMD that are not estrogen dependent (e.g., alendronate, calcitonin) presumably will not increase this risk.

D.B. Reuben, M.D.

Smoking History in Middle Age and Subsequent Cognitive Performance in Elderly Japanese-American Men: The Honolulu-Asia Aging Study

Galanis DJ, Petrovich H, Launer LJ, et al (Univ of Hawaii, Honolulu; NIH, Bethesda, Md; Kuakini Med Ctr, Honolulu, Hawaii; et al)

Am J Epidemiol 145:507–515, 1997 1–14

Introduction.—Although cigarette smoking has been linked to many different diseases, little is known about its potential influence on cognitive impairment in the elderly. There is some epidemiologic evidence to suggest that smoking may be associated with a lower risk of Alzheimer's disease. There have been few community-based or longitudinal studies of smoking and cognitive function. Data from a large, longitudinal study were used to analyze the link between smoking history and later cognitive performance.

Methods.—The analysis included data on 3,429 Japanese-American men who were participants in the Honolulu Heart Program and its extension, the Honolulu-Asia Aging Study (HAAS). As part of the HAAS, all men underwent measurement of cognitive performance using the Cognitive Abilities Screening Instrument (CASI). Mean age at this examination was 77.7 years. The men had provided information on smoking history previously, at a mean age of 58.6 years.

Results.—Cognitive scores were significantly lower for men who had smoked continuously and for those who had recently quit than for men who had never smoked. The relationship between CASI scores and smoking held after adjustment for age, education, Japanese acculturation, and recent alcohol intake. On multiple logistic regression analysis, the risk of cognitive impairment was higher for men who had smoked continuously (odds ratio 1.36, 95% confidence interval 1.10–1.69) and for those who had quit since the start of the study (odds ratio 1.36, 95% confidence interval 1.03–1.80). Further analysis suggested that men who had not smoked for a longer time were at lower risk of cognitive impairment.

Conclusions.—This study of Japanese-American men suggests that those who smoke continuously during middle age are at elevated risk of cognitive impairment in old age. Long-term cessation of smoking appears to reduce this risk. The findings contradict previous case-control studies suggesting that smoking has a protective effect against Alzheimer's disease. Future analyses will assess the effects of smoking on the outcomes of Alzheimer's disease and vascular dementias in the study subjects.

▶ This article presents support for the notion that there is an increased risk of poor cognitive performance associated with long-term smoking. It is a secondary analysis of the Honolulu Heart Program and its extension, the Honolulu-Asia Aging Study. This clearly presents data that contradict some epidemiologic studies which have suggested that cigarette smoking may be associated with a lower risk of Alzheimer's disease.[1, 2] The presence of cognitive impairment is at the moment projected to increase, and thus it is important to identify as many risk factors for cognitive decline as possible, particularly those that are potentially modifiable. The evidence in the present study suggests that continuous smoking in middle age is associated with an increased risk of cognitive impairment in later life among Japanese-American men. In the smokers group, there appears to be a cognitive benefit associated with long-term cessation of smoking. The authors also present some preliminary evidence that smoking influences both vascular dementia and dementia of the Alzheimer's type and suggest that further analyses directed at clarification of these preliminary findings are underway.

The major strengths of this study are the well-documented assessment of smoking history, not relying on long-term retrospective recall as other studies have done; the large sample and its longitudinal nature; and the availability of objective measures of vascular conditions that might confirm associations between smoking history and cognitive performance. The limitations of the study include the fact that only a single cognitive examination was carried out; the sample was confined to Japanese-American men, and thus its generalizability to European populations and women is unclear; and that there were many possible confounders which were unmeasured, such as genetic susceptibility, comorbidity, behavioral habits, psychological conditions, etc.

J.C. Beck, M.D.

References

1. Launer LJ, Feskens EJM, Kalmijn S, et al: Smoking, drinking, and thinking: The Zutphen Elderly Study. *Am J Epidemiol* 143:219–227, 1996.
2. Hebert LE, Scherr PA, Beckett LA, et al: Relation of smoking and low-to-moderate alcohol consumption to change in cognitive function: A longitudinal study in a defined community of older persons. *Am J Epidemiol* 137:881–891, 1993.

A Prospective Study of Cigarette Smoking and Age-related Macular Degeneration in Women

Seddon JM, Willett WC, Speizer FE, et al (Harvard Med School, Boston; Harvard School of Public Health, Boston)

JAMA 276:1141–1146, 1996 1–15

Objective.—To develop effective preventive strategies and treatments for age-related macular degeneration (AMD), it is essential to determine the causes of the disease. Proposed factors include oxidative stress and vascular abnormalities, both of which are related to cigarette smoking. There have been no prospective studies of the possible link between smoking and AMD. This relationship was addressed with data from the Nurses' Health Study.

Methods.—The study cohort consisted of 31,843 female registered nurses who were in their 50s in 1980 and had no diagnosed cancer or AMD at that time. At baseline, 28% of the women were current smokers, 28% were ex-smokers, and 44% had never smoked. Other subjects entered the analyses as they reached age 50. In the Nurses' Health Study protocol, the women were followed up every 2 years through 1992. Total follow-up was 556,338 person-years. The link between AMD with visual loss and smoking was assessed.

Results.—Two hundred fifteen women received a new diagnosis of AMD during follow-up. The relative risk of AMD for women who currently smoked 25 or more cigarettes/day was 2.4, compared with never-smokers and after adjustment for other AMD risk factors. Ex-smokers had a relative risk of 2.0, and this risk did not fall significantly even 15 years after smoking cessation. As the number of pack-years smoked increased, so did the women's risk of AMD—risk was 240% higher for women who had smoked for 65 or more pack-years, compared with those who had never smoked. The findings were similar for analysis of dry and exudative types and other definitions of AMD.

Conclusions.—Women who smoke cigarettes are at increased risk of AMD. The prospective analysis finds smoking to be an independent and avoidable risk factor for AMD. The findings provide yet another reason to discourage patients from smoking.

▶ Age-related macular degeneration (AMD) is the leading cause of severe visual impairment among older persons. The disorder is largely confined to the white population and has been associated with advancing age and dietary and serum carotenoids. Using the Nurses' Health Study cohort, the investigators identified cigarette smoking as an independent risk factor for development of AMD. Among those who smoked at least 1¼ packs per day, the relative risk of AMD was 2.4 compared with those who never smoked, even after adjusting for known and potential risk factors. The authors were also able to establish a dose-response relationship by associating the risk with increasing number of pack-years of smoking, representing lifetime exposure. Although the data for subgroup analyses are based on few cases, the study also indicates that past smoking has nearly as powerful an effect. At 15 years after cessation, the risk had not significantly attenuated. Moreover, the effect of smoking is consistent with two of the leading hypotheses for the pathogenesis of the disorder: vascular insufficiency or increased oxidative stress (perhaps as the result of reduced levels of antioxidants). The Australian Blue Mountains Eye Study found similar associations between current and ever smoking and late AMD.[1] Thus, this common eye disease can be added to the long list of diseases associated with smoking. In this case, the importance of never taking up the habit is particularly important as cessation later in life may be too late.

D.B. Reuben, M.D.

Reference

1. Smith W, Mitchell P, Leeder SR: Smoking and age-related maculopathy: The Blue Mountains Eye Study. *Arch Ophthalmol* 114:1518–1523, 1996.

Age-related Macular Degeneration and Smoking

Vingerling JR, Hofman A, Grobbee DE, et al (Erasmus Univ, Rotterdam, The Netherlands; Academic Med Ctr, Amsterdam, The Netherlands)

Arch Ophthalmol 114:1193–1196, 1996 1–16

Objective.—Because there is evidence to suggest that smoking increases the risk of age-related macular degeneration (AMD), the relation between these 2 variables was investigated with data from a population-based Rotterdam study.

Methods.—A single-center, cross-sectional, community-based, prospective follow-up study of individuals 55 and older in Rotterdam, The Netherlands, involved ophthalmic examinations of 6,174 individuals for atrophic or neovascular AMD. Smoking status and number of smoking years was determined for participants.

Results.—Neovascular AMD was diagnosed in 65 individuals and atrophic AMD in 36 individuals. The prevalence of AMD was 1.1% in individuals younger than 85 and 11.0% in individuals older than 85. Current and former smoking status was associated with an increased risk of 6.6-fold and 3.2-fold, respectively, in individuals younger than 85 only. Individuals who had quit smoking 10–19 years or 1–9 years before the study were 4.2 times and 7.2 times more likely to have neovascular AMD, respectively.

Conclusion.—Smokers and former smokers younger than 85 who quit less than 20 years before the study were at significantly increased risk for neovascular AMD. Smoking possibly reduces the levels of retinal antioxidants that protect the retina against light exposure that generates oxygen radicals. There was no association between smoking and atrophic AMD, possibly because of small sample size. These findings have not been previously reported. Reports of smoking history were subjective, and therefore the diminishing effect of smoking after cessation of more than 20 years may be overestimated.

▶ There is a good deal of uncertainty as to whether the previously reported association between smoking and AMD is a true relation.[1–7] This report presents baseline data on a large population-based Dutch study that clearly emphasizes an association between smoking status and neovascular AMD, but not atrophic AMD. The relation between the length of the period since smoking cessation and the risk of neovascular AMD has never been reported before.

The other important contribution of this study is the fact that efforts were made to gain insight into the role of atherosclerotic changes in the development of AMD; these data suggest that it is unlikely to be the mechanism of the relation.

There are a number of limitations to this study: (1) the data elements on which this paper is based were available for only 60% of the total population-based study, but it seems highly unlikely that a special selection would have occurred on this basis and thus biased the data that are reported; (2) the observation that the effect of smoking diminishes after 20 years may be an overestimate because of the method of the calculation of the period since the last cigarette was smoked, which assumes that no long cessation periods had occurred previously; and (3) the mechanism of this association, although atherosclerosis seems less likely, still remains to be elucidated.

J.C. Beck, M.D.

References

1. Paetkau MD, Boyd TA, Grace M, et al: Senile disciform macular degeneration and smoking. *Can J Ophthalmol* 13:67–71, 1978.
2. Hyman LG, Lilienfeld AM, Ferris FL, et al: Senile macular degeneration: A case-control study. *Am J Epidemiol* 118:213–227, 1983.
3. Vinding T, Appleyard M, Nyboe J: Risk factor analysis for atrophic and exudative AMD. *Acta Ophthalmol Scand* 70:66–72, 1992.
4. Eye Disease Case-Control Study Group: Risk factors for neovascular age-related macular degeneration. *Arch Ophthalmol* 110:1701–1708, 1992.
5. Klein R, Klein BE, Linton KL, et al: The Beaver Dam Eye Study: The relation of age-related maculopathy to smoking. *Am J Epidemiol* 137:190–200, 1993.
6. Kahn HA, Leibowitz HM, Ganley JP, et al: The Framingham Eye Study, II: Association of ophthalmic pathology with single variables previously measured in the Framingham Heart Study. *Am J Epidemiol* 106:33–41, 1977.
7. West SK, Rosenthal FS, Bressler NM, et al: Exposure to sunlight and other risk factors for age-related macular degeneration. *Arch Ophthalmol* 107:875–879, 1989.

The Five-Year Incidence and Progression of Age-related Maculopathy: The Beaver Dam Eye Study

Klein R, Klein BEK, Jensen SC, et al (Univ of Wisconsin—Madison)

Ophthalmology 104:7–21, 1997 1–17

Objective.—The incidence of age-related macular degeneration (ARM) has rarely been studied in individuals free of the condition in both eyes. Results of the 5-year incidence, progression, regression, disappearance, and interrelationships of lesions associated with early and late ARM in a large population-based cohort were reported.

Methods.—Fundoscopic examinations using the Wisconsin Age-Related Maculopathy Grading System and drusen and other lesion characterizations were performed in a population of 3,583 individuals, age 43–86, living in Beaver Dam, Wisconsin. Individuals were followed for an average of 5 years.

Results.—Results are presented for right eyes only because the correlation of all parameters between eyes was high. Age-related macular degeneration increased significantly with age. Over the 5-year study period, compared with individuals age 43–54, individuals older than 75 had significantly increased drusen size (125–249 μm), were significantly more likely (16 times) to have large areas of confluence of soft drusen, significantly more likely to have abnormal retinal pigment changes (12.9% vs. 0.9%), and significantly more likely to have geographic atrophy or exudative macular degeneration. Compared with individuals age 43–54, individuals 75 and older were 10.7 times as likely to receive a diagnosis of ARM. Women were significantly (2.2 times) more likely to receive such a diagnosis as men. The condition was significantly more likely to develop in eyes with soft indistinct drusen than in eyes without (6.5% vs. 0.1%) and in eyes with increased pigment abnormalities than in eyes without (7.1% vs. 0.1%). The incidence of exudative macular degeneration in this population was slightly higher than the 5-year incidence found in the Chesapeake Bay Waterman Study, probably because the population in the former study was older.

Conclusion.—The incidence (and severity) of ARM increases with age, approaching 7.1% in individuals 75 and older. The number of people at risk will probably increase because of the aging of the population. Development of soft indistinct drusen and retinal pigmentation abnormalities increase the risk of late age-related macular degeneration. Because there is no treatment for the condition, research into prevention is important.

▶ This descriptive study examines the natural history of the incidence and progression of retinal drusen, retinal pigmentary abnormalities, and signs of late ARM. The paper was selected because there are no other population-based reports of the incidence of late ARM. All other studies have been based in ophthalmology clinics or comparable surroundings, except for the Chesapeake Bay Waterman Study, which included a younger cohort. The overall incidence of ARM in persons over age 75 is 7.1%. Thus as the American population ages still further, the overall number of people at risk of late ARM will undoubtedly increase, emphasizing the critical importance of understanding the pathogenesis of this disease.

J.C. Beck, M.D.

Does Estrogen Prevent Skin Aging?: Results From the First National Health and Nutrition Examination Survey

Dunn LB, Damesyn M, Moore AA, et al (Univ of California, San Francisco; UCLA School of Public Health, Los Angeles)

Arch Dermatol 133:339–342, 1997 1–18

Background.—Skin problems are common among older people and may adversely affect quality of life. Aging is associated with dry skin, wrinkling, and decreased collagen content. Although the findings of some studies suggest that estrogen treatment in postmenopausal women helps prevent these problems, the effects of estrogen on skin aging are uncertain. In this study, conducted at multiple community sites throughout the United States, the relationship between noncontraceptive estrogen and skin atrophy was examined.

Methods.—Data were obtained from the First National Health and Nutrition Examination Survey (NHANES I), in which 28,000 participants were enrolled between 1971 and 1974. (This study was limited to 3,875 postmenopausal women who were at least 40 at the time of the survey.) Dermatology residents conducted examinations and assessed sun exposure. Body mass index was calculated for all women, and a smoking history was taken from 1,862 members of the group. Follow-up studies of the NHANES I cohort were conducted between 1982 and 1984 and in 1986.

Results.—Participants had a mean age of 61.6 and were a mean of 15.6 years past menopause; 83.7% were white and 15.9% were black. Skin characteristics associated with aging included dryness (36.2%), wrinkling (28.2%), and atrophy (16.2%). The prevalence of all 3 of these conditions was lower in black women than in white women. Information on hormone use was available for 88% of the study group. After adjustment for age, body mass index, and sun exposure, the use of estrogen was associated with a statistically significant decrease in the likelihood of age-related dry skin (odds ratio, 0.76). Skin wrinkling and skin atrophy were also less common among women who had used estrogen.

Conclusions.—The use of estrogen appears to prevent dry skin and wrinkling in postmenopausal women. The findings of previous studies have suggested such a benefit, but few were adjusted for confounding factors or involved clinical dermatologic examinations. Although sun protection and skin hygiene also must be emphasized, estrogen treatment may protect against some aspects of cutaneous aging.

► The decision to take or refuse estrogen therapy after menopause should be made by each woman after weighing the potential benefits and risks of hormone therapy. Accordingly, physicians who present hormone therapy as an option to their patients should be well versed in the pros and cons of taking estrogen. To date, the most convincing evidence supporting therapy stems from epidemiologic evidence suggesting strong benefit in protecting against heart disease and osteoporosis. This epidemiologic study adds protective effects against skin disorders—specifically, decreased likelihood of wrinkling and drying—as other benefits of estrogen therapy. These advantages of estrogen therapy must then be considered in light of the adverse consequences, particularly the increased risk of uterine cancer in women taking unopposed estrogen and the increased risk of breast cancer. A thorough discussion of such pros and cons will lead to informed decisions by women who stand to gain or lose from this treatment.

D.B. Reuben, M.D.

The Significance of Subnormal Serum Vitamin B_{12} Concentration in Older People: A Case Control Study

Metz J, Bell AH, Flicker L, et al (Royal Melbourne Hosp, Australia; North West Hosp, Melbourne, Australia; Baylor Research Inst, Dallas, Tex)

J Am Geriatr Soc 44:1355–1361, 1996 1–19

Objective.—Because of the tendency in some older adults for intermediates of vitamin B_{12} to accumulate before serum vitamin B_{12} levels reach subnormal values, interpretation of these low normal results is difficult. Whereas in healthy young adults, about 20% of serum vitamin B_{12} is found on its carrier transcobalamin II (TCII), the amount of TCII-bound B_{12} (holoTCII) in older adults is often low. The hematologic, biochemical, and neurologic features associated with low B_{12} levels in older people compared with those of age-matched controls with serum B_{12} levels above 150 pmol/L (measured by both total B_{12} and holoTCII) were presented.

Methods.—Fasting blood samples were drawn from 43 patients (18 males) with an average age of 79.8 and serum B_{12} levels above 150 pmol/L and from 51 patients (22 males) with an average age of 80.7 years and normal serum B_{12} levels. Complete blood, red cell folate, and serum vitamin B_{12} tests; neutrophil lobe counts; and holoTCII, folate, gastrin, total homocysteine (Hcy), urea, creatinine, parietal cell antibody, and intrinsic factor antibody determinations were made. Neurologic testing and cognitive assessments were also done.

Results.—Compared with controls, patients with low serum B_{12} levels had a significantly increased incidence of elevated percent hypersegmented neutrophils ($r = 0.221$) and a significantly increased mean serum Hcy level (25.01 vs. 17.50 μmol/L). Forty percent of control patients and 76% of test patients had elevated serum Hcy, and 75% of control patients and 88% of test patients had increased levels of 1 or more of the following: serum total Hcy, mean cell volume, or percent of hypersegmented neutrophils. Including patients with borderline B_{12} levels (150–250 pmol/L) in the low B_{12} group eliminated many of these hematologic and biochemical overlaps. Of the 83% of test and control patients with very low TCII values, the fact that most had almost no B_{12} on TCII may suggest that this group may be more susceptible to the effects of vitamin B_{12} deficiency.

Conclusion.—Low serum B_{12} concentrations in older individuals indicate B_{12} deficiency at the tissue level and are often accompanied by low levels of holoTCII, particularly in those with B_{12} levels in the 150 to 250 pmol/L range.

▶ This Australian study gives further insight into the interpretation of low serum B_{12} concentrations in older people. Lindenbaum and his associates[1] have previously suggested that clinical B_{12} deficiency should be expected in the elderly when serum B_{12} levels fall below 256 pmol/L. This case-control study supports this suggestion and that subnormal serum B_{12} concentrations most often indicate tissue B_{12} deficiency. These 2 observations suggest that serum B_{12} be measured in all older patients with neurologic changes suggestive of B_{12} deficiency or with impairment of cognitive function, and that a therapeutic trial of B_{12} be undertaken if subnormal serum concentrations are found. The authors suggest that this be carried out at serum B_{12} levels below 250 pmol/L. The failure to demonstrate a relationship between the presence or severity of neurologic changes or cognitive function impairment and indices of B_{12} deficiency remain an enigma, although this lack of correlation may be attributable to the high degree of neurologic abnormalities found in the older population.

Finally, the mechanisms for these findings remain unclear. Twenty percent of serum B_{12} is found on transcobalamin II, which is the carrier that transfers B_{12} to sites of utilization. It is well established that the amount of B_{12} on TCII is low, and this results in a possible defect of delivery of B_{12} to tissues. This hypothesis is worthy of more extensive research.

J.C. Beck, M.D.

Reference

1. Lindenbaum J, Savage DG, Stabler SP, et al: Diagnosis of cobalamin deficiency: II. Relative sensitivities of serum cobalamin, methylmalonic acid, and total homocysteine concentrations. *Am J Hematol* 34:99–107, 1990.

Body Height, Cardiovascular Risk Factors, and Risk of Stroke in Middle-aged Men and Women: A 14-Year Follow-up of the Finnmark Study

Njølstad I, Arnesen E, Lund-Larsen PG (Univ of Tromsø, Norway; Natl Health Screening Service, Oslo, Norway)

Circulation 94:2877–2882, 1996 1–20

Objective.—Taller height has been shown to be inversely related to risk of all-cause and cardiovascular mortality. Results of a study investigating height as a risk factor for stroke in a free-living population were presented.

Methods.—A population-based study of the incidence of stroke and its relationship to height was conducted with 13,266 northern Norwegian individuals (47% women) age 35–52. Participants were followed for an average of 14 years. The outcome measure was first stroke. Stroke incidence and its relationship to cardiovascular risk factors and to height were analyzed statistically.

Results.—There were 144 first strokes in men and 97 first strokes in women. The overall stroke incidence was 36% higher in men. Risk factors for stroke included height, systolic blood pressure, and smoking 10 or more cigarettes/day. Hypertension was a risk factor for men. Body mass index was a significant risk factor in the univariate but not in the multivariate analysis. There was a significant inverse dose-response–type relationship between height and stroke. The tallest men had half the stroke risk of the shortest men. The tallest women had a stroke risk reduction of 66% over that of the shortest women. Because height is inversely related to heart rate, the lower stroke risk could be the result of physiologic mechanisms.

Conclusion.—Height for both men and women was significantly and inversely related in a dose-response manner to stroke risk independent of cardiovascular risk factors in this population-based study. Studies of stroke in relation to nutrition and other health factors in pregnancy, childhood, and adulthood are necessary.

► There is an increasing body of evidence relating height to a variety of disease patterns, including cardiovascular and all-cause mortality. This very large population based sample (13,266 men and women) demonstrates a clear inverse relationship between height and stroke incidence. The report contradicts the findings on height and stroke in 2 large cohort studies among United States physicians[1] and nurses.[2] The explanation for this inverse relationship is either related to some as yet unrecognized physiologic mechanisms or, alternatively, to the fact that final attained height is a marker for a sum of factors that are operative in early life (prenatal as well as postnatal), including a series of unfavorable factors such as socioeconomic status and social class. The discordance in the observations in 2 countries would suggest that the socioeconomic conditions of the physicians and nurses in the large cohort study was more optimal and, thus, this relationship was not demonstrable.

J.C. Beck, M.D.

References

1. Hebert PR, Rich-Edwards JW, Manson JAE, et al: Height and incidence of cardiovascular disease in male physicians. *Cirulation* 88:1437–1443, 1993.
2. Rich-Edwards JW, Manson JE, Stampfer MJ, et al: Height and the risk of cardiovascular disease in women. *Am J Epidemiol* 142:909–917, 1995.

Bone Mineral Density and Aortic Calcification: The Study of Osteoporotic Fractures

Vogt MT, Valentin RS, Forrest KY-Z, et al (Univ of Pittsburgh, Pa; Univ of California, San Francisco)

J Am Geriatr Soc 45:140–145, 1997 1–21

Objective.—Increasing osteoporosis and arterial calcification in older women has been linked to deposition on arterial walls of calcium from resorbed bone, hemodynamic changes that result in bone loss and independent progression of osteopenia and arterial calcification. The relationship between bone mineral density and the presence of aortic calcification in a large cohort of older women enrolled in the Study of Osteoporotic Fractures was investigated.

Methods.—Aortic calcification was assessed using a consecutive sample of lateral spine radiographs. Bone mineral density (BMD) was measured at the hip, spine, calcaneus, and proximal and distal radius using an OsteoAnalyser in 2,051 women age 65 and older. Demographic characteristics, medical and smoking histories, medication use, exercise, dietary history, weight, height, blood and pulse pressure, and functional status were obtained. Differences between those with and without aortic calcification were compared statistically.

Results.—The prevalence of aortic calcification increased from 60% at ages 65–69 to 96% at ages 85 and older. Women with aortic calcification tended to be older and to have statistically, but not clinically significantly, lower BMD at all sites except the lumbar spine. Bone mineral density at hip, spine, and calcaneus was not correlated with the presence of arterial calcification, whereas former and current smoking history, coffee intake, current thiazide or other diuretic use, systolic blood pressure, pulse pressure, body mass index greater than waist/hip ratio above 0.84 were. Calcification risk was less for women who exercised more and took calcium supplements, vitamin D, or estrogen. There was no relationship between the type of bone measured and the presence of aortic calcification.

Conclusion.—Osteopenia and aortic calcification appear to be independent processes that affect women as they age. The same mechanism involved in bone mineralization may be responsible for arterial calcification. Others suggest that stimulation of smooth muscle in arterial walls may result in arterial osteogenesis. As yet, there are no community-based epidemiologic studies that can definitively link osteopenia and aortic calcification. One Mayo Clinic study found no relationship between BMD and aortic calcification. However, the prevalence of plaques in postmenopausal women increases from 15% at ages 50–55 to 80% at age 80.

▶ Aging is associated with increased prevalence of osteopenia and calcification in the walls of large arteries, particularly aortic calcification and mitral annular calcification. The relationship between these 2 processes is unclear, and this paper lends some insight into the 3 hypotheses that have been put forward over the years to explain this relationship. It has been postulated that the mobilization of ionized calcium during bone resorption is a promoter for the deposition of calcium in damaged areas of the arterial wall. It has also been postulated by others that arterial wall calcification by some humoral mechanism may facilitate bone loss; and, finally, it has been suggested that the 2 processes are totally independent and are age related.

There is a good deal of evidence that arterial tissue is calcified by mechanisms similar to those involved in the mineralization of bone. The mineral deposited in the arterial wall is hydroxyapatite, and it can be seen to be organized structurally with trabeculae and lacunae visible in the deposits. This suggests that arterial osteogenesis is a highly organized process and that smooth muscle cells in the arterial wall may be stimulated to participate in local osteogenesis.

This study, which derives from a multicenter observational study entitled "Study of Osteoporotic Fractures," is the first definitive community-based epidemiologic study which, to my knowledge, has been published. It confirms a Mayo Clinic study of an age-stratified random sample of 200 women over the age of 50 years, and the reported prevalences of calcific aortic plaques are very similar. There is a striking increase in the percentage of women with aortic calcification as they age, and at 80 years of age, it may be as high as 80%.[1]

J.C. Beck, M.D.

Reference

1. Witteman JC, Kok FJ, van Saase JL, et al: Aortic calcification as a predictor of cardiovascular mortality. *Lancet* 2:1120–1122, 1986.

Epidemiology of Insulin-like Growth Factor-I in Elderly Men and Women: The Rancho Bernardo Study

Goodman-Gruen D, Barrett-Connor E (Univ of Calif, San Diego)
Am J Epidemiol 145:970–976, 1997 1–22

Background.—Insulin-like growth factor-I (IGF-I) is structurally similar to insulin, abundant in the circulation, and associated with protein, carbohydrate, and bone metabolism. It may be involved in the pathophysiology of cancer, diabetes mellitus, cerebral ischemia, osteoporosis, and renal disease. There has been only one small study of IGF-I in adults, and no large studies of the epidemiology of IGF-I in older adults.

Methods.—Individual, laboratory, diurnal, and seasonal variation in serum IGF-I concentrations, and the association of age, gender, body size, fat distribution, grip strength, use of alcohol and tobacco, physical activity, and medications with IGF-I concentration were studied in 419 consecutive women not receiving hormone replacement therapy and 420 consecutive men. All patients were between the ages of 50 and 97, white, community-dwelling, and ambulatory.

Results.—No evidence of diurnal or seasonal variation was seen. The IGF-I concentrations decreased linearly with age in men and women. Men had significantly lower levels. Insulin-like growth factor-I was not associated with height, total or central body fat, lean body mass, current use of tobacco, physical activity, or common medications in age-adjusted analyses. In men and women who reported alcohol use, IGF-I was significantly higher than in those who reported no use of alcohol. Alcohol as a continuous variable had a significant positive linear trend in men.

Discussion.—The decrease in IGF-I with age in these older subjects was less significant than previously reported in younger subjects. Other studies that have reported a significant correlation between IGF-I and total body fat and lean body mass examined only younger men or obese women. An increase in IGF-I with increased use of alcohol was seen in both men and women. No association between IGF-I and physical activity or grip strength was found. Insulin-like growth factor-I can be used in epidemiologic studies of the effect of IGF-I and growth hormone on morbidity and mortality in older adults.

▶ This article raises the important issue of using IGF-I for epidemiologic studies linking possible effects of decreased growth hormone secretion with aging with morbidity and mortality in future studies of older adults. Insulin-like growth factor-I is a growth hormone dependent peptide, and there is abundant evidence for its association with protein, carbohydrate, and bone metabolism. It thus may play a possible role in the pathophysiology of a number of problems common to older individuals, such as cancer, diabetes melitus, and osteoporosis.

The paper is a description of a large sample of older men and women and thus is the first observation of IGF-I concentrations in an adult population, the only previous study of this type being a very small one.[1] In this older cohort, IGF-I levels decreased with age and were lower in men than in women, although the rate of decline with age in the Rancho Bernardo population seems less steep than those reported for younger adults. It is also important that there were no significant seasonal or diurnal variations, the latter being a major problem in measurement of plasma growth hormone. In contrast to other reported studies, there was no association with height, total or central body fat, lean body mass, or physical activity. The failure to confirm previous associations with body fat may be because of the small number of obese persons in the Rancho Bernardo study—no other obvious explanation exists. An intriguing observation is that increased alcohol is associated with increased IGF-I levels in both sexes and the mechanism of this remains obscure. The previous observation that a decrease in

IGF-I with age may be the result of a sedentary lifestyle[2] is not confirmed in this study, although this population seemed to be physically active. If an association exists, then perhaps these older adults were exercising below the threshold of benefit.

J.C. Beck, M.D.

References

1. Landin-Wilhelmsen K, Wilhelmsen L, Lappas G, et al: Serum insulin-like growth factor I in a random population sample of men and women: Relation to age, sex, smoking habits, coffee consumption and physical activity, blood pressure and concentrations of plasma lipids, fibrinogen, parathyroid hormone and osteocalcin. *Clin Endocrinol* 41:351–357, 1994.
2. Rudman D, Drinka PJ, Wilson CR, et al: Relations of endogenous anabolic hormones and physical activity to bone mineral density and lean body mass in elderly men. *Clin Endocrinol* 40:653–661, 1994.

The Effects of Alpha Tocopherol Supplementation on Monocyte Function: Decreased Lipid Oxidation, Interleukin 1β Secretion, and Monocyte Adhesion to Endothelium

Devaraj S, Li D, Jialal I (Univ of Texas, Dallas)

J Clin Invest 98:756–763, 1996 1–23

Purpose.—Low alpha-tocopherol levels have been linked to an increased risk of cardiovascular disease. Increasing the intake of alpha-tocopherol may protect against cardiovascular disease. Alpha-tocopherol acts to decrease low-density lipoprotein oxidation; in addition, it may have intracellular effects on monocytes and other cells involved in atherogenesis, such as monocytes. The effects of alpha-tocopherol supplementation on monocyte function were investigated.

Methods.—Twenty-one healthy adults were studied before and after 8 weeks of alpha-tocopherol supplementation, 1,200 IU/day, and again after a 6-week washout period. Changes in monocyte function relevant to atherogenesis were studied.

Results.—During alpha-tocopherol supplementation, plasma lipid-standardized and monocyte alpha-tocopherol levels increased by 2.5-fold. At the same time, there were significant reductions in release of reactive oxygen species, i.e., hydrogen peroxide and superoxide anion; lipid oxidation; interleukin-1β-secretion; and monocyte-endothelial cells. These changes were noted in both resting and activated cells. The effect of alpha-tocopherol in inhibiting release of reactive oxygen species and oxidation of lipids appeared to result from inhibition of protein kinase C activity.

Conclusions.—Alpha-tocopherol appears to have an intracellular anti-atherogenic effect in monocytes. The changes observed with alpha-tocopherol supplementation, including inhibition of reactive oxygen species and lipid oxidation, appear to be mediated by inhibition of protein kinase C.

Although clinical trials are needed, the findings add evidence for an intracellular effect to the scientific basis for alpha-tocopherol supplementation.

► This important paper lends further mechanistic evidence to the relationship between alpha-tocopherol and cardiovascular disease. There are now several lines of evidence that support a relationship between low levels of alpha-tocopherol and increased cardiovascular morbidity and mortality,[1–3] as well as an increased intake of alpha-tocopherol leading to decreased cardiovascular morbidity.[4–6] This article examines the role of alpha-tocopherol supplementation on monocyte function because there is evidence that the monocyte is a critical cell in early atherogenesis and fatty streak modification. One of the mechanisms discovered in this study with respect to alpha-tocopherol is that it causes an intracellular effect on the monocyte that is anti-atherogenic. It decreases the ability of the monocytes to release both hydrogen peroxide and superoxide anion and reduces lipid oxidation by monocytes. The authors further suggest that this appears to be mediated by an inhibition of protein kinase C activity. Other effects that are observed is a suppression of a potentially atherogenic cytokine (interleukin-1β) and an inhibition of a crucial event in atherogenesis, namely, monocyte-endothelial cell adhesion. These observations therefore strengthen the scientific basis for alpha-tocopherol supplementation, but the final answer as to the protective effect of alpha-tocopherol must await a large randomized clinical trial.

J.C. Beck, M.D.

References:

1. Gey KF, Puska P, Jordan P, et al: Inverse correlation between plasma vitamin E and mortality from ischemic heart disease in a cross-cultural epidemiology. *Am J Clin Nutr* 53:326–335, 1992.
2. Riemersma R, Wood D, McIntyre C, et al: Risk of angina pectoris and plasma concentrations of vitamins A, C, E and carotene. *Lancet* 337:1–5, 1991.
3. Manson JE, Gaziano JM, Jonas MA, et al: Antioxidants and cardiovascular disease: a review. *J Am Coll Nutr* 12:426–432, 1993.
4. Stampfer MJ, Hennekens CH, Manson JE, et al: Vitamin E consumption and the risk of coronary disease in women. *N Engl J Med* 328:1444–1449, 1993.
5. Rimm EB, Stampfer MJ, Ascherio A, et al: Vitamin E consumption and the risk of coronary disease in men. *N Engl J Med* 328:1450–1456, 1993.
6. Hodis HN, Mack WJ, LaBree L, et al: Serial coronary angiographic evidence that antioxidant vitamin intake reduces progression of coronary artery atherosclerosis. *JAMA* 273:1849–1854, 1995.

Geriatric Syndromes

Osteoporosis

The Economic Cost of Hip Fractures in Community-dwelling Older Adults: A Prospective Study

Brainsky A, Glick H, Lydick E, et al (Univ of Pennsylvania, Philadelphia; Merck Research Labs, West Point, Pa; Merck-Medco Managed Care Inc, Montvale, NJ; et al)

J Am Geriatr Soc 45:281–287, 1997 1–24

Objective.—The annual incidence of hip fracture in United States adults 65 and older is 6.6 per 1,000. The incidence increases with age and will cost the health care system an estimated $16 billion in 2040. Hip fracture cost studies have been based mainly on survey and other cross-sectional data rather than prospective information and have not taken into account co-morbid conditions that contribute to the cost of treatment. Results of a prospective study of the costs of medical, nonmedical, and informal services used by a cohort of community-dwelling subjects in the 6 months before and after hip fracture were reported.

Methods.—Resource use and costs, nursing home care, rehabilitation, outpatient visits, formal home care, use of special devices, use of special types of transportation, and informal care costs were estimated for 759 patients (79.4% female), age 65–100, admitted to Baltimore area hospitals for hip fracture. Costs were tallied for the 6 months before hip fracture, hospital admission, 2 months after discharge, 4 months between the 2- and 6-month follow-up interviews, and the 6 months between the 6- and 12-month interviews.

Results.—There were 17 deaths in hospital and 112 more deaths during the year after discharge. Another 56 patients were lost to follow-up. The annualized costs per patient in the year preceding the fracture were $20,928 without accounting for mortality and $18,523 when mortality was included. The cost of initial hospitalization for the fracture averaged $11,480, and for the year after discharge it was $37,250. Incremental costs ranged from $16,322 to $18,727, depending on whether mortality was considered.

Discussion.—Annualized costs after fracture were similar to annualized costs before fracture. Incremental costs were lower in this study because it compared before and after fracture costs. These estimates were based on costs rather than on charges and included indirect costs and service costs. The patients lived in the community, not in nursing homes, and served as their own controls. These data were collected before implementation of the Federal Prospective Payment System, which resulted in decreased use of hospital services and increased use of nursing homes and rehabilitation services. The minimum wage was used to price the services of family and friends. Proxy information was used to obtain follow-up data.

Conclusion.—The incremental cost of a hip fracture ranged from $16,322 to $18,727 for community-dwelling elderly patients.

▶ To my knowledge, this is the first article to address the incremental cost of resource utilization after a fracture. It includes medical and nonmedical costs and the costs of informal care, which have not been assessed previously in a prospective study. The study is an analysis of data obtained from the Baltimore Hip Fracture Study. The costs addressed are for community-dwelling older persons in the 6 months before and the year after the hip fracture. They demonstrate that the monthly costs increased substantially for the first 6 months after the fracture and then decreased, approaching the prefracture levels by the end of the first year.

It is of interest that because this paper addresses incremental costs of a fracture, the estimates reported are generally lower than those found in the literature. This is because most older persons who sustain hip fractures have substantial co-morbidities which are already costly before the event takes place. Other unique features of this study are the fact costs were used rather than charges; only community-dwelling older persons, not nursing home patients, were included; and a variety of nonmedical and informal care costs were measured by proxy interview.

There are some limitations to this study which the reader should be aware of. The first is that the patients were used as their own controls; the second is that this study was carried out before the Federal Prospective Payment System was implemented; the third is that the authors used the federal minimum wage when costs were assigned to family and friends for their time in helping with patients, instead of considering the opportunity costs that might have been incurred, which would have increased the incremental costs substantially; finally, the authors used proxies for the patients in the interviews. However, the reliability of proxy responses for many of the measures used in this study have been demonstrated and are particularly good regarding the items that were objective and observable.

J.C. Beck, M.D.

Meta-analysis of How Well Measures of Bone Mineral Density Predict Occurrence of Osteoporotic Fractures

Marshall D, Johnell O, Wedel H (Swedish Council on Technology Assessment in Health Care, Stockholm; Malmö General Hospital, Sweden; Nordic School of Public Health, Gothenburg, Sweden)

BMJ 312:1254–1259, 1996 1–25

Objective.—Osteoporosis increases the risk and consequences of fractures, particularly for women over 50, 30% of whom have a bone mineral density 2.5 SDs below that of young healthy women. Scandinavia has an unexplainably high prevalence of osteoporotic fractures. Bone density measurements, as a screening measure, fail because there is a large overlap between patients with a fracture and those without. Results of a review of prospective studies to determine the ability of bone density measurements in women to predict later fractures are presented.

Methods.—Results of a meta-analysis of prospective cohort studies published between 1985 and 1995 were compared with case-control studies of hip fractures published between 1990 and 1994. Patients were monitored for 1.8 to 24 years.

Results.—Results in prospective cohort studies showed no association between length of follow-up and risk of decrease in bone mineral density of 1 SD. Most measuring sites were equally able to predict a bone mineral density of 1 SD (relative risk [RR] = 1.5), with spine measurements better predictors of spinal fractures (RR = 2.3) and hip measurements better predictors of hip fractures (RR = 2.6). These findings agreed with those of the case-control studies. The ability of a decrease in bone mineral density of 1 SD as a predictor of fracture was similar to a 1 SD increase in blood pressure as a predictor of stroke or a 1 SD increase in serum cholesterol as a predictor of cardiovascular disease.

Conclusion.—Measurements of bone mineral density can predict an increased risk of fracture but cannot be used to identify individuals who will have a fracture. Because there are no clear cut-off values, the risks of screening should be considered. However, because the risk gradient is steeper at the lower ranges, the risk of a 1 SD decrease in bone mineral density may underestimate the risk for women with low bone densities.

▶ This article represents a meta-analysis of 11 study populations with approximately 90,000 person-years of observation time and more than 2,000 fractures. It thus represents a unique contribution to a discussion of the use of the measurements of bone mineral density as a screening procedure for predicting fracture risk. The conclusion, for the moment, which can be drawn from this elegant study, is that measurement of bone mineral density can predict a risk factor but cannot identify individuals who will have a fracture. Because one is dealing with continuous predictors, there is no obvious cut-off value that can be determined, and thus it would seem unwise to recommend using bone density measurements as a routine screening procedure. There are obviously other risk factors that contribute importantly to the occurrence of fracture, and at best, bone mineral density might be used for selective screening. There is much too little known about compliance rates for attending screening programs and compliance with an effective intervention. And the data on the effectiveness of treatment from the point of view of a significant reduction of fractures are still to come.

It is of interest that the investigators were able to examine the predictive value related to a specific site, and the results of this analysis demonstrate that most measuring sites had virtually the same predictive ability in bone density with two exceptions: measurement at the spine seemed to be a better predictor for spine fractures, whereas measurement at the hip was better for predicting hip fractures.

J.C. Beck, M.D.

Effect of Calcium and Vitamin D Supplementation on Bone Density in Men and Women 65 Years of Age or Older
Dawson-Hughes B, Harris SS, Krall EA, et al (Tufts Univ, Boston)
N Engl J Med 337:670–676, 1997 1–26

Objective.—Inadequate intake of calcium and vitamin D may increase the risk of bone loss in older individuals. The effect of combined calcium and vitamin D supplements on bone loss, biochemical measures of bone metabolism, and incidence of nonvertebral fractures was studied in community-living men and women age 65 or older.

Methods.—The 389 (176 men and 213 women) healthy community-dwelling seniors, ages 65 or older, were enrolled in a 3-year, double-blind, placebo-controlled trial and received either placebo or 500 mg of calcium and 700 IU of vitamin D_3 daily. Bone mineral density, which was measured by dual photon absorptiometry, as well as blood and urine measures of bone metabolism, were analyzed every 6 months. All nonvertebral fractures were recorded.

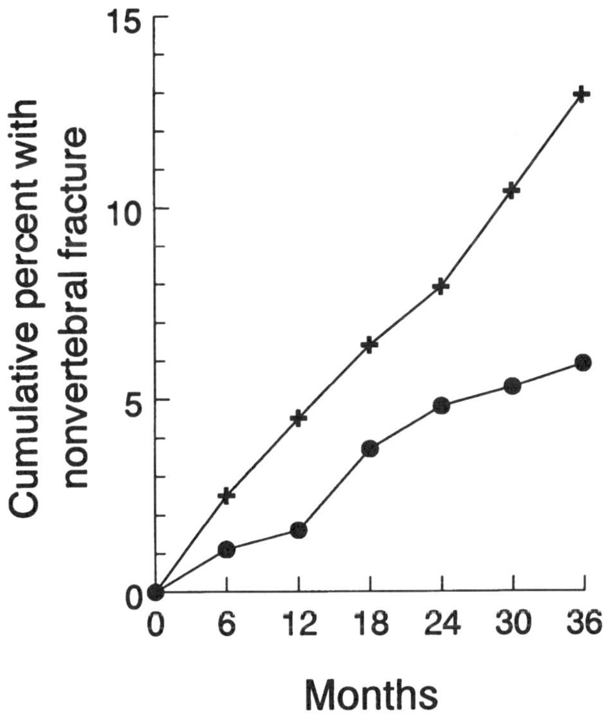

FIGURE 1.—Cumulative percentage of all 389 subjects with a first nonvertebral fracture, according to study group. By 36 months, 26 of 202 subjects in the placebo group and 11 of 187 subjects in the calcium–vitamin D group had had a fracture ($P = 0.02$). (Reprinted by permission of *The New England Journal of Medicine,* from Dawson-Hughes B, Harris SS, Krall EA, et al: Effect of calcium and vitamin D supplementation on bone density in men and women 65 years of age or older. *N Engl J Med* 337:670–676, 1997.)

Results.—At 3 years, changes in bone mineral density were better for the supplemented group than for the placebo group. Changes were as follows: femoral neck, +0.50% vs. −0.70%; spine, 2.12% vs. 1.22%; and total body +0.06% vs. −1.09%. Compared with the placebo group, the supplemented group showed significantly less bone loss in all areas measured during the first and second years. In the third year, only total body bone loss was significantly less in the supplemented group. A total of 37 nonvertebral fractures were reported, 5 in men and 32 in women (Fig 1). At 3 years, there was a significantly higher incidence of fractures in the placebo group than there was in the supplemented group (12.9% vs. 5.9%). The 3-year incidence for women was 19.6%. The 3-year incidence of osteoporotic fractures was significantly lower in the supplemented group than it was in the placebo group (relative risk = 0.4).

Conclusion.—Vitamin D and calcium supplementation reduced bone loss and the incidence of nonvertebral fractures in a 3-year study in community-dwelling individuals age 65 or older.

► Calcium and vitamin D are commonly prescribed for prevention of osteoporosis in older individuals, although the evidence supporting their effectiveness has been inconsistent. In this trial, community-dwelling elderly male and female subjects received either calcium (500 mg) plus vitamin D_3 (700 IU per day) or a placebo. After 1 year, differences in changes in bone mineral density were significant, indicating benefit of treatment among all subjects at the femoral neck, spine, and total body, but after 3 years the only significant difference was in total body bone density. Although the number of fractures at each individual skeletal site was small, when pooled, the number of nonvertebral fractures in the treated group was significantly less than that occuring in the placebo group. Although the study was well designed and implemented, the regimen utilized was somewhat unconventional in that it did not meet the recommended calcium intake, and the vitamin D dose differed from other studies. Nevertheless, this study supports the continued prescription of calcium and vitamin D to prevent osteoporosis. It still remains uncertain whether this regimen is effective in reducing the rate of fractures, especially of the hip, that have the most dramatic impact on mortality and functional status.

D.B. Reuben, M.D.

► Dietary calcium supplementation prescribed to limit or replace bone loss in postmenopausal women is commonly practiced medical therapy. Support for this was recommended by the 1994 NIH Consensus Conference on Optimal Calcium Intake. Those recommendations included a 1,000 mg daily intake for perimenopausal women and 1,500 mg daily intake for postmenopausal women.[1] Moreover, 1,500 mg calcium intake was recommended (with little supporting data) for men.

In a previous study, Dr. Dawson-Hughes reported that dietary calcium supplementation in elderly subjects with low dietary calcium, increased bone density and lowered fracture rate.[2] Here, subjects whose dietary intake (748 ± 391 mg/day) was, on average, near the RDA recommended level of

800 mg, demonstrated a modest increase (but no loss) in bone mass and a 50% decrease in non-vertebral fracture rate when supplemented daily with 500 mg of calcium and 700 IU of vitamin D (Fig 1). As indicated in an accompanying editorial, 1,200 mg/day is the minimum daily intake considered to be effective.[3] The current recommendation for supplemental vitamin D is only 400 IU; the rationale for using 700 IU is not clear.

We do not know the effect of this regimen on vertebral fracture rate. An additional question involves whether the response was dependent on initial levels of calcium and vitamin D intake. Finally, how does the statistically insignificant increase in bone density relate to the significant decrease in non-vertebral fracture rate? Recall that bisphosphonate therapy typically increases spine bone density approximately 8% over 36 months but also leads to a 50% reduction in fracture rate. Why this disparity exists is not known at this time.

J.R. Shapiro, M.D.

References

1. NIH Consensus Conference on Optimal Calcium Intake. *JAMA* 272:1942–1948, 1994.
2. Dawson-Hughes B, Dallal GE, Krall EA, et al: A controlled trial of the effect of calcium supplementation on bone density in postmenopausal women. *N Engl J Med* 323:878–893, 1990.
3. Prince RL: Diet and the prevention of osteoporotic fractures. *N Engl J Med* 337:701–702, 1997.

Randomised Trial of Effect of Alendronate on Risk of Fracture in Women With Existing Vertebral Fractures

Black DM, for the Fracture Intervention Trial Research Group (Univ of California San Francisco; et al)

Lancet 348:1535–1541, 1996 1–27

Objective.—Although studies have shown that alendronate reduces the risk of vertebral fracture in women with low bone mineral density (BMD) by increasing BMD, its effect on non-vertebral fractures was not convincingly determined. The double-blind Fracture Intervention Trial was designed to assess the effect of alendronate on vertebral and nonvertebral fractures in postmenopausal women with low BMD and at least 1 vertebral fracture at recruitment.

Methods.—Either placebo (n – 1005) or 5 mg daily of alendronate (n – 1022), increased to 10 mg daily at 24 months, was administered to 2,027 postmenopausal women age 55–81 for at least 2 years. All the women had a femoral neck BMD of no more than 0.68 g/cm^2 and at least 1 vertebral fracture. None of the women had taken estrogen or calcitonin within the last 6 months. Lateral spine radiographs were obtained at baseline, 24 months, and 36 months. New vertebral and nonvertebral fractures were

TABLE 2.—Participants With New Vertebral Fractures

	Women with vertebral fractures*		Relative risk
	Placebo	Alendronate	(95% CI)
Morphometric fractures			
One or more	145 (15·0%)	76 (6·0%)	0·53 (0·41–0·68)
Two or more	47 (4·9%)	5 (0·5%)	0·10 (0·05–0·22)
Clinical vertebral fractures	50 (5·0%)	23 (2·3%)	0·45† (0·27–0·72)

*Among the 965 women in the placebo group, there were 240 morphometric fractures in 145 of them. Among the 981 women in the alendronate group, there were 86 morphometric fractures in 78 of them.

†Relative hazard.

(Courtesy of Black DM, for the Fracture Intervention Trial Research Group: Randomized trial of effect of alendronate on risk of fracture in women with existing vertebral fractures. *Lancet* 348:1535–1541, 1996. Copyright by The Lancet Ltd., 1996.)

confirmed radiographically, vertebral height was calculated. Patients were monitored for an average of 2.9 years.

Results.—Compared with placebo, alendronate significantly increased average bone mass and BMD and significantly decreased the risk of new vertebral fractures (Table 2). Alendronate patients lost significantly less vertebral height in 36 months than the placebo patients did (6.1 mm versus 9.3 mm). Similar numbers of women in both groups discontinued the medication because of adverse effects. Alendronate patients had significantly fewer hip and wrist fractures than placebo patients did (Table 3).

Conclusion.—Alendronate significantly reduces the risk of vertebral and nonvertebral fractures in postmenopausal women with low BMD and existing vertebral fractures.

► Alendronate, the first of a new generation of bisphosphonates, previously has been demonstrated to increase BMD in the lumbar spine, femoral neck, and trochanter and to reduce the risk of vertebral fractures[1] Now in a new randomized clinical trial that studied women age 55–81 who had at

TABLE 3.—Participants With Clinical Fractures

	Women with at least one fracture		Relative hazard (95% CI)
	Placebo	Alendronate	
Any clinical fracture*	183 (18·2%)	139 (13·6%)	0·72 (0·58–0·90)
Type of fracture			
Any non-vertebral	148 (14·7%)	122 (11·9%)	0·80 (0·63–1·01)
Hip	22 (2·2%)	11 (1·1%)	0·49 (0·23–0·99)
Wrist	41 (4·1%)	22 (2·2%)	0·52 (0·31–0·87)
Other†	99 (9·9%)	100 (9·8%)	0·99 (0·75–1·31)

*Includes clinical vertebral fracture.

†Placebo versus alendronate: shoulder, 3 vs. 2; arm, 22 vs. 21; hand, 7 vs. 5; fingers, 6 vs. 7; other small wrist bones, 0 vs. 3; ribs, 12 vs. 15; chest and sternum, 1 vs. 3; pelvis, 9 vs. 6; coccyx and sacrum, 0 vs. 2; leg, 12 vs. 9; ankle, 10 vs. 15; foot and metatarsal, 17 vs. 14; toes, 9 vs. 10; periprosthetic, 1 vs. 0.

(Courtesy of Black DM, for the Fracture Intervention Trial Research Group: Randomized trial of effect of alendronate on risk of fracture in women with existing vertebral fractures. *Lancet* 348:1535–1541, 1996. Copyright by The Lancet Ltd., 1996.)

least 1 vertebral fracture at baseline, this medication has been shown to reduce new clinically apparent or radiologically determined vertebral fractures by about half, over an average of approximately 3 years of follow-up. More importantly, perhaps, it also was able to reduce wrist and hip fractures by the same amount. Unfortunately, this report presents only half the findings of this major study. Subjects who had abnormal femoral neck BMD without vertebral fractures at baseline also were recruited into the study and given the same treatment. The findings of that subgroup will have important implications on the treatment of those who are at high risk for fractures but who have not yet experienced this outcome at any site.

D.B. Reuben, M.D.

Reference

1. Lieberman UA, for the Alendronate Phase III Osteoporosis Treatment Study Group: Effect of oral alendronate on bone mineral density and the incidence of fractures in postmenopausal osteoporosis. *N Engl J Med* 333:1437–1443, 1995. (1997 YEAR BOOK OF GERIATRICS AND GERONTOLOGY, pp 84–86.)

Effects of Hormone Therapy on Bone Mineral Density

Bush TL, and the Writing Group for the PEPI Trial (Parke-Davis, Morris Plains, NJ)
JAMA 276:1389–1396, 1996 1–28

Background.—Estrogen protects against bone loss fracture and appears to be one of the best treatments for preventing postmenopausal osteoporosis. However, there are still many unanswered questions about the effect of this hormone on bone mineral density (BMD). The effects of hormone therapy on BMD in the spine and hip of postmenopausal women were investigated.

Methods.—Eight hundred seventy-five healthy women, age 45–64, seen at 7 clinical centers were included in the 3-year, randomized, double-blind, placebo-controlled clinical trial. The women were assigned to placebo; conjugated equine estrogens (CEE), 0.625 mg/day; CEE, 0.625 m/day, and medroxyprogesterone acetate (MPA), 10 mg/day for 12 day/m; CEE, 0.625 mg/day, and MPA, 2.5 mg/day; or CEE, 0.625 mg/day, and micronized progesterone, 100 mg/day for 12 day/mo. BMD was determined before treatment and after 12 and 36 months of treatment.

Findings.—By the 36-month evaluation, women receiving placebo lost a mean 1.8% of spine BMD and 1.7% of hip BMD. Women assigned to the active regimens gained BMD at both sites, ranging from 3.5% to 5% mean total increases in spinal BMD and an average increase of 1.7% of BMD in the hip. The differences in BMD changes between the placebo and active treatment groups were significant. Women receiving CEE plus continuous MPA had significantly greater spinal BMD increases (5%) than did women in the other 3 active treatment groups, whose mean increase was 3.8%. Among women adhering to treatment, there were no significant differences in BMD changes among the 4 active treatment groups. The gain in bone was significantly greater in older women, women with low initial BMD, and women with no previous hormone use than in younger women, those with higher initial BMD, and those who had previously taken hormones, respectively.

Conclusions.—Postmenopausal women receiving placebo had reduced BMD at the spine and hip, whereas those receiving estrogen treatment had increased BMD during the 36 months of the study. Estrogen replacement therapy results in BMD increases at clinically important sites.

▶ Despite the introduction of nonhormonal medications to treat and prevent osteoporosis (e.g., alendronate, calcitonin), estrogen is the most commonly used agent to prevent bone loss among postmenopausal women. Because of estrogen's other beneficial effects in preventing coronary artery disease and skin changes associated with aging (Abstract 1–18), the choice of this hormone is probably appropriate for most women. However, it is unclear whether administration of estrogen to postmenopausal women merely prevents further bone loss or actually increases BMD. Moreover, the additive effect of a progestin (which is prescribed for women who are using estrogens and have an intact uterus) on BMD is unknown. The Postmenopausal Estrogen/Progestin Interventions trial, which assigned women to 1 of 5 treatment regimens and monitored them for 36 months, provides some convincing answers to these questions. Not only did estrogen increase BMD compared with placebo, but this effect persisted throughout the entire 3 years. The combination of estrogen plus a progestin (with any of 3 regimens) did not result in further gains in BMD. This study adds credence to the current practice of using estrogen for prevention and therapy of osteoporosis. Whether estrogen combined with one of the new nonhormonal therapies confers additional benefit is a question that remains to be answered.

D.B. Reuben, M.D.

Influence of Physical Activity on Vertebral Deformity in Men and Women: Results From the European Vertebral Osteoporosis Study

Silman AJ, for the European Vertebral Osteoporosis Study Group (Univ of Manchester, England; et al)

J Bone Miner Res 12:813–819, 1997 1–29

Background.—Vertebral deformity is associated with back pain and disability, but little is known of its lifestyle risk factors. Cross-sectional and short-term prospective studies have shown an association between high levels of physical activity and increased bone density in men and women. Other studies have indicated that excessive physical activity may be associated with hormonal disturbances and decreased bone density in young and premenopausal women. Although there have been many studies of the effects of physical activity on bone density in the spine, there is little information on the relationship between physical activity and vertebral deformity.

Methods.—Subjects between the ages of 50 and 79 were enrolled by 36 centers in 19 European countries. Subjects had lateral radiographs taken of the lumbar and thoracic spine, and completed an interviewer-administered questionnaire. The questionnaire identified the level of occupational and leisure time physical activity at age 15–24, age 25–49, and age 50 and older. Subjects were also asked about time spent walking or cycling outdoors everyday.

Results.—Data from 14,261 subjects were analyzed. There were 1,693 subjects with vertebral deformity and 12,568 subjects with no vertebral deformity. In men, very high levels of physical activity at all 3 periods in life were associated with higher risk of vertebral deformity, after adjustment for age, center, smoking, and body mass index. In women, very high levels of physical activity were not associated with vertebral deformity. In women, walking or cycling more than 0.5 hr/day was associated with a lower risk of vertebral deformity.

Discussion.—The relationship between physical activity and vertebral deformity is affected by gender and intensity of activity. Regular exercise is associated with a lower risk of vertebral deformity in women age 50–79. Heavy physical activity in early and middle adult life is associated with a higher risk of vertebral deformity in men. It was difficult to obtain independent validation of physical activity, and the measures used must be considered crude. The mechanism of the negative effect of heavy activity on men needs further study. Walking and cycling should be incorporated into a population prevention strategy for osteoporosis.

▶ This article was selected because it is one of the first that addresses the issue of the effect of physical activity on the risk of vertebral deformity in contrast to bone mineral density. It represents a multicenter trial involving 19 European countries using a population survey method with a subject total of 14,261, of which more than 800 men and women had one or more vertebral deformities. Selecting vertebral deformity as an important health problem is related to its association with back pain and disability in older subjects. It is of interest that very heavy levels of activity were associated with an increased risk of vertebral deformity in men, whereas no such increased risk was observed in women, perhaps because their levels of physical activity were relatively less. The observation that current walking or cycling more than one-half hour per day was associated with a reduced risk of vertebral deformity in women has important public health implications. In men, the data might suggest that the deformity is related to trauma earlier in adult life, whereas in women, walking or cycling out of doors exerted a moderate protective effect.

There are a number of limitations to this study of which the most important are: (1) vertebral morphometry may be classified as positive suggesting a vertebral fracture, but other pathologic entities may also be included; and (2) the data were self-reported using an interviewer-administered questionnaire and the instrument used was one that was translatable across multiple

European languages and cultures without detailed performance data in each cultural group. However, neither the interviewers, nor the subjects were aware of their case-control status at the time. I believe this paper contributes substantially to our understanding of the epidemiology of vertebral deformity and thus the planning of appropriate interventions.

J.C. Beck, M.D.

Drug Prescribing

Sedative-Hypnotic Use and Increased Hospital Stay and Costs in Older People

Zisselman MH, Rovner BW, Yuen EJ, et al (Jefferson Med College, Philadelphia)

J Am Geriatr Soc 44:1371–1374, 1996 1–30

Objective.—Sedative-hypnotic drugs are administered to 41% of older hospitalized patients, often without proper documentation. Although these drugs can calm anxieties and treat sleep disorders, they also can cause confusion and can predispose the patient to falls or motor vehicle accidents. The Health Care Financing Administration (HCFA) guidelines were applied to the use of sedatives and hypnotics in hospitalized older patients and to the association of use with duration of hospitalization and costs.

Methods.—Drug type and dose were obtained from computerized pharmacy and administrative records at Thomas Jefferson University Hospital, a 717-bed tertiary care facility in Philadelphia. Of the 856 (54.3%, female) consecutive patients, average age 74.5, admitted between November 1993 and March 1994, 170 of them received doses of sedative-hypnotic drugs in excess of HCFA guidelines. A total 283 patients received doses of medication within the guidelines, and 403 did not receive any sedative-hypnotic medication. Severity of illness, demographics, duration of hospitalization, and costs were recorded.

Results.—Patients were hospitalized an average of 11.5 days. Patients who received an excess of sedative-hypnotic drugs had significantly more severe illnesses and significantly longer hospital stays (21.5 days) than the patients receiving doses within the HCFA guidelines (12.3 days) or the patients receiving no sedative-hypnotic drugs (6.7 days). Patients receiving an excess of sedative-hypnotic drugs also had significantly higher hospital costs ($29,245), compared with patients receiving doses within HCFA guidelines ($15,219), or patients receiving no sedative-hypnotic drugs ($7,561). Two separate multivariate stepwise regression models showed that duration of hospitalization was determined by severity of illness, followed by any use of sedative-hypnotic drugs, older age, and race. Determinants of hospital costs, according to the stepwise model, were severity of illness, followed by surgery, any use of sedative-hypnotic drugs, older age, and race.

Conclusion.—Older patients receiving sedative-hypnotic drugs have longer hospital stays, more severe illnesses, and higher hospital costs than patients not receiving them. Doses of sedative-hypnotic drugs often exceed HCFA guidelines. Increased scrutiny of sedative-hypnotic use in older hospitalized patients is recommended.

▶ Iatrogenic complications of hospitalization are tragedies in the care of older persons. In this study, the investigators examined one source of potential hospital-induced problems, the inappropriate use of sedative-hypnotic drugs. Their standard for inappropriateness was the HCFA guidelines that specify "optimum" starting and total daily doses for nursing home residents. In fact, these guidelines can be considered quite liberal because they do not judge the appropriateness of prescribing the sedative-hypnotic, versus using other treatments for insomnia or anxiety.

In this study, more than 50% of hospitalized elderly patients received 1 of these drugs, and 20% of elderly hospitalized patients received doses outside the HCFA guidelines. Moreover, those who had greater severity of illness and those who had cancer were more likely to receive doses that exceeded the guidelines. Although severity of illness was the most powerful determinant of length of hospital stay and hospital costs, excessive doses of sedative-hypnotic drugs remained an independent predictor. The lesson is simple and clear: when writing a hospital admission order, first consider whether a patient needs a hypnotic-sedative at all, and, if so, use the lowest dose that is effective.

D.B. Reuben, M.D.

Diseases Affecting Organ Systems

CARDIOLOGY

Randomised Trial of Losartan Versus Captopril in Patients Over 65 With Heart Failure (Evaluation of Losartan in the Elderly Study, ELITE)
Pitt B, on behalf of ELITE Study investigators (Univ Hosp, Ann Arbor, Mich; et al)
Lancet 349:747–752, 1997 1–31

Background.—Angiotensin-converting enzyme (ACE) inhibitors are useful in the treatment of chronic heart failure and left ventricular dysfunction. However, probably because of their preservation of bradykinin, these drugs (such as captopril) are associated with significant side effects like cough, angioedema, renal dysfunction, and hypotension. Angiotensin II type 1 receptor antagonists exert their effects without increasing bradykinin levels, and thus these drugs (such as losartan) may avoid the side effects of ACE inhibitors. The safety and efficacy of captopril and losartan were compared in the treatment of heart failure in elderly patients.

Methods.—This prospective, double-blind, randomized study involved 722 patients age 65 and older with New York Heart Association classes II–IV heart failure, decreased (40% or less) left-ventricular ejection fraction, and no history of previous ACE inhibitor use. Patients received

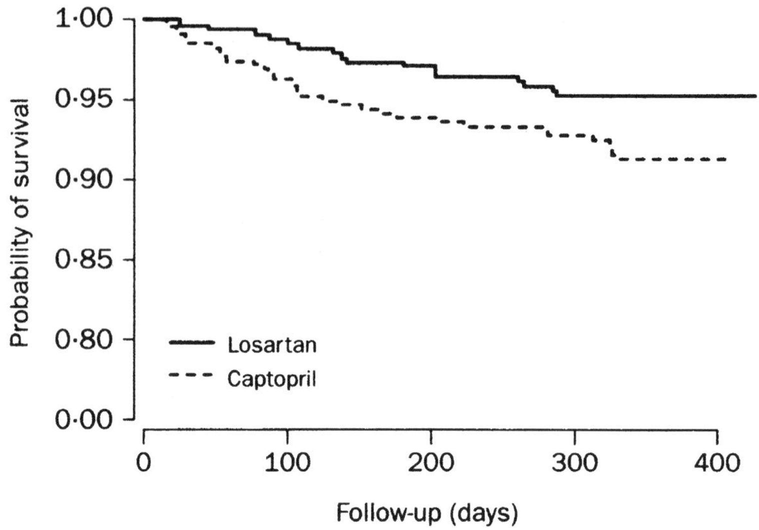

FIGURE 2.—Kaplan-Meier survival curves among patients with chronic heart failure in losartan and captopril groups. Patients in the losartan group had a 46% lower risk of death than patients in the captopril group ($P = 0.035$). Patients were followed up for 48 weeks. (Courtesy of Pitt B, on behalf of ELITE Study investigators: Randomised trial of losartan versus captopril in patients over 65 with heart failure [Evaluation of Losartan in the Elderly Study, ELITE]. *Lancet* 349:747–752, 1997. Copyright by the Lancet Ltd, 1997.)

48 weeks of therapy with either captopril (titrated to 50 mg 3 times daily; $n = 370$) or losartan (titrated to 50 mg once a day; $n = 352$). End points for discontinuing therapy included a persistent increase in serum creatinine levels of 0.3 mg/dL or more (indicating renal dysfunction); hospitalization for heart failure, myocardial infarction, or angina; worsening of heart failure; hypotension-related symptoms; adverse reaction to the study drugs; and death.

Findings.—The 2 groups were similar at baseline with respect to demographics, other drug therapies, and hemodynamic parameters. After treatment, both groups were also similar in the increases in serum creatinine (10.5% in each group) and symptoms related to hypotension. However, the losartan group experienced fewer all-cause deaths (4.8%) than the captopril group (8.7%), primarily because of fewer sudden cardiac deaths in the losartan group (Fig 2). Significantly more patients discontinued therapy or died while taking captopril (30%) than while taking losartan (18.5%).

Conclusions.—Neither renal dysfunction nor hospitalizations and deaths because of heart failure were more common with either drug. Similarly, both drugs improved cardiac function after long-term treatment. However, losartan was associated with less all-cause mortality, mainly because of fewer sudden cardiac deaths. Losartan was also associated with fewer drop-outs as a result of drug intolerance. Whether the effects of losartan on reducing cardiac deaths are specific to this drug, or are general to all angiotensin II type 1 receptor antagonists, remains to be determined.

► Angiotensin-converting enzyme (ACE) inhibitors have had a dramatic impact in reducing morbidity and mortality in patients who have chronic congestive heart failure and systolic dysfunction. However, some patients have not been able to tolerate ACE inhibitors because cough or other side effects have developed. Recently, angiotensin II type 1 receptor antagonists have been developed that are not associated with cough and have comparable hemodynamic effects to ACE inhibitors. However, it is unknown whether angiotensin antagonists have similar benefits on health outcomes and whether they are actually better tolerated in clinical practice. This randomized clinical trial compared an ACE inhibitor with an angiotensin receptor antagonist in elderly patients with symptomatic congestive heart failure and left-ventricular ejection fraction of 40% or less.

The findings of the study, in some respects, were somewhat expected and reassuring. There were no differences between the 2 groups with respect to persistent renal dysfunction (10.5% overall) and no subject discontinued losartan because of cough. Overall, fewer subjects in the losartan group discontinued drug therapy because of adverse side effects. However, the study had an important unexpected finding; survival was significantly better in the losartan group, primarily as a result of a reduction in sudden cardiac deaths. The mechanism for this benefit is uncertain and may relate to more complete blockade of angiotensin II or a specific property of this medication. Nevertheless, if this difference in mortality is confirmed, it may lead to a preference for ACE antagonists over ACE inhibitors in this subgroup of patients. For the present, clinicians can feel comfortable that losartan provides at least as much benefit as an ACE inhibitor for patients with symptomatic heart failure and is an acceptable alternative for those who cannot tolerate ACE inhibitors.

D.B. Reuben, M.D.

Double-blind, Placebo-controlled Study of the Effects of Carvedilol in Patients With Moderate to Severe Heart Failure: The PRECISE Trial
Packer M, for the PRECISE Study Group (Columbia Univ, New York, et al)
Circulation 94:2793–2799, 1996 1–32

Introduction.—In the treatment of patients with heart failure, β-adrenergic blocking drugs have emerged as a promising approach. A decrease in the risk of progression to end-stage disease was shown with long-term treatment with bisoprolol, carvedilol, and metoprolol. Less is known, however, regarding the effects of these drugs on the symptoms of heart failure. To assess the efficacy of carvedilol in patients with moderate-to-severe heart failure, a large number of clinical variables were evaluated because of uncertainties regarding the most appropriate end points to use for the evaluation of a β-blocker.

Methods.—There were 278 patients with moderate-to-severe heart failure and a left ventricular ejection fraction 0.35 or less. There were 145 patients randomly assigned to placebo and 133 assigned to carvedilol, with a target dose of 25–50 mg twice a day for 6 months. The background therapy with an angiotensin-converting enzyme (ACE) inhibitor, diuretics, and digoxin remained constant. Patients were evaluated by New York Heart Association functional class or by a global assessment of progress by either themselves or by a physician.

Results.—A greater frequency of symptomatic improvement and a lower risk of clinical deterioration was found in the patients taking carvedilol compared with the patients taking placebo. A significant increase in ejection fraction and a significant decrease in the combined risk of morbidity and mortality was seen in patients treated with carvedilol. Little effect, however, was seen in the indirect measurements of patient benefit, such as quality-of-life scores or exercise tolerance in patients taking carvedilol. Patients with ischemic heart disease or idiopathic dilated cardiomyopathy as the cause of heart failure had similar effects when taking carvedilol.

Conclusion.—In patients with moderate-to-severe heart failure treated with digoxin, diuretics, and an ACE inhibitor, carvedilol produces important clinical benefits and has favorable effects on survival. Benefits include ameliorating the symptoms, diminishing the disability, and reducing the morbidity.

Carvedilol Inhibits Clinical Progression in Patients With Mild Symptoms of Heart Failure

Colucci WS, for the US Carvedilol Heart Failure Study Group (Boston Univ, et al)

Circulation 94:2800–2806, 1996 1–33

Introduction.—Most patients with heart failure have only mild symptoms and are usually not considered candidates for additional treatment, yet they still remain at risk for clinical progression. Activation of the sympathetic nervous system is often responsible for progression of heart failure, suggesting that drugs that interfere with the actions of the sympathetic nervous system, such as β-blockers, may reduce the risk of disease progression. The potential use of carvedilol, a nonselective β-adrenergic receptor antagonist that also blocks α_1-adrenergic receptors, was assessed in clinically stable, well-compensated patients with mildly symptomatic heart failure.

Methods.—There were 366 patients with mildly symptomatic heart failure and a left ventricular ejection fraction of 0.35 or less. There were 134 patients randomized to placebo and 232 randomized to carvedilol and followed for 12 months. All had minimal functional impairment and were receiving optimal standard therapy, including angiotensin-converting enzyme (ACE) inhibitors. A sustained increase in heart failure medications, hospitalization for heart failure, or death caused by heart failure were the primary end points.

Results.—In 11% of carvedilol patients and in 21% of placebo patients, clinical progression of heart failure occurred. In the primary end point of heart failure progression, there was a 48% reduction. Sex, age, race, cause of heart failure, or baseline left ventricular ejection fraction did not influence the effect of carvedilol. Several secondary end points—such as heart failure score, physician and patient global assessments, New York Heart Association functional class, and left ventricular ejection fraction—were also improved with carvedilol and all-cause mortality was reduced. The Minnesota Living with Heart Failure scale, the distance walked in 9 minutes on a self-powered treadmill, and the cardiothoracic index were not improved by carvedilol.

Conclusion.—In patients who are only mildly symptomatic with well-compensated heart failure, carvedilol reduces clinical progression when added to standard therapy, including an ACE inhibitor. In the therapeutic regimen of patients with mild heart failure, carvedilol may play an important part.

Carvedilol Produces Dose-related Improvements in Left Ventricular Function and Survival in Subjects With Chronic Heart Failure

Bristow MR, for the MOCHA Investigators (Univ of Colorado, Denver; et al)

Circulation 94:2807–2816, 1996 1–34

Background.—Carvedilol is a β-blocker that does not cause myocardial depression or reduced cardiac output in patients with heart failure. Although previous short-term, smaller trials have documented the drug's effectiveness in treating symptoms of heart failure, its effectiveness over a longer term remains to be determined. This multicenter, placebo-controlled study evaluated the drug's effectiveness over 6 months.

Methods.—Patients with stable, symptomatic, chronic heart failure (New York Heart Association [NYHA] class II or III) underwent a 2-week challenge with 6.25 mg of carvedilol twice daily. Those who tolerated this challenge were then assigned to 1 of 4 treatment groups and given placebo (n = 84) or low-dose (n = 83), medium-dose (n = 89), or high-dose (n = 89) carvedilol (6.25, 12.5, or 25 mg bid, respectively). After titration to the desired dose, patients were monitored at regular intervals for 6 months. Electroencephalograms and submaximal exercise tests were performed at regular intervals. The left ventricular ejection fraction was measured at baseline and at the end of treatment.

Findings.—Most patients (92%) tolerated the 2-week drug challenge; those who stopped taking the drug had symptoms related to orthostatic hypotension or myocardial depression. Patients in the 4 study groups showed no changes in blood pressure over the course of the study, but there was a minimal decrease in heart rate as the carvedilol dose was increased. The results of submaximal exercise tests did not differ between the placebo and active drug groups, but the left ventricular ejection fraction was significantly improved in a dose-dependent manner in patients taking carvedilol. Hospitalization and mortality rates were significantly reduced in patients taking carvedilol. The only side effects reported significantly more often by carvedilol-treated patients were dizziness and bradycardia. However, withdrawal from the study because of adverse effects was more common in patients taking placebo than in those taking any dose of carvedilol.

Conclusions.—Over 6 months of follow-up, carvedilol was well tolerated and resulted in improved left ventricular ejection fraction, lower hospitalization rates, and fewer deaths, compared with placebo. Beneficial effects were greater with greater doses of the drug.

▶ Carvedilol is a third-generation β-blocking agent that also has α-blocking and antioxidant effects. These 3 randomized clinical trials (Abstracts 1–32, 1–33, and 1–34) of patients with congestive heart failure and various degrees of symptoms provide important information about the effectiveness of this new drug. All 3 studies included subjects with poor ventricular function (left ventricular ejection fraction, 0.22–0.23). In 1 trial, the majority of participants were categorized as NYHA class II. In the other 2 trials, there was a fairly even split between participants who were categorized as NYHA class II and those classified as NYHA class III. There were also a few NYHA class IV participants. Patients remained on constant background therapy with digoxin, diuretics, and angiotensin-converting enzyme inhibitors. All 3 of the studies indicated substantial benefits of the new agent. Among the benefits were improvements in survival, left ventricular function, and specific symptoms. Hospitalizations also were reduced. There were no differences in most quality-of-life measures or performance-based (e.g., treadmill or 6-minute walk) tests. However, 6% to 8% of research subjects who were otherwise eligible for the study could not tolerate the medication in an open-label challenge. The most common side effects were dizziness, fatigue, congestive heart failure, and hypotension. Although not all elderly patients may be able to tolerate carvedilol, it appears that this medication represents a major addition to the pharmacotherapy of congestive heart failure.

D.B. Reuben, M.D.

A Comprehensive Management System for Heart Failure Improves Clinical Outcomes and Reduces Medical Resource Utilization

West JA, Miller NH, Parker KM, et al (Veterans Affairs Palo Alto Health Care System, Calif; Stanford Univ, Calif; Kaiser Permanante Med Care Program of Northern California, Haywood)

Am J Cardiol 79:58–63, 1997 1–35

Background.—The management of chronic heart failure requires vigilance by both physician and patient. Suboptimal prescription practices (such as the underprescribing of angiotensin-converting enzyme [ACE] inhibitors), poor outpatient monitoring, and poor patient adherence to behavioral (sodium lowering) and drug regimens can detract from effective disease control. Can improvements in these factors be made, and if so, will they improve clinical outcomes?

Methods.—The study group consisted of patients hospitalized with heart failure who had no significant comorbid conditions or psychosocial factors that limited their capacity to participate fully. A total of 51 patients with heart failure were enrolled in the MULTIFIT intervention for an average of 138 ± 44 days (range, 55–196 days). This intervention had the following 3 goals: (1) use of optimal doses of ACE inhibitors or isosorbide dinitrate or hydralazine therapy, (2) salt restriction to less than 2 g/day, and (3) recognition of worsening symptoms and initiation of efficient treatment. A nurse manager educated patients about their disease, the roles of salt restriction and drug compliance, the warning signs of adverse effects, and how to improve adherence. At frequent intervals, nurse managers followed up with scheduled patient phone calls and questionnaires regarding salt intake, drug compliance, and any adverse effects.

Findings.—Only 3 patients were hospitalized for heart failure during the study, and only 8 patients went to an emergency department for treatment of heart failure. Patients in the MULTIFIT intervention had significant decreases in the number of medical and cardiology visits, emergency department visits (for heart failure, as well as other causes), and hospitalizations (for heart failure or any other cause), compared with rates 6 months before the study began, which were normalized to address different amounts of follow-up. Functional status improved significantly, as did symptoms of cough, dyspnea on exertion, orthopnea, and fatigue. The percentage of patients taking their target dose of an ACE inhibitor increased from 45% to 83%. Self-reported salt intake declined by 38% over the course of the intervention. Nurse managers and patients interacted an average of 7 hours over 4.5 months of follow-up.

Conclusions.—Although physicians maintained overall responsibility for management of the patient's condition, involvement of the nurse managers resulted in improved functional status and reduced utilization of medical resources by home-living patients with heart failure. Compliance with both pharmacologic and behavioral therapies improved significantly, as did the clinical outcomes.

▶ Congestive heart failure (CHF) is a common, serious, and chronic disease for which there are beneficial interventions that are underutilized. The reasons for lack of optimal management of CHF relate to physician factors (e.g., not prescribing ACE inhibitors) and patient factors (e.g., not taking prescribed medications or maintaining low-sodium diets). Moreover, the sometimes haphazard system of health care delivery frequently does not permit adequate monitoring of persons with chronic diseases. This case–series describes an intervention to address some of these problems.

The intervention focused on attempting to titer patients to optimum doses of medication, lowering sodium intake, and surveillance and prompt intervention if patients demonstrated instability. To achieve these goals, nurse educators were used to teach self-management to patients and to monitor patients frequently by telephone. Primary physicians retained overall responsibility for patient management.

The results of this study were impressive, demonstrating reductions in dietary sodium; increases in medications for CHF; improvements in functional status and exercise capacity; and reductions of medical visits, emergency department visits, and hospitalizations. Because of the absence of a control group, these striking findings must be considered preliminary. Nevertheless, similar to the intervention described by Rich et al.,[1] paying meticulous attention to the details of managing this chronic illness can result in major benefits.

D.B. Reuben, M.D.

Reference

1. Rich MW, Beckham V, Wittenberg C, et al: A multidisciplinary intervention to prevent the readmission of elderly patients with congestive heart failure. *N Engl J Med* 333:1190–1195, 1995. (1997 Year Book of Geriatrics and Gerontology, pp 36–38.)

Infectious Diseases

Hospitalization for Pneumonia Among Older Adults

Callahan CM, Wolinsky FD (Indiana Univ, Indianapolis; Saint Louis Univ)
J Gerontol 51A:M276–M282, 1996 1–36

Objective.—There are 4 million cases of pneumonia in the United States annually, and hospitalization rates increase with age from 5.1/1,000 for ages 60–64 to 56/1,000 for those age 85 and older. This risk of death from pneumonia is higher among men and among those with malnutrition or a history of stroke, cancer, or diabetes. Risk increases in the elderly because of decreased ability to clear secretions, a decline in the immune system, and more frequent upper respiratory infections. The frequency and costs of hospitalization for pneumonia over an 8-year period among a nationally representative sample of community-dwelling Americans age 70 and older, together with the risk factors for hospitalization for pneumonia with the possibility of functional impairment were investigated.

Methods.—Functional status, health, living arrangements, demographics, social structure, behaviors, medical history, and case findings were examined in 7,527 subjects (62% women), age 70–99 in 1984, who participated in the Longitudinal Study of Aging. The Cox regression analysis was used to determine the risk for pneumonia hospitalization.

Results.—By 1991, 2,867 (38.1%) had died. Between 1984 and 1991, 617 participants were hospitalized 813 times for pneumonia. There were 84 participants with 2 bouts of pneumonia, 31 with 3, 13 with 4 or more, and the remainder with 1. Ninety percent of hospitalized participants had a co-morbid condition. The frequency of hospitalization for pneumonia increased from 0.6% in 1984 to 2.4% in 1994. Older participants had longer hospital stays than younger participants (49 vs. 27 days) and incurred greater hospital charges ($34,259 vs. $21,345). Those hospitalized tended to be older, male, have less than 8 years of education, live in the South, live in nonmetropolitan areas, receive Medicaid, have malnutrition, have a history of hip fracture and hospitalizations, and have impaired functional status of the legs. Over the study period, hospital charges for patients with pneumonia increased, whereas hospital stays decreased.

Conclusion.—This prospective 8-year study of community-dwelling elderly patients found that hospitalization for pneumonia was common, particularly among males, those in poorer health, those with lower body limitations, and those receiving Medicaid. These hospitalizations resulted in significant costs to Medicare. More than 80% of patients survived their first hospitalization. Hospitalization for pneumonia was age-related.

▶ The data presented in this article differ from previous reports[1] by focusing on a much older community-dwelling population and by prospectively following the patients over an 8-year period. It is of interest that lower body limitations, but not limitations in activities of daily living or instrumental activities of daily living, were associated with hospitalization for pneumonia among the participants in the study. This may be because the functional status data were those at baseline rather than those just before admission for pneumonia. The chronic illness indicators that were important included malnutrition and a history of hip fracture, whereas none of the other associations had significance. One other limitation to this study is that there were no indicators of self-reported pulmonary disease, or tobacco or alcohol consumption.

J.C. Beck, M.D.

Reference

1. Graves EJ: Detailed diagnoses and procedures: National hospital discharge survey, 1991. *Vital Health Stat* 13:115, 1994.

Community-acquired Pneumonia in the Elderly: A Multivariate Analysis of Risk and Prognostic Factors

Riquelme R, Torres A, El-Ebiary M, et al (Universitat de Barcelona)

Am J Respir Crit Care Med 154:1450–1455, 1996 1–37

Introduction.—The occurrence of pneumonia in the elderly population is a substantial public health problem. Hospitalizations due to pneumonia increase dramatically in persons over age 55, and the prevalence and fatality rates are higher in the elderly when compared with the younger populations. The risk factors for older persons developing community-acquired pneumonia have been insufficiently studied. Over an 8-month period, the risk and prognostic factors of community-acquired pneumonia were studied in an elderly population requiring hospitalization.

Methods.—One hundred and one patients with community-acquired pneumonia, age 78.5 ± 7.9 years, were studied. Risk factors were analyzed by matching each patient with a pneumonia-free control subject admitted to the hospital through the emergency room. Each match was made on the basis of age, sex, and date of admission.

Results.—In 43 of 101 pneumonia patients (42%), etiologic diagnosis was obtained. *Streptococcus pneumoniae* (44%) and *Chlamydia pneumoniae* (21%) were the main microbial agents causing pneumonia. It was uncommon to find gram-negative bacilli (5%). Independent risk factors associated with the development of pneumonia were large volume aspiration and serum albumin of less than 30 mg/dL. The pneumonia-related mortality rate was 20%, the crude mortality rate was 26%, and the attributable mortality rate was 23%. Prognosis was worse for patients who had 3 or more affected lobes on chest radiography, respiratory frequency greater than 30 breaths/min, a body temperature on admission of less than 37°C, prior swallowing disorders, or if they were previously bedridden. Prognosis was not significantly related to age.

Conclusion.—Some risk factors associated with the development of community-acquired pneumonia in the elderly population are potentially remediable. Once pneumonia has developed few of the prognostic factors are modifiable.

▶ Despite the availability of pneumococcal vaccine, pneumonia is still a major cause of morbidity and mortality among community-dwelling older persons. This study of older persons with pneumonia requiring hospitalization provides insight into the causes (by far, *Streptococcus pneumoniae* was the leading organism), risk factors for the development of pneumonia (clinical suspicion of large-volume aspiration and low serum albumin), and the prognosis for this infection (26% overall mortality, and 20% pneumonia related). Independent prognostic factors for death included the following characteristics at the time of hospital admission: bedridden, temperature of 37°C or less, respiratory rate of 30/min or more, and 3 or more affected lobes. The findings of this study suggest several steps that can be taken to prevent pneumonia, particularly the administration of pneumococcal vaccine, methods to reduce aspiration risk, and the maintenance of adequate nutrition. In contrast, the study sheds little light on correctable factors that might improve the prognosis of pneumonia once it is present.

D.B. Reuben, M.D.

Clinical and Bacteriological Characteristics of Infective Endocarditis in the Elderly

Selton-Suty C, Hoen B, Grentzinger A, et al (CHU Brabois, Nancy, France)

Heart 77:260–263, 1997 1–38

Background.—The incidence of infective endocarditis is increasing among older people, but it remains difficult to diagnose. The potential age-related features of the presentation of infective endocarditis were examined in this prospective study.

Methods.—From 1990 to 1991, 114 patients with the diagnosis infective endocarditis treated in the Lorraine region of France were studied prospectively. The patients were divided into 2 groups: group 1, patients older than 70; and group 2, patients older than 15-years-old but younger than 70. Age, sex, preexisting heart disease, previous infective endocarditis, fever, echocardiographic data, blood cultures, microorganisms, portal of entry, duration of hospital stay, surgery, and death were recorded.

Results.—The location of endocarditis clinical signs, and symptoms were not significantly different between the 2 groups. The older patients had a lower occurrence of embolic episodes. The rate of infective endocarditis on intracardiac prosthetic devices was higher in the older patient group. The older patients had more infections with bacteria from the gastrointestinal tract such as group D streptococci and enterococci. The presumed portal of entry was more often digestive among the older patients. Older patients were less often treated with surgery and had higher mortality than younger patients with infective endocarditis.

Conclusions.—The diagnosis of infective endocarditis remains difficult. In older patients, infective endocarditis often occurs in those with intracardiac prosthetic devices and is more often caused by gastrointestinal bacteria. The prognosis is worse in older patients. Better prophylaxis in older patients—such as detection of colonic lesions, antibiotic prophylaxis during gastrointestinal investigations, and prevention of nosocomial infection—should be developed. Increased use of surgery may also improve prognosis in older patients with infective endocarditis.

► Endocarditis is rare in older persons but is frequently considered in the differential diagnosis for patients hospitalized with fever without a clear source. This case series reports some interesting findings comparing endocarditis in older and younger persons. Older persons were more likely to have prosthetic valve infection. Although embolic events and echocardiographic vegetations occur less frequently in older persons, diagnostic clinical findings were no more likely to occur in either age group. However, group D streptococci and enterococci were more common among older persons, and a gastrointestinal source was more often implicated. Such information is valuable in deciding on an antibiotic if empiric treatment is being considered. Unfortunately, in any age group the diagnosis of infective endocarditis remains difficult.

D.B. Reuben, M.D.

Rheumatology

A Randomized Trial Comparing Aerobic Exercise and Resistance Exercise With a Health Education Program in Older Adults With Knee Osteoarthritis: The Fitness Arthritis and Seniors Trial (FAST)

Ettinger WH, Burns R, Messier SP, et al (Wake Forest Univ, Winston-Salem, NC; Univ of Tennessee, Memphis)
JAMA 277:25–31, 1997 1–39

Background.—Osteoarthritis of the knee is a common cause of pain and activity limitation among the elderly. There is no cure, and the goals of therapy are pain reduction and improved quality of life. The American College of Rheumatology has recently recommended that exercise should be part of the treatment for osteoarthritis. The Fitness and Arthritis in Seniors Trials (FAST) examined the effect of structured exercise programs on self-reported disability in older adults with documented knee osteoarthritis.

Study Design.—A randomized, single-blind, 18-month clinical trial of 439 elderly participants with osteoarthritis was conducted at 2 academic medical centers. The patients were randomized to aerobic exercise, resistance exercise, or a health education program. The primary outcome was self-reported disability, and knee pain scores, physical performance measures, radiographs, aerobic capacity, and knee muscle strength were secondary assessments.

Results.—There were a total 365 volunteers who completed the trial. The overall compliance was 68% in the aerobic group and 70% in the resistance training group. After the 18-month trial period, the aerobic exercise group had a 10% lower adjusted mean score on physical disability and a 12% lower score on the knee pain questionnaire; the aerobic exercise group performed better on the 6-minute walk test and had better times when it came to climbing and descending stairs, lifting and carrying 10 pounds, and getting in and out of a car than the health education group. The resistance exercise group had an 8% lower score on the physical disability questionnaire, an 8% lower pain score, greater distance on the 6-minute walk, faster times on the lift and carry test, and faster times on the car test than the health education group. There were no significant differences in x-ray scores among these 3 groups.

Conclusions.—The results of this large 18-month study of older patients with osteoarthritis demonstrated that those who participated in either an aerobic or resistance training program had modest improvements in tests of disability, physical activity, and pain compared with those who participated in a health education program. Exercise appears to be a safe and effective treatment that improves both pain and function in older patients with osteoarthritis. A program of moderate exercise should be included in the treatment program for elderly patients with osteoarthritis.

► Osteoarthritis is the most commonly reported disease among older individuals. When affecting the knee, osteoarthritis often causes pain and functional impairment. Although analgesics and nonsteroidal anti-inflammatory agents have been the mainstay of treatment for osteoarthritis of the knee, increasing attention has been paid to the use of exercise as an adjunct or a primary therapy. This randomized clinical trial of elderly individuals with knee osteoarthritis with resultant pain and functional impairment evaluated 2 types of exercise: aerobic exercise via walking and resistance training using weights; an attention-control education group was also enrolled. At 18 months, self-reported disability scores were lower (better) by approximately 10% in both exercise groups compared with the education group. There were no differences between the 2 types of exercise. Although overall compliance with the exercise regimens was approximately 70%, by 18 months it was only 50%. Those who had higher levels of compliance had more benefit from the exercise regimens. Although the magnitude of benefit from the exercise programs was not large, the programs had few adverse effects. This study provides further evidence of the importance of exercise in the management of osteoarthritis in older individuals. Further research needs to be conducted on developing and testing strategies to improve compliance with the exercise prescription.

D.B. Reuben, M.D.

► Osteoarthritis of the knee is one of the most important causes of pain and limitation in activities in older persons but many questions remain about the effects of exercise. This particular paper addresses what types of exercise are most beneficial; what is the compliance/adherence rate of older persons with long-term exercise programs; what are the additional effects of exercise above and beyond the effects of patient education, attention and socialization, and if there are any harmful effects of exercise associated with long term exercise programs.

This is the first randomized trial of an exercise intervention in knee osteoarthritis to last for 18 months. Other studies in both osteoarthritis and rheumatoid arthritis have shown improvements in pain and disability, but the interventions have never lasted more than 2–3 months.[1, 2] This study shows modest but significant reductions in disability and pain associated with 2 levels of exercise with a maximum improvement seen at the end of the 3-month supervised exercise period. Subgroup analyses showed that benefit existed in both sexes, in black persons as well as white persons, in individuals with obesity, and in individuals over the age of 70.

It seems clear that in the absence of a definitive therapy for osteoarthritis treatment should include both a moderate intensity exercise program and standard pharmacologic therapy. Further research is clearly needed on increasing the compliance of the older person with exercise since these data clearly showed a dose-response effect of the exercise program related to compliance.

J.C. Beck, M.D.

References

1. Kovar PA, Allegrante JP, MacKenzie CR, et al: Supervised fitness walking in patients with osteoarthritis of the knee. *Ann Intern Med* 116:529–534, 1992.
2. Minor MA, Hewett JE, Wevel RR, et al: Efficacy of physical conditioning exercise in patients with rheumatoid arthritis and osteoarthritis. *Arthritis Rheum* 32:1396–1405, 1989.

ENDOCRINOLOGY

Does Treatment With L-Thyroxine Influence Health Status in Middle-aged and Older Adults With Subclinical Hypothyroidism?

Jaeschke R, Guyatt G, Gerstein H, et al (McMaster Univ, Hamilton, Ont; St Joseph's Hosp, Hamilton, Ont)
J Gen Intern Med 11:744–749, 1996 1–40

Introduction.—Thyroid replacement therapy in patients with subclinical hypothyroidism is controversial. Thirty-seven patients who were middle-aged and older were evaluated to determine whether L-thyroxine replacement therapy improved health-related quality of life (HRQL).

Methods.—Patients were randomized in double-blind, placebo-controlled fashion to receive either L-thyroxine replacement therapy or placebo. The mean daily dose of L-thyroxine replacement was 68 µg in the treatment group. Patients completed HRQL questionnaires, participated in a battery of cognitive function tests, underwent bone mineral density measurement using dual photon absorptiometry of the lumbar spine, and had serum drawn for thyroid studies and lipid levels.

Results.—In the treatment group, thyroid-stimulating hormone decreased by 8.6 mIU/L and T_4 increased by 27.9 nmol/L. Significant improvements were observed in psychometric memory scores in treated patients, compared to controls. There were no between-group differences in all other outcome measures. No measure of symptoms of subclinical hypothyroidism or HRQL questionnaires indicated clinically important trends in favor of treatment.

Conclusion.—Findings indicate that it may not be harmful to follow biochemical and clinical status in middle-aged and older patients with elevated thyroid stimulating hormone and normal T_4, even in the presence of nonspecific clinical symptoms potentially associated with hypothyroidism.

► Subclinical (or biochemical) hypothyroidism, characterized by an elevated thyroid-stimulating hormone level with a normal thyroxine level, is an exceptionally common disorder among older individuals, particularly older women in whom the prevalence may exceed 15%. Accordingly, clinicians are frequently confronted with the question of whether to treat or watch for symptoms or a drop in the thyroxine level that would indicate overt hypothyroidism. In older patients, this decision is complicated by the desire not to add another medication to a list that is often long and cumbersome, but by the realization that symptoms of hypothyroidism, particularly cognitive symptoms, may be subtle. Furthermore, there have been few data to indicate a preferred strategy. In this study, Jaeschke et al. report the result of a small, randomized clinical trial that provides some useful information but cannot be considered conclusive. As the authors note, the study's major limitation was its sample size (N=37), but the differences in change of most measures between groups do not suggest that a larger sample would have led to different outcomes. The overall results do not indicate clinical improvement from treating subclinical hypothyroidism. A sole exception was a composite measure of memory, which indicated a small but statistically significant benefit from thyroid replacement. Most clinicians will decide about treatment on a case-by-case basis, but the results of this study may reassure clinicians that watchful waiting is probably a reasonable choice for some.

D.B. Reuben, M.D.

Prevalence of Undiagnosed Non–Insulin-dependent Diabetes Mellitus and Impaired Glucose Tolerance in a Cohort of Older Persons With Hypertension

Johnson KC, Graney MJ, Applegate WB, et al (Univ of Tennessee, Memphis; Gen Clinical Research Ctr, Memphis, Tenn)

J Am Geriatr Soc 45:695–700, 1997 1–41

Background.—Hypertension is associated with hyperinsulinemia and insulin resistance. Insulin resistance leading to hyperinsulinemia may be the etiologic connection between hypertension and glucose intolerance. The incidence of undiagnosed non–insulin-dependent diabetes mellitus or impaired glucose tolerance in older adults with essential hypertension is unknown.

Methods.—An ancillary study was conducted of 95 randomly chosen subjects from the Trial of Nonpharmacologic Interventions in the Elderly. All subjects were between the ages of 60 and 80. The relation of the baseline glycemic state to insulin and C-peptide levels was examined to learn the prevalence of undiagnosed non–insulin-dependent diabetes mellitus and impaired glucose tolerance. At baseline, subjects were given a 75-gm glucose solution. Blood specimens were drawn 30, 60, 90, and 120 minutes after ingestion.

Results.—Of the 95 subjects, 43 had normal glucose tolerance, 41 had impaired glucose tolerance, and 11 had undiagnosed non–insulin-dependent diabetes mellitus. The positive predictive value for non–insulin-dependent diabetes mellitus of a fasting glucose of 115 mg/dL or more was 57%. Only 1 subject had hyperinsulinemia; this subject also had impaired glucose tolerance.

Discussion.—Non–insulin-dependent diabetes mellitus and impaired glucose tolerance are common in elderly individuals taking medication for essential hypertension. There was a correlation between higher fasting glucose levels and higher risk for diabetes mellitus and impaired glucose tolerance. Female gender, higher diastolic blood pressure, and older age may be risk factors for non–insulin-dependent diabetes mellitus. Hypertension may not be related to fasting hyperinsulinemia in older adults. It is unclear whether screening for diabetes should be performed before symptoms or complications develop. Evidence indicates that undiagnosed diabetes and impaired glucose tolerance are not benign, and that outcome can improve with treatment. The American Diabetes Association recommends screening for individuals at current or future risk of having diabetes.

▶ This article was identified because it is the first to report on the prevalence of undiagnosed diabetes in patients with hypertension. The report focuses on baseline glycemic states in relation to blood glucose, insulin, and C-peptide levels identified after a standardized oral glucose tolerance test. The data demonstrate that impaired oral glucose tolerance in this population is seen in 43.2% of the sample and that using the standard criteria, 11.6% had undiagnosed non–insulin-dependent diabetes mellitus (NIDDM). The data further show that there is an increased prevalence of the disease in women and an increased prevalence as persons age. It is intriguing that the majority of the persons did not have an associated fasting hyperinsulinemia, and that additional analyses would suggest that hypertension is not associated with fasting hyperinsulinemia in this particular older cohort, in contrast to previously reported findings. This may be related to the method for insulin assay, because previous studies have often measured both pro insulin and insulin, whereas this study used a monoclonal antibody technique that cross-reacted only with insulin.

It would seem that, from a public health standpoint, older individuals deserve a screening procedure to exclude undiagnosed NIDDM, and if the new criteria utilized by the American Diabetes Association are considered, an even higher proportion of older individuals have NIDDM. There are several limitations to this study, the first being that it represented a substudy in a larger study addressing nonpharmacologic treatment of essential hypertension in older persons and that 60% of the sample was obese as part of the recruitment effort for the primary study. It is also possible that the failure to confirm the apparent relationship between hypertension and glucose intolerance may be because the Trial of Nonpharmacologic Interventions in the Elderly excluded subjects whose fasting blood sugars were greater than 160 mg/dL. The sample size in this study was small, and the racial distribution was such that there was inadequate power to examine possible racial differences. Finally, although the report suggests that antihypertensive medication use was not associated with impaired glucose tolerance, it is clearly impossible to be certain that the study completely differentiated a drug effect from a metabolic effect.

J.C. Beck, M.D.

GENITOURINARY/GYNECOLOGY

Replens Versus Dienoestrol Cream in the Symptomatic Treatment of Vaginal Atrophy in Postmenopausal Women

Bygdeman M, Swahn ML (Karolinska Hosp, Stockholm)

Maturitas 23:259–263, 1996 1–42

Background.—Estrogen is often used both systemically and topically to treat the effects of vulvovaginal atrophy. However, this hormone also has effects on organs other than the vagina, including the endometrium. This study compared the effectiveness and safety of an estrogen gel (Dienestrol) with a nonhormonal gel (Replens) in treating vaginal dryness.

Methods.—Thirty-nine postmenopausal women, age 43–76, were randomized to receive either Replens, 1 vaginal application 3 times a week for 3 months (n = 20) or Dienestrol vaginal cream (0.01%), 0.5 mg/day for 2 weeks, then 3 times a week for up to 3 months (n = 19). Patients were examined regularly for pH level, vaginal dryness, itching, irritation, dyspareunia, length of moisturizing effects, and satisfaction.

Findings.—Although the effect was more significant with the hormonal gel, both Replens and Dienestrol significantly improved vaginal dryness within 1 week. Both drugs improved itching and dyspareunia, and neither drug caused adverse events or a change in pH. Patient satisfaction was good to excellent for 60% of the patients taking Replens and for 84% of those taking Dienestrol.

Conclusions.—Both treatments successfully managed vaginal dryness, itching, and dyspareunia, yet Replens did so without any of the side effects inherent in the use of estrogen gels. Thus, nonhormonal gels such as Replens should be considered for women seeking nonhormonal relief from vaginal atrophy.

► Symptoms associated with vaginal atrophy include dryness, itching, irritation, and dyspareunia. Although topical estrogens can relieve these symptoms, many women cannot (e.g., because of breast cancer) or will not use estrogens. This small, randomized trial supports the effectiveness of using a nonhormonal, bioadhesive vaginal gel to provide some relief of these symptoms, in particular, itching and dyspareunia. Although vaginal dryness also improved, the estrogen preparation was more effective than the gel. Topical estrogen remains the preferred treatment for atrophic vaginitis, but Replens may provide symptomatic relief for those women who cannot or will not use estrogen.

D.B. Reuben, M.D.

The Predictive Value of Microscopic Haematuria in Patients With Lower Urinary Tract Symptoms and Benign Prostatic Hyperplasia

El Din KE, Koch WFRM, de Wildt MJAM, et al (Nijmegen Univ, The Netherlands)

Eur Urol 30:409–413, 1996 1–43

Objective.—Benign prostatic hyperplasia (BPH) is the most common cause of bladder outlet obstruction in elderly men. Although urinalysis is a standard test performed when the patient has lower urinary tract symptoms, it is not a useful screening procedure. Although the finding of erythrocyturia is disturbing, the correlation between this result and any clinical parameter is not known. The clinical implications of finding erythrocyturia in patients with prostate-related voiding problems, was examined in this case series.

Methods.—Among 750 consecutive men, age 40–85, screened at an outpatient department for benign prostatic enlargement and lower urinary tract symptoms, there were 238 with erythrocyturia.

Results.—There was no correlation between presence or grade of erythrocyturia and age, symptoms score, prostate volume, postvoid volume, hematuria, renal cysts, stones, tumors, or findings on urethrocystoscopy, cytology, or histology. There was no correlation between hematuria and degree of bladder obstruction.

Conclusion.—Findings of hematuria in men with BPH and lower urinary tract symptoms are common but are unrelated to any specific clinical parameters. Additional tests should be performed on these patients only if other indications warrant them.

▶ Hematuria is often noted in older men with BPH. The question becomes whether all of these men need to have a full evaluation to exclude genitourinary tract tumors. In this case series, men with BPH and hematuria (one third of all men with BPH and lower urinary tract symptoms) were systematically evaluated. The evaluation included urine culture, transrectal ultrasonography, renal US, abdominal x-ray examination, and flexible cystoscopy. The majority of men with hematuria had 1–5 RBCs per high-power field. Serious disease was uncommon. Only 0.4% had bladder tumors, and fewer than 7% had renal stones. Moreover, there was no relationship between the amount of hematuria and any specific urologic disease. In fact, most men with tumors or stones had little or no hematuria. Among men with BPH and lower urinary tract symptoms, a complete diagnostic evaluation of hematuria will yield little. However, a small percentage of these men will have serious disease. The findings do not support performing a complete diagnostic evaluation in this group of men.

D.B. Reuben, M.D.

Health Care Delivery

Relationship Between the Volume of Total Hip Replacements Performed by Providers and the Rates of Postoperative Complications in the State of Washington

Kreder HJ, Deyo RA, Koepsell T, et al (Univ of Washington, Seattle)

J Bone Joint Surg Am 79A:485–494, 1997 1–44

Objective.—In addition to patient age, disease severity, and comorbidity, the rate of adverse outcomes after surgery may be affected by the experience of the surgeon and hospital. High-volume providers are known to achieve excellent results in total hip arthroplasty, but there are few data on the outcomes of patients treated by lower volume providers. Any valid comparison of providers must consider variations in case mix. A computerized administrative database was used to determine how provider volume affects the rate of complications after elective total hip arthroplasty.

Methods.—The study used Washington State hospital discharge data on 7,936 patients undergoing 8,774 primary total hip replacements between 1988 and 1991. For each hospital and surgeon involved, the average number of hip replacements performed per year was determined. The complication rate was analyzed in terms of the volume of procedures performed, with adjustment for relevant factors.

Results.—On analysis of case mix, the patients treated by lower volume providers—below the 40th percentile—had a more adverse risk profile in terms of age, comorbidity, and diagnosis. However, even after adjustment for these factors, outcomes were worse for surgeons who performed an average of less than 2 hip replacements per year. Patients of low-volume surgeons had higher mortality, more infections, more revision surgeries, and more serious inhospital complications. An inverse relationship was noted between length of hospitalization and surgeon's volume, and a direct relationship between length of stay and hospital volume. There was also an inverse relationship between hospital charges and hospital volume, even after adjustment for length of stay, year of operation, and discharge destination.

Conclusions.—The outcomes of primary hip replacement surgery appear to be related to provider volume. Patient outcomes seem to be influenced by surgeon volume, whereas resource utilization is influenced by hospital volume. The findings must be interpreted cautiously, given the drawbacks of using administrative datasets. However, if confirmed, the results suggest that some types of elective total hip replacements may be best performed at regional centers.

▶ This article adds to the mounting body of evidence that demonstrates an association between outcome and provider volume.[1] This suggests that the experience of the surgeon and the hospital with a specific procedure is an additional factor that affects the rate of operative complications in addition to those such as age, severity, and comorbidity. The results show that the group of patients having total hip replacements managed by a surgeon who averages fewer than 2 hip replacements a year fared worse with regard to most of the outcomes evaluated after adjustment for hospital volume, age, comorbidity, gender, and operative diagnosis. Hospital volume, in contrast to surgeon volume, was related only to hospital charges and the duration of hospitalization, the low-volume hospital charging more for an elective hip replacement. Interestingly, the duration of stay in the low-volume hospitals tended to be shorter. It thus appears that the outcomes are more closely related to surgeon volume, whereas the use of resources is related to hospital volume. This analysis included administrative data from the whole state of Washington, and secondary analyses of administrative datasets always deserve caution. This is because clinically relevant information is often not collected, the coding of the information may be inaccurate, and there are well-known limitations to hospital discharge datasets.

This increasing evidence demonstrating an association between outcome and provider volume suggests that the time is approaching when firm policy recommendations might be made regarding certain patient populations that deserve referral to more specialized centers for management.

J.C. Beck, M.D.

Reference

1. Luft HS, Garnick DW, Mark DH, et al: *Hospital Volume, Physician Volume, and Patient Outcomes: Assessing the Evidence*. Ann Arbor, Mich, Health Administration Press Perspectives, 1990.

Collaborative Systematic Review of the Randomised Trials of Organised Inpatient (Stroke Unit) Care After Stroke

Langhorne, P, for the Stroke Unit Trialists' Collaboration (Royal Infirmary, Glasgow, Scotland)

BMJ 314:1151–1159, 1997 1–45

Background.—The role of organized care of inpatients with stroke has been debated for more than 30 years. The moderate benefits of such care can be detected only in large randomized trials or with proper review of smaller trials. A review of randomized trials through 1993 indicated that specialized stroke units may reduce mortality and the rate of institutionalization after stroke. New information has now become available.

Methods.—A meta-analysis was conducted of 19 prospective randomized trials comparing organized stroke units and conventional care. Twelve trials had 2,060 patients treated in a dedicated stroke unit or general medical ward, 6 trials had 647 patients treated in a mixed assessment and rehabilitation unit with a general medical ward, and 4 trials had 542 patients treated in a dedicated stroke unit and a mixed assessment and rehabilitation unit.

Results.—Organized inpatient stroke unit care was characterized by coordinated multidisciplinary rehabilitation, stroke education and training, and specialized staff. The stroke unit was usually housed in a separate ward. Stroke unit care was associated with a long-term reduction in death only, death or dependency, and death or institutionalization. Benefits were independent of age, gender, stroke severity, and variation in stroke unit organization. Length of hospital stay was reduced by 8% compared to conventional care, but results were very heterogeneous.

Discussion.—This review showed that organized stroke unit care resulted in lower mortality, dependency, and institutionalization. The benefits were not restricted to any patient subgroups or model of care. Organized stroke unit care did not result in greater use of resources. All patients with acute stroke should be given early multidisciplinary care in an organized stroke unit.

► I believe this article puts to rest the long-standing controversy as to whether organized care for stroke supplies any benefit with respect to outcomes. It represents a further supplement to an analysis that had previously been published by the Cochrane Group.[1] This particular meta-analysis includes all literature until late 1995, and because of the extensiveness of the additional data collection that was carried out, I believe it to be a definitive statement on this controversial problem.

Important new observations obtained primarily by subgroup analyses are: (1) that the important characteristics of stroke unit care are a provision of coordinated multidisciplinary rehabilitation, specialization of all staff in stroke or rehabilitation, and improved education and training as compared to routine care; (2) patients managed in stroke units were more likely to survive, and more likely to regain independence and return home than those that received conventional care; and (3) the benefits were not restricted to any subgroup of stroke patients (mild, moderate, or severe) or model of stroke unit care. In terms of cost-effectiveness, the data are relatively crude in the sense that there was no systematic increase in length of stay; in fact, the length of stay in a hospital or rehabilitation unit was reduced by 8% compared to conventional care, but these data show enormous heterogeneity across studies.

J.C. Beck, M.D.

Reference

1. Stroke Unit Trialists' Collaboration: A systematic overview of specialist multidisciplinary team (stroke unit) care for stroke inpatients. *Cochrane Database of Systematic Reviews*. Disk Issue 1, 1995.

The Impact of Payor/Provider Type on Health Care Use and Expenditures Among the Frail Elderly

Experton B, Li Z, Branch LG, et al (HUMETRIX, Inc, San Diego, Calif; Duke Univ, Durham, NC; MEDSTAT Group, Ann Arbor, Mich)
Am J Public Health 98:210–216, 1997 1–46

Background.—Older people consume a disproportionate share of health care resources. In an attempt to reduce associated costs, the Health Care Financing Administration introduced Medicare health maintenance organizations (HMOs) in 1983. In an attempt to assess the effectiveness of this program, differences in health care use and cost were examined in a group of frail older subjects enrolled in Medicare fee-for-service, Medicare HMO, and dual Medicare-Medicaid programs.

Methods.—This study was conducted at the largest health care organization in San Diego County, Sharp HealthCare, which comprises 6 acute care hospitals, 4 skilled-nursing centers, 15 ambulatory clinics, a rehabilitation center, and a large home health agency. The study population was derived from 700 over-65 patients of Sharp Home HealthCare, a Medicare-certified home health agency. There were 220 patients enrolled in Medicare fee for service, 310 enrolled in the Medicare HMO, and 170 enrolled in both Medicare and Medicaid. All Medicare HMO patients were members of Secure Horizons. Patients were included if they re-

TABLE 3.—Regression Results of the Effect of Payor/Provider on Specific Service Use* by Frail Older Persons (n = 450)

Variable	Medicare FFS vs Medicare–Medicaid Coefficient	OR†	HMO vs Medicare–Medicaid Coefficient	OR†	Medicare FFS vs HMO Coefficient	OR†
Hospital inpatient						
Any admission(s)	−0.7071	0.49‡	−0.4087	0.66	−0.2984	0.74
≥2 admissions	−0.7002	0.50	0.1432	1.15	−0.8434	0.43‡
Ln of no. of user days	−0.2545		−0.2466		−0.0080	
Emergency room						
Any visit(s)	−0.2917	0.75	−0.7217	0.49‡	0.4301	1.54
≥2 visits	−0.9165	0.40	−1.1589	0.31	0.2424	1.27
Nursing home						
Long-term stay(s) (≥100 days)	−1.6201	0.20‡	−1.6848	0.19‡	0.0648	1.07
Subsequent home health care						
Any admission(s)	−0.0728	0.93	0.2903	1.34	−0.3630	0.70
Ln of no. of user visits	0.2584		−0.9788‡		−1.2372‡	

Note: All multivariate regression analyses were conducted for a total sample of 450 subjects, except for the regression on the natural logarithm (*Ln*) of the number of hospital days, which was based on a subsample of 190 users, and the regression on the Ln of the number of subsequent home health visits, which was based on a subsample of 143 users.

*Data were obtained from logistic-regression analyses with adjustment for factors related to sociodemographic features, physical and mental health status, diagnosis, and perceptions of unmet service needs.

†ORs for total number of hospital days and total number of subsequent home health visits are not provided because the coefficients are the result of ordinary least-squares regression.

‡Significant coefficients ($P < 0.05$).

Abbreviations: FFS, fee for service; *HMO*, health maintenance organization; *Ln*, natural logarithm.

(Courtesy of Experton B, Li Z, Branch LG, et al: The impact of payor/provider type on health care use and expenditures among the frail elderly. *Am J Public Health* 98:210–216, 1997. Copyright by the American Public Health Association.)

sponded to all baseline and follow-up surveys, did not change payor type, and survived the 18-month study period between November 1990 and May 1993. The final study group comprised 400 patients. Statistical analysis indicated no significant differences in 50 demographic variables between patients who left the study and those who remained. The survey data were collected during in-home interviews conducted by home health nurses at baseline and at 6-month intervals for 18 months.

Results.—No differences were found in expenditures between fee-for-service and HMO patients, but Medicare–Medicaid patients had significantly higher expenditures. Fee-for-service patients were half as likely to have a hospital admission or emergency department visit as the other 2 groups. Medicare–Medicaid beneficiaries were more likely to use long-term nursing home care than the other 2 groups. There was no difference in access to home health care between these groups, but HMO members received significantly fewer home health care services than the other 2 groups (Table 3).

Conclusions.—This study examined the costs of care and the services provided to a population of frail older patients by 3 payor-provider types: Medicare fee for service, Medicare HMO, and dual Medicare–Medicaid. Little difference was found among these groups in total expenditure per patient and provision of most services, but significantly fewer home health services were provided to HMO members and use of services was significantly greater by dual enrollees. Further research will be necessary to relate differences in service provision to outcome, to determine the effect of these differences on the frail older population.

Differences in 4-Year Health Outcomes for Elderly and Poor, Chronically Ill Patients Treated in HMO and Fee-for-Service Systems: Results From the Medical Outcomes Study

Ware JE Jr, Bayliss MS, Rogers WH, et al (Tufts Univ, Boston; Harvard School of Public Health, Boston)

JAMA 276:1039–1047, 1996 1–47

Background.—Enrollment in HMOs has increased 10-fold since 1976, and government policies now seek to shift publicly insured patients to HMOs. The Medical Outcomes Study (MOS) compared 4-year health outcomes for chronically ill patients treated in well-established HMOs and fee-for-service (FFS) plans serving the same medical marketplaces in Boston, Chicago, and Los Angeles. Only those with hypertension, non-insulin-dependent diabetes mellitus, recent acute myocardial infarction, congestive heart failure, and depressive disorder were studied. This study focused on patients aged at least 65 years covered by Medicare and those with near or below poverty-level income.

Methods.—The study group consisted of 2,235 adult patients with 1 of the 5 index conditions who were included in the study sample in 1986 and followed up through 1990. Medicare and low-income patients were analyzed separately. The Short-Form Health Survey was used to determine differences in physical and mental health during the 4-year study period.

Results.—Overall, physical health declined and mental health remained stable for the 4-year follow-up period of this study. These physical declines were significantly larger for the elderly than for the nonelderly in the study group. For the average patient, physical and mental health outcomes were not different between the HMO or FFS systems. For elderly Medicare patients, physical health declines were significantly more common in HMOs than in FFS plans. For patients with incomes near or below the poverty level, outcomes were more favorable in the FFS system than in HMOs.

Conclusions.—The MOS observed adult patients treated in HMO and FFS systems for 4 years to determine changes in medical status. Although for the average patient there was no difference in medical outcome between these two systems, for poor and elderly patients health outcomes were worse in HMOs than in FFS systems. These results indicate that vulnerable subgroups need to be separately monitored by health care plans to ensure that their needs are being adequately met.

▶ As costs of caring for older persons have increased, there has been a progressive shift of Medicare enrollees into capitated plans. Although these plans frequently have attractive incentives for older persons who enroll (e.g., no premiums, pharmacy and eyeglass benefits), there have been concerns that these plans select healthier older persons and create impediments to receiving some services (e.g., easy access to specialists, wide choice of physicians) that are readily available under fee-for-service (FFS) Medicare. Although it would be valuable to have the results of a clinical trial that randomly assigned older persons to one of the two types of reimbursement system, such a trial is unlikely. Accordingly, other methods must be used to examine the differences in the care received in capitated vs FFS systems. Two studies published in the past year shed some light on how older persons fare under different systems of reimbursement. In 1 study (Abstract 1–46), Experton et al. interviewed older persons who were frail (as indicated by their receiving home care) under 3 systems of health care: FFS Medicare, HMO Medicare, and Medicare-Medicaid. They found that compared with the other 2 systems, the dually insured had considerably more health care expenditures. Although in most respects, FFS and Medicare HMOs were similar, HMO enrollees were more likely than those in FFS plans to have 2 or more admissions during the follow-up period. These data suggest that capitation may not result in cost savings for Medicare for the frail elderly population.

In the other study (Abstract 1–47), Ware et al. conducted analyses of the MOS, an observational study of variations in practice styles and outcomes for chronically ill adults reimbursed under a variety of systems. Under prepaid HMO care, older persons were more likely to experience a decline in physical health during 4 years compared with those cared for by FFS Medicare; in contrast, HMO enrollees were more likely to have better mental health within the same time period. Together, these 2 studies do not provide support for a major effort to induce Medicare beneficiaries to enroll in capitated at-risk health care plans. Nevertheless, other research published this year and cited in this volume (Abstract 1–48) demonstrates that because of their flexibility in determining how health care dollars are spent, HMOs have the potential to develop and implement programs that reduce health care utilization, are cost-effective, and lead to high patient satisfaction.

D.B. Reuben, M.D.

► I selected the article by Ware (Abstract 1–47) because of its major policy implications as well as its importance to the large number of consumers who are considering moving from a FFS plan to an HMO system. It is also of major importance because it raises the urgency of further research into why the differences that are reported in this article have taken place.

In summary, this article clearly shows that elderly and poor, chronically ill patients of all ages have poorer physical health outcomes in a prepaid system as contrasted with a FFS system. Equally important is that mental health outcomes varied by study site and patient characteristics, raising important questions about what were the ingredients of the care package that led to improvement in mental health outcomes in some sites and not in others.

There are a number of limitations to this study, of which the most important is whether the observations reported here (1986 to 1990) apply to the current health care received by older and poorer individuals at this time. Because efforts to reduce health service use have become even more active since these data were collected, one would suspect that the situation for high-risk individuals might actually be worse than what is reported in this study. The second limitation is that the study was not randomized, although the authors make major efforts to correct for this deficiency. The third limitation is that the study monitored outcomes in 3 large, urban cities and, because there was a difference in some outcomes according to site, their generalizability may be in question. Finally, the outcomes concerned those attached to 5 common, chronic conditions and may not reflect the outcomes from conditions that were not studied, although I believe this to be unlikely.

The results reported here are different from those of previous reports, in which it has been shown that there are no differences in health outcomes between FFS and HMO plans.[1–4] One of these studies actually dealt with the same population but only addressed 2 of the 5 diseases that are reported here. In the latter case, averages were reported across all age groups for hypertension and non-insulin-dependent diabetes, which may well explain the differences in results. Even more important is that the other studies showing no difference had short follow-up (1 year), emphasizing the importance of a much longer follow-up period in addressing health outcomes as it applies to these 2 subcategories of patients.

J.C. Beck, M.D.

References

1. Greenfield S, Rogers W, Mangotich M, et al: Outcomes of patients with hypertension and non–insulin-dependent diabetes mellitus treated by different systems and specialties: Results from the Medical Outcomes Study. *JAMA* 274:1436–1474, 1995.
2. Lurie N, Moscovice IS, Finch M, et al: Does capitation affect the health of the chronically mental ill?: Results from a randomized trial. *JAMA* 267:3300–3304, 1992.
3. Retchin SM, Clement DG, Rossiter LF, et al: How the elderly fare in HMOs: Outcomes from the Medicare competition demonstrations. *Health Serv Res* 27:651–669, 1992.
4. Clement DG, Retchin SM, Brown RS, et al: Access and outcomes of elderly patients enrolled in managed care. *JAMA* 271:1487–1492, 1994.

A Randomized Trial of Group Outpatient Visits for Chronically Ill Older HMO Members: The Cooperative Health Care Clinic

Beck A, Scott J, Williams P, et al (Colorado Permanente Medical Care Program, Denver)

J Am Geriatr Soc 45:543–549, 1997 1–48

Objective.—New models of ambulatory care for the elderly are needed to prepare for the coming "senior boom." In the authors' HMO, elderly people consume a disproportionately high share of inpatient and outpatient resources, while not necessarily having their needs met in routine outpatient visits. These problems led to the development of the Cooperative Health Care Clinic, a group outpatient visit model of comprehensive care delivered by a team of health care providers of various disciplines. This model was compared with the traditional physician visit on several relevant outcome measures such as resource utilization, costs, self-reported health status, and patient and physician satisfaction.

Methods.—The randomized trial included 321 HMO members age 65 or older. All had at least 1 of the 4 following chronic illnesses: heart disease, lung disease, joint disease, or diabetes, with relatively high levels of health care utilization. Patients were assigned to usual care or the group visit model for a 12-month period. In the group model, the patients met in groups with their primary care physician and nurse on a monthly basis. Each visit included health education and preventive information, opportunities for socialization and mutual support, and one-to-one visits with the physician, as needed. Educational sessions included professionals from many different disciplines, such as pharmacists, physical therapists, and dietitians. Each patient received a summarized medical record to keep and to bring for updating at future visits. Outcome measures were compared at 1-year follow-up for the usual care and group models.

Results.—At 1 year, the group model scored lower on indicators of health services utilization, including emergency department visits, subspecialist visits, and repeat hospital admissions. Although patients in the group model made more visits and calls to nurses, they made fewer calls to physicians. Patients in the group model were more likely to receive influenza and pneumonia vaccinations. Patient and physician satisfaction were both higher with the group model. The 2 groups were similar in terms of self-reported health and functional status. The group model reduced the monthly cost of care per HMO member by $15.

Conclusion.—A group model of outpatient visits for elderly HMO members appears to have some important advantages over traditional outpatient visits. The group model can reduce key markers of health services utilization, including repeat admissions and resource utilization; reduce the monthly costs of care; improve delivery of preventive interventions; and increase patient and physician satisfaction. This type of care model may be useful in meeting the increasing demand for health care resources by the elderly.

▶ A major limitation of fee-for-service Medicare is that it is based on purchasing discrete services rather than providing comprehensive, well-integrated medical care. Because of their flexibility in determining how capitated dollars will be spent, HMOs have the potential for improving care for older persons by providing innovative types of services that better meet the needs of their members. Beck et al. conducted a randomized clinical trial of the effectiveness of the Cooperative Health Care Clinic, which consisted of monthly group sessions aimed at meeting the informational needs of healthier (although with at least 1 chronic illness) community-based older persons.

As the trial's results indicate, the program led to reduced health care utilization (particularly fewer urgent visits, emergency department visits, and specialist visits) and costs, while having no adverse effects on functional status. Intervention group patients were also more satisfied with the quality of care they received. Unfortunately, because of current Medicare guidelines, which do not include reimbursement for these services, dissemination of this type of program into fee-for-service settings will be extremely difficult.

D.B. Reuben, M.D.

▶ The concept of group visits for patients with similar chronic diseases has become increasingly popular. This study shows in an HMO setting a clear benefit in the hospitalization and emergency care use in those who participated in a group visit program. There is also benefit in the cost of care, some preventive strategies, and inpatient and physician satisfaction.

These models of care frequently are multidisciplinary with a very heavy nursing component. This design, in my view, makes enormous sense and once established is clearly cost effective. In this study, the patient population was not particularly frail. My guess is that a population of more frail patients would likely show benefit, but this, of course, needs to be carefully studied.

J.R. Burton, M.D.

2 Long-term Care

Introduction

The tradition in this chapter has been to define long-term care in broad terms. Therefore, articles appearing in this chapter may be reflective of any aspect of the health care of the elderly that is provided for extended periods. Obviously, this approach results in overlap with other chapters, but articles are kept in separate chapters to provide consistency in the editorial comments.

New and valuable scientific information in the published literature relating to the care of the elderly is appearing increasingly frequently. More and more articles are reviewed yearly. This year, several hundred were reviewed before those appearing in this chapter were selected. Those that were selected provide a new idea or concept or have moved the field forward. For easier reference, the chapter is divided into sub-sections on incontinence, infections, ethics and advance directives, nursing home issues, falls, physical restraints, pressure sores, managed care, Alzheimer's disease, and several miscellaneous articles that I thought were of interest and value.

This year, I added several papers on managed care. I thought these articles had valuable information for clinicians who are struggling with the evolving health care system. Again, this year, there is a series of articles on ethics and advance directives, as each is increasingly an issue in clinical settings.

All in all, I am pleased that there is a balance of articles focused on clinical care of older persons. My hope is that it will provide a quick review of some of the significant advances in this field over the last 12 months.

John R. Burton, M.D.

Incontinence

Urinary Incontinence in Rural Older Women: Prevalence, Incidence and Remission

Nygaard IE, Lemke JH (Univ of Iowa, Iowa City)

J Am Geriatr Soc 44:1049–1054, 1996 2–1

Background.—Urinary incontinence is a common problem among older women. It has been presumed that urinary incontinence is a static state, but the natural history of this condition has not been well studied. To explore the natural history of urinary incontinence in older women, a longitudinal cohort study was done with data from the Iowa 65+ Rural Health Study of Establishment of Populations for Epidemiologic Studies of the Elderly.

Methods.—The study group consisted of 2,025 noninstitutionalized women aged at least 65 years who resided in 2 rural Iowa counties. The participants were interviewed in person each year for 6 years. Questions about urinary incontinence were answered at baseline and at 3 and 6 years.

Results.—The baseline prevalence of urge incontinence was 36.3% and of stress incontinence was 40.3%. For urge incontinence, the 3-year incidence rate was 28.5% and the 3-year remission rate was 22.1% (Fig 5). For stress incontinence, the 3-year incidence rate was 28.6% and the 3-year remission rate was 25.1% (Fig 4). Of those women who reported no urge incontinence at baseline, 76% were continent at both follow-up interviews. Of those women who reported no stress incontinence at baseline, 84% were continent at both follow-up interviews. Increased age was significantly associated with increased incidence of urge incontinence. Improvement in activities of daily living was associated with increased remission of urge incontinence.

Conclusions.—Contrary to the commonly held static view of urinary incontinence in elderly women, this longitudinal cohort studied showed that urinary incontinence can be a dynamic state, with older women moving back and forth along the continuum between continence and incontinence. More study is required to prospectively examine the multiple

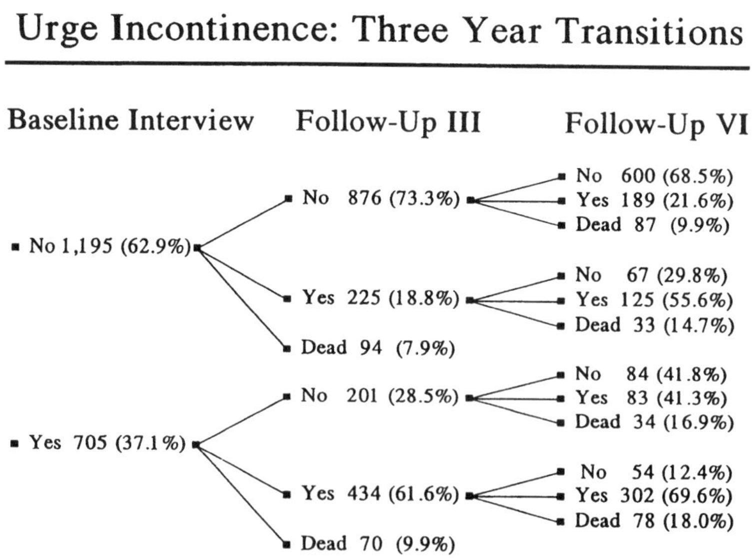

FIGURE 5.—Three-year transition tree for urge incontinence. (Courtesy of Nygaard IE, Lemke JH: Urinary incontinence in rural older women: Prevalence, incidence and remission. *J Am Geriatr Soc* 44[9]:1049–1054, 1996.)

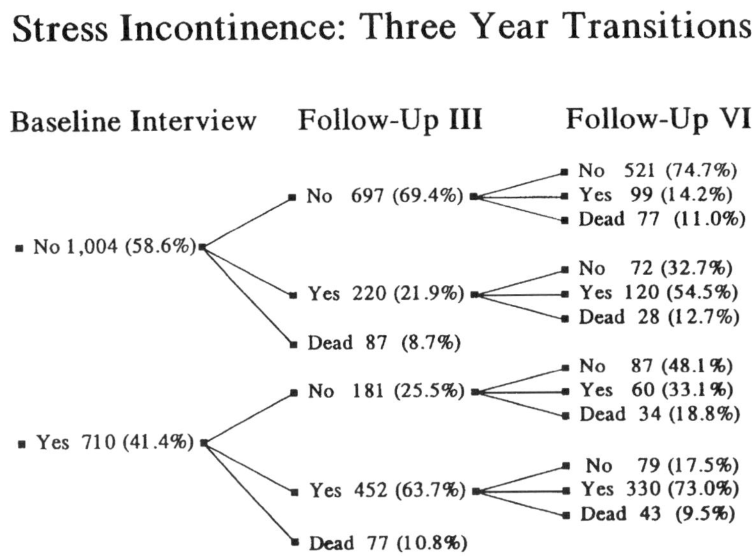

FIGURE 4.—Three-year transition tree for stress incontinence. (Courtesy of Nygaard IE, Lemke JH: Urinary incontinence in rural older women: Prevalence, incidence and remission. *J Am Geriatr Soc* 44[9]:1049–1054, 1996.)

factors that contribute to the incidence and remission of urinary incontinence in older women.

▶ This is an important article because it is the first report to present a 6-year study of the incidence and remission rate or urinary incontinence in a large group of community-based women. The data set consisted of 2,025 women older than age of 65 living in rural Iowa. The baseline prevalence of urge incontinence was 36% and stress incontinence, 40%. What is unique about this study is that it shows that urinary incontinence is a dynamic state and that women move in both directions along a continuum of continence and incontinence.

There are clearly some limitations to the study in that nonsurgical treatments could not be fully tracked. The figures show the transitions of these patients. Additional research will be necessary to define precisely the flux from continence to incontinence and the reasons for change. At least, this study alerts us that urinary incontinence may not always be a static disorder.

J.R. Burton, M.D.

A Study of Female Urinary Incontinence in General Practice: Demography, Medical History, and Clinical Findings

Seim A, Eriksen BC, Hunskaar S (Trondheim Univ, Norway; Univ of Bergen, Norway)

Scand J Urol Nephrol 30:465–471, 1996 2–2

Objective.—Urinary incontinence (UI) has an estimated prevalence of 16% to 60% in perimenopausal women, although only about 25% of women with the problem consult their doctors. Little is known about the extent of the problem at the primary care level. Results of a prospective study of female UI in a general practice community is presented.

Methods.—A total of 105 women, aged 20 to 87, consulted their general practitioners (GPs) about UI in Rissa, Norway, during 1990 through 1993.

TABLE 2.—Characteristics of Urinary Incontinence Among the 105 Women

Duration of UI	%	%
<2 years	19	
2–5 years	32	
5–10 years	21	
>10 years	28	
Frequency of leakage	Day	Night
Never	7	74
A few times per month	18	11
A few times per week	31	8
1–2 times per day	33	7
More often	12	1
Amount of leakage		
Drops	23	
Little	62	
More	15	
Severity		
Slight	8	
Moderate	28	
Severe	64	
Use of protective pads or garments		
Not using	41	
Use during day	30	
Use during night	5	
Both day and night	24	
Use of different types of pads or garments	Ever used	Using now
Sanitary towels	17	49
UI protective pads	4	17
Towels	7	6
Toilet paper	10	6
Special clothes	3	2
Cotton	1	2
Baby napkins	4	1
Plastic	2	2

Note: Because of missing data, each category is based on answers from 101 to 105 women.

(Courtesy of Seim A, Eriksen BC, Hunskaar S: A study of female urinary incontinence in general practice. *Scand J Urol Nephrol* 30:465–471, 1996.)

Standardized guidelines were developed, thorough medical histories and examinations were documented, and demographic information was included. A 48-hour frequency and 48-hour pad test were conducted at home, pelvic muscle floor contractility was measured, and cystocele, rectocele, or prolapse of the uterus was determined and categorized. Incontinence was classified as stress, urge, or mixed. The women assessed the impact of incontinence on a VAS 100 mm scale from "absolutely no bother" to "cannot imagine anything worse."

Results.—About two thirds of the women were postmenopausal, 20% were also fecal incontinent, and 35% had consulted a doctor about UI before. Many patients had significant comorbid conditions. Duration, frequency, and leakage parameters were reported (Table 2). Almost half the women had experienced incontinence for more than 5 years. Clinical results showed that 28% had moderate and 4% had considerable cystocele, 8% had moderate and 1% had considerable rectocele, 4% had moderate and 3% had considerable prolapse of portio, and 38% had significant genital prolapse. No association was found between prolapse and leakage. Perianal insensibility was weak or absent in 17% of women in whom fecal incontinence was also frequent, 88% had a positive stress provocation test, and 28% had weak contractility of the pelvic floor muscles. Stress incontinence was found in 50% of women, urge incontinence in 10%, and mixed incontinence in 40%. Incontinence was bothersome to 42% of women, although those with stress incontinence were less bothered than those with urge or mixed incontinence, despite the fact that more than 60% of patients have been diagnosed with severe UI. It appears that many patients do not want treatment.

Conclusion.—Women are frequently bothered by UI, and many have severe disease. A general physician can evaluate and manage many patients, although some may need to be referred for specialized treatment.

▶ I selected this article for this edition of the YEAR BOOK because it has great generalizability to a typical community practice situation. This study represents a survey of all women with urinary incontinence who were cared for by a general practice group in which no one had particular experience or expertise in the area of UI. Although it was conducted in Norway, I believe it does provide insights into the patterns of incontinence and comorbidities of patients seen by generalists in this country. The study includes only women who consulted their general practitioner for UI. Of course, the survey could miss those individuals who never mentioned the problem to their physicians. The evaluation of these patients was done entirely in the generalist's office and included a perfectly acceptable, noninvasive approach to the office evaluation of patients with incontinence. One hundred five women were included in the study. Almost 50% of women with incontinence had symptoms for greater than 5 years, two thirds of subjects believed the problem was severe, and nearly 60% used protective pads or garments. The study clinicians classified the incontinence as stress in 50%, urge in 10%, and mixed pattern in 40%. Also 20% of these women describe concomitant fecal incontinence and—as is typical in earlier studies—a third of the women had previously consulted a physician for the problem, but little or nothing was done. The study does not provide data on therapy or the need for referral, but it is hoped that these data will be forthcoming. My guess is that more than 90% of patients with UI can be effectively evaluated and managed by the generalist physicians who are willing to take a minimal interest in the problem of UI in their elderly patients. The addition of an office nurse to the evaluation and management team for patients with UI can be extremely effective.

J.R. Burton, M.D.

Urodynamic and Rectomanometric Findings in Urinary Incontinence

Pannek J, Haupt G, Sommerfeld H-J, et al (Ruhr-Univ Bochum, Germany)

Scand J Urol Nephrol 30:457–460, 1996 2–3

Background.—Embryologically, both bladder and rectum derive from the cloaca. They share the same innervation from the pelvic parasympathetic outflow, and the external sphincters are both innervated by the pudendal nerve. In addition, the external sphincter muscle slings are both part of the pelvic floor. These similarities suggested a possible correlation between urinary and fecal incontinence in patients with urinary incontinence.

Methods.—Fifty-two patients with urinary incontinence undergoing cystometry and rectomanometry were studied. Twenty-five had stress incontinence; 20, urge incontinence; and 7, overflow urinary incontinence.

Findings.—Rectomanometry findings were normal in 29 patients. Five had a compensated and 18 a partially compensated sphincter incompe-

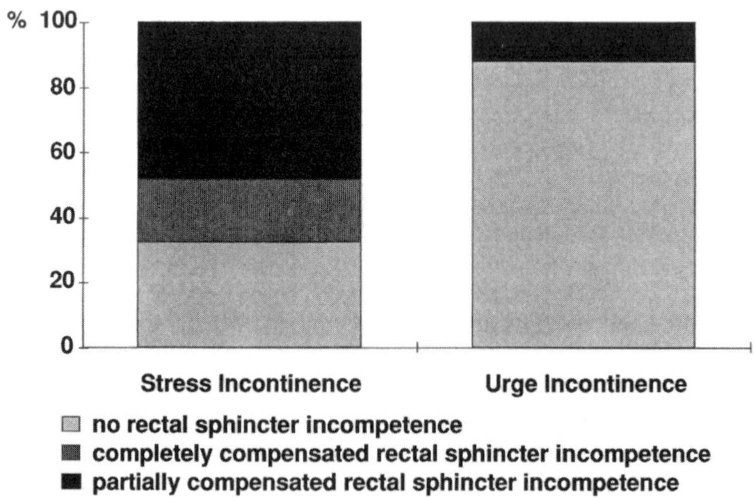

FIGURE 1.—Correlation urinary incontinence and rectal sphincter incompetence. (Courtesy of Pannek J, Haupt G, Sommerfeld H-J, et al: Urodynamic and rectomanometric findings in urinary incontinence. *Scand J Urol Nephrol* 30:457–460, 1996.)

tence. Normal rectal sphincter function was identified in 18 of 20 patients with urge incontinence. By contrast, 16 of 25 patients with stress incontinence had rectal sphincter incompetence.

Conclusions.—A marked correlation exists between stress urinary incontinence and rectal sphincter incompetence (Fig 1). These findings support the notion that a weakness in the entire pelvic floor is a typical feature of urinary incontinence.

► By using rectomanometry (a test of anal sphincter function by instilling 400 mL of saline into the rectum), the authors show a very high correlation of anal sphincter weakness with urinary sphincter insufficiency. While patients in this study didn't complain spontaneously of anal incompetence, most on questioning did have symptoms suggesting sphincter weakness when they had a diarrheal illness. There is not yet much for the clinician to do therapeutically based on this 1 study, but it is certainly an eye opener. I suspect this problem of anal sphincter weakness may be an important issue particularly in older women. It is worth our inquiring about fecal incontinence particularly in women with sphincter inadequacy. If it is identified, fecal incontinence would not be expected to be improved with surgery directed at stress incontinence. It could well be that pelvic muscle exercises would improve the symptoms or prevent anal sphincter weakness from becoming a problem. However, much more research is necessary.

J.R. Burton, M.D.

Evaluation and Treatment of Urinary Incontinence: Report of a Physician Survey

McFall S, Yerkes AM, Bernard M, et al (Univ of Oklahoma, Oklahoma City; Oklahoma State Dept of Health, Oklahoma City)

Arch Fam Med 6:114–119, 1997 2–4

Background.—The practice patterns of physicians responsible for assessing and treating urinary incontinence (UI) are not well documented. The patterns of identification, evaluation, and treatment of UI used by Oklahoma physicians in family and general practice, internal medicine, obstetrics/gynecology, and urology were reported.

Methods.—Lists were obtained from the Oklahoma State Medical Association and the Oklahoma Osteopathic Medical Association, and 274 family practitioners, internists, gynecologists, and urologists were selected. Eighty were subsequently determined to be ineligible; the remainder received a questionnaire. The response rate was 80%.

Findings.—The respondents' replies indicated that they missed opportunities to identify patients with UI. In addition, UI treatment varied markedly. Gynecologists and, to a lesser extent, family physicians were more likely to prescribe pelvic muscle exercises, presumably for stress UI. A less frequently used treatment was bladder training, which may be beneficial in patients with urge UI and urge accompanied by stress. Non-urologists were less likely to use medications for UI, compared with other treatments. More than 40% of the family physicians and internists said they frequently recommended absorbent pads.

Conclusion.—There are several ways to improve practice patterns for the identification and treatment of UI. The physicians surveyed in this study expressed great interest in continuing medical education for this condition. Also, efforts to disseminate Agency for Health Care Policy and Research clinical guidelines need to be improved.

▶ This is an important and practical study regarding the identification and treatment of patients with UI. The study reports on the analysis of a self-administered questionnaire sent to a random sample of generalist physicians as well as urologists and gynecologists in Oklahoma. I find it especially valuable because it essentially compares the standard practice in the community with the ideal suggested in the clinical guidelines of the Agency for Health Care Policy and Research. Some salient points from this study:

1. Less than 20% of the physicians surveyed had any knowledge of the available guidelines, although, clearly, most wanted to gain information about UI.
2. Less than one third generalist physicians always, or often, asked new patients about UI. In general, about 80% of ambulatory patients identified as having UI and given appropriate treatment can be cured or substantially improved.
3. One third to one half of generalist physicians felt ill prepared to treat patients with UI. This should be a wakeup call for directors of training programs.
4. Early in discussions with patients, approximately 40% of generalist physicians routinely recommend the use of absorptive pads. These should be used only after all other treatments fail, and, frankly, are uncommonly required with available treatments in nondemented, nondisabled community-dwelling elders.

This situation regarding urinary incontinence is quite amazing. It is a condition that affects nearly 25% of ambulatory, community-dwelling older persons and one in which substantial improvement or cure could be achieved in about 80% of individuals. Yet, patients don't tell and physicians don't ask about the problem. Clearly, physician and public education are desperately needed. All the wonderful guidelines really don't mean a thing unless physicians and patients are aware of and use them.

J.R. Burton, M.D.

Primary Degeneration of the Internal Anal Sphincter as a Cause of Passive Faecal Incontinence

Vaizey CJ, Kamm MA, Bartram CI (St Mark's Hosp, Harrow, England)

Lancet 349:612–615, 1997 2–5

Purpose.—In the past, pudendal nerve damage was believed to be the main cause of fecal incontinence. Now, with the availability of anal endosonography, 90% of patients with fecal incontinence are found to have structural damage to the external or internal anal sphincter. Still, some patients with neither structural damage nor neurologic impairment have signs and symptoms of internal sphincter dysfunction. The cause of this type of passive fecal incontinence was investigated.

Methods.—The retrospective study included 45 patients with passive fecal incontinence, intact internal and external sphincter muscles on anal endosonography, and normal results on pudendal nerve latency testing. There were 35 women and 10 men (median age, 63). None had urge incontinence. Anal pressure at rest was normal (less than 60 cm H_2O) in all patients. Endoanal ultrasound films were available for review in 38 patients.

Findings.—The films showed thinning of the internal anal sphincter, median thickness was only 1.8 mm, compared with a normal value of 2.8 mm. In some cases, the internal sphincter showed increased echogenicity with a poorly defined edge. The patients lacked the normal age-related increase in internal anal sphincter thickness. This condition was subsequently identified in 8 of 230 newly referred patients (4%).

Conclusion.—Passive fecal incontinence may result from primary degeneration of the smooth muscle of the internal anal sphincter. Treatment with loperamide may be successful, although this can cause constipation. Prospective studies of primary internal anal sphincter degeneration in the nonreferred population are needed.

▶ Fecal incontinence is much less common than urinary incontinence, but it has even greater devastating effects on functional and social outcomes. Generalist physicians are, for the most part, ill prepared to evaluate the condition and prescribe therapy for patients with this problem. This study is abstracted because it focuses on and identifies a patient population with a potentially new cause of fecal incontinence. This new cause is primary degeneration of the internal anal sphincter. The problem is diagnosable by endoanal ultrasound, as displayed in the figure included with the original article.

Generalists will need to explore resources in their own communities to effectively identify help for such patients. My guess is that a gastrointestinal motility specialist is likely to provide the greatest help. Studies on treatment are desperately needed, but I predict that many patients will benefit from biofeedback. In this study, however, only medical and surgical therapies are recommended. The bottom line is that generalist geriatricians should be on the lookout for patients with fecal incontinence and try to get appropriate help for them.

J.R. Burton, M.D.

Morbidity and Mortality of Incontinence Surgery in Elderly Women: An Analysis of Medicare Data

Sultana CJ, Campbell JW, Pisanelli WS, et al (Case Western Reserve Univ, Cleveland, Ohio)

Am J Obstet Gynecol 176:344–348, 1997 2–6

Introduction.—In the last few decades, the proportion of surgery performed among the elderly has grown from 19% of all operative procedures in 1980 to 29% in 1989. Little data are available on surgery for urinary incontinence in older women. In women 65 or older, surgical mortality rates and causes of mortality for needle urethropexies, retropubic suspensions, and anterior vaginal repairs were determined, as well as specific complications and causes of postoperative morbidity.

Methods.—A review was conducted of surgical procedures done for incontinence from data obtained from Medicare billing forms in the Medicare Provider Analysis and Review Record database. The procedures were performed from 1984 and 1991 for 66,478 women, with a mean and median age of 71, and the population was overwhelmingly white. A review of secondary diagnosis codes helped reveal co-morbidities and reasons for readmission.

Results.—There was 0.33% 30-day surgical mortality (Table 7). Age affected length of stay and was associated with an increase in mortality. Death was associated with the acute events of cerebrovascular accident (stroke) (14.6%); myocardial infarction (14.2%); pulmonary embolism or deep vein thrombosis (9.7%); and pneumonia (2.7). Higher rates of diabetes and heart failure were seen with patients who died, but they did not have higher rates of hypertension (Table 6). Patients older than 80 had higher rates of 30-day readmission than their younger counterparts, who had a 4.8% rate of readmission (Table 5). The most frequent diagnoses on readmission were urinary tract infection (12.2%), hypertension (16%), and unspecific complications (9%). In only 1% of the population were myocardial infarction, pulmonary embolism, cerebrovascular accident, deep vein thrombosis, and pneumonia noted. One admission for surgery for incontinence was seen with 97.7% of patients, 2.2% had 2 visits, and 0.12% had 3 or more procedures.

TABLE 7.—Number of Deaths Within 30, 60, and 90 Days of Surgery

Age group (yr)	*30 days* No.	%*	*60 days* No.	%*	*90 days* No.	%*
65–74	106	0.2	148	0.3	177	0.4
75–84	91	0.5	126	0.7	160	0.9
≥85	28	1.6	34	2.0	40	2.3
TOTAL	225	0.3	298	0.5	377	0.6

*Percentage of total in age group.

(Courtesy of Sultana CJ, Campbell JW, Pisanelli WS, et al: Morbidity and mortality of incontinence surgery in elderly women: An analysis of Medicare data. *Am J Obstet Gynecol* 176:344–348, 1997.)

TABLE 6.—Comorbidities and Readmissions

Comorbidities	*No. with comorbidities not readmitted*	*No. with comorbidities readmitted (n = 3176)*	*Odds ratio and 95% CI*
HTN	10,182	514	1.0 (0.9–1.1)
COPD	3,362	245	1.5 (1.3–1.7)
DM	3,428	255	1.5 (1.3–1.7)
Dementia	75	10	2.7 (1.4–5.0)
CHF	684	100	3.0 (2.4–3.7)
Pneumonia	223	33	3.0 (2.1–4.2)
MI	113	17	3.0 (1.9–4.9)
CVA, stroke	241	43	3.5 (2.5–4.9)
PE, DVT	159	25	2.6 (1.7–3.9)

Abbreviations: CI, Confidence interval; *HTN*, hypertension; *COPD*, chronic obstructive pulmonary disease; *DM*, diabetes mellitus; *CHF*, congestive heart failure; *MI*, myocardial infarction; *CVA*, cerebrovascular accident; *PE*, pulmonary embolism; *DVT*, deep venous thrombosis.

(Courtesy of Sultana CJ, Campbell JW, Pisanelli WS, et al: Morbidity and mortality of incontinence surgery in elderly women: An analysis of Medicare data. *Am J Obstet Gynecol* 176:344–348, 1997.)

Conclusion.—In the "young elderly" or, those younger than 80, incontinence surgery is safe. Increased risks are apparent with those older than 80 and those with certain chronic illnesses.

► This is a huge national dataset that defined the morbidity and mortality among elderly women undergoing surgery for urinary incontinence. Table 7 shows the increasing mortality in parallel with increasing age. It is of value as a resource when advising patients who are considering such surgery. Because these data are derived from the Medicare data tapes, no information is available on the benefit of the surgery performed in these patients.

J.R. Burton, M.D.

TABLE 5.—Percentage of Women Readmitted for Any Reason Within 30, 60, and 90 Days of Surgery, by Age

Age group (yr)	*30 days (n = 3176) (%)**	*60 days (n = 4789) (%)**	*90 days (n = 6250) (%)**
65–69	4.1	6.0	7.9
70–74	4.5	6.8	8.9
75–79	5.5	8.5	11.1
80–84	7.1	10.5	13.7
85–89	7.9	11.8	15.1
90–99	7.9	12.0	16.2
TOTAL	4.8	7.2	9.4

*Percentage of total in age group.

(Courtesy of Sultana CJ, Campbell JW, Pisanelli WS, et al: Morbidity and mortality of incontinence surgery in elderly women: An analysis of Medicare data. *Am J Obstet Gynecol* 176:344–348, 1997.)

Infections

Sequential Outbreak of Influenza A and B in a Nursing Home: Efficacy of Vaccine and Amantadine

Libow LS, Neufeld RR, Olson E, et al (Jewish Home and Hosp for Aged of New York; Mount Sinai School of Medicine, New York)
J Am Geriatr Soc 44:1153–1157, 1996 2–7

Background.—Influenza outbreaks remain an important health problem in nursing homes, despite efforts to administer vaccine to all older individuals. The failure of influenza vaccine to achieve its desired effect has been attributed to insufficient vaccine potency, inadequate immune response by debilitated nursing home residents, low levels of vaccination, and antigenic drift from the strain included in the vaccine. In this report of an influenza epidemic in a skilled nursing facility, investigators evaluated the effectiveness of the vaccine, amantadine treatment, or both.

Methods.—At the onset of the epidemic, the facility contained 514 beds and 499 residents. All residents as of October 1987 (except some who refused vaccination) had received the 1987 trivalent influenza vaccine, which contained virus antigens from 2 A strains and a B strain. The period of the epidemic extended from February 8 to April 5, 1988 (Fig 1). At the onset, 77.4% of residents had a known positive immunization status. Data were collected from a chart review of 175 residents with influenza-like

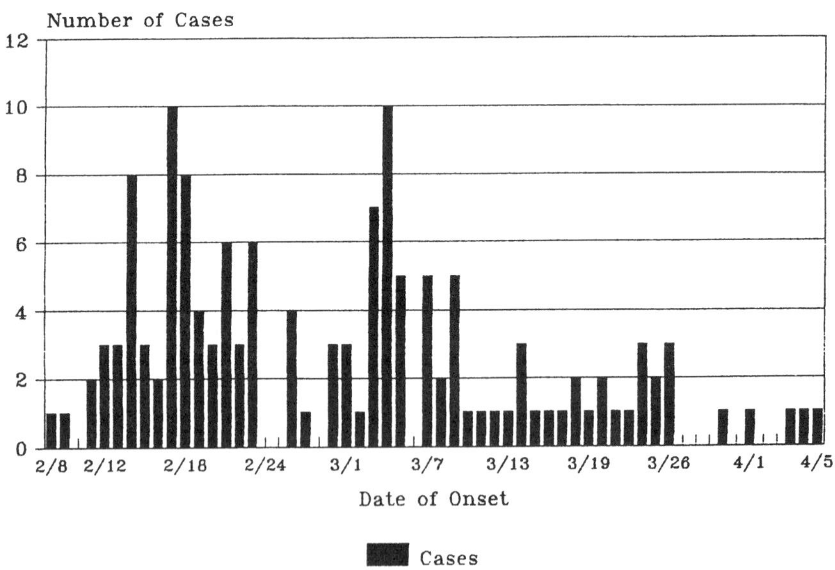

FIGURE 1.—Influenza outbreak of February through April 1988 at The Jewish Home and Hospital for the Aged. The histogram shows the spread of the epidemic. (Courtesy of Libow LS, Neufeld RR, Olson E, et al: Sequential outbreak of influenza A and B in a nursing home: Efficacy of vaccine and amantadine. *J Am Geriatr Soc* 44[10]:1153–1157, 1996.)

TABLE 1.—Comparison of Vaccinated Group With Those Not Vaccinated

	Vaccine	No Vaccine	Total
Mean age (SD)*	87.8 (6.7)	86.4 (6.5)	87.5 (6.7)
Median days ill (range)†	5 (1–29)	3.5 (1–13)	5 (1–29)
Death, pneumonia, and hospitalization associated with influenza A (n = 68)‡	35% (19/55)	38% (5/13)	36% (24/68)
Death, pneumonia, and hospitalization associated with influenza B (n = 71)§	30% (17/56)	67% (10/15)	38% (27/71)
N	111‖	28¶	139

*$P_{t\ test}$ = 0.313.
†$P_{Wilcoxon}$ = 0.190.
‡P = 0.790.
§P = 0.010.
‖Of whom 50 received vaccine only and 61 received vaccine and amantadine.
¶Of whom 16 received amantadine and 12 received neither vaccine nor amantadine.
(Courtesy of Libow LS, Neufeld RR, Olson E, et al: Sequential outbreak of influenza A and B in a nursing home: Efficacy of vaccine and amantadine. *J Am Geriatr Soc* 44[10]:1153–1157, 1996.)

illness. One hundred thirty-nine patients met study criteria for influenza, including 111 who had received vaccine and 28 who were not vaccinated.

Findings.—The attack rate for the nursing home was 27.9%. After the start of the outbreak, 257 of 499 residents completed an effective course of amantadine therapy. Neither the vaccine nor amantadine therapy had a significant effect on the influenza attack rate. The mean age of the residents with influenza was 87.5; the median duration of illness was 5 days. Influenza A was predominant in the first phase of the epidemic and influenza B in the second phase. Vaccine reduced the rate of pneumonia secondary to influenza A and B. Although amantadine was associated with decreased mortality and shorter duration of influenza A illness, this treatment did not affect the rate of pneumonia secondary to influenza. The combination of vaccine and amantadine was associated with a significantly lower incidence of pneumonia, hospitalization, or death (Table 1).

Discussion.—Over a period of 2 months, the influenza epidemic spread rapidly through the nursing home, affecting nearly 30% of residents. A bimodal pattern was observed, with influenza caused sequentially by the A virus and the B virus. The combination of vaccine and amantadine was successful in reducing the rate of sequelae.

▶ Over the years, I have selected many articles focused on nursing home epidemics, particularly those of influenza. There is something to learn from each of these epidemics. This article shows a sequential outbreak of influenza A, then B, in a nursing home and is the first to reflect that problem. The benefits with respect to the occurrence of death and of pneumonia, hospitalization, or both for those vaccinated and nonvaccinated are significantly different, as shown in Table 1. Also, amantadine was effective in shortening the length of time with influenza A from an average of 6–3.5 days for those who had been treated.

Nursing homes should immunize all patients except those who have an allergy or a religious objection. Amantadine is beneficial in reducing the symptoms, shortening the course, and reducing serious sequelae of influenza A. The dose should be low and monitored carefully in patients in nursing homes because of the side-effect profile.

J.R. Burton, M.D.

Influenza Vaccination of Health Care Workers in Long-term–Care Hospitals Reduces the Mortality of Elderly Patients

Potter J, Stott DJ, Roberts MA, et al (Univ of Glasgow, Scotland; Greater Glasgow Health Board, Scotland; Western Infirmary Glasgow, Scotland)

J Infect Dis 175:1–6, 1997 2–8

Objective.—Because of the health risks to elderly patients caused by influenza, the Centers for Disease Control recommend vaccination. Vaccination of health care workers (HCWs) caring for the elderly has been suggested to reduce the transmission to patients. Results of a study assessing whether vaccination of HCWs caring for elderly patients in long-term care reduces the incidence of influenza, lower respiratory tract infection, and death are presented.

Methods.—On October 31, 1994, the vaccination status of 1,059 patients (302 men), in 12 geriatric long-term care hospitals in Glasgow was assessed. The number of patients per site ranged from 55 to 119. Six hospitals had "opt-out" policies where patients were vaccinated unless they refused or had a contraindication, and 6 hospitals had "opt-in" policies, where patients were vaccinated only if relatives requested it. Staff vaccination status was also recorded. Four groups resulted: staff and patients unvaccinated (S0P0), staff vaccinated and patients not vaccinated (SVP0), staff unvaccinated and patients vaccinated (S0PV), and staff and patients vaccinated (SVPV). Vaccination began in October 1994, and patients were monitored for symptoms and signs through the end of March 1995. Deaths were recorded.

Results.—There was a significant reduction in mortality from 17% in the S0PV and S0P0 groups to 10% in the SVPV and SVP0 groups (Fig 1). There was no significant difference in mortality between hospitals that offered or did not offer vaccination to patients. There was a significant difference in the prevalence of influenza-like illnesses in patients in sites that vaccinated HCWs.

Conclusion.—Although influenza vaccination of HCWs reduced mortality in long-term care elderly patients, vaccination of the patients themselves did not decrease mortality.

▶ This study from the United Kingdom study suggests that there is value in the annual vaccination (every fall) of HCWs who are employed in long-term care institutions. There appears to be a reduction of nearly 40% in total patient mortality and almost 60% in influenza-like illness among the patients in the institution. The authors suggest that the vaccination of the HCWs is far more important than the vaccination of the patients at risk. The study design, however, is flawed, thereby weakening these conclusions. The ma-

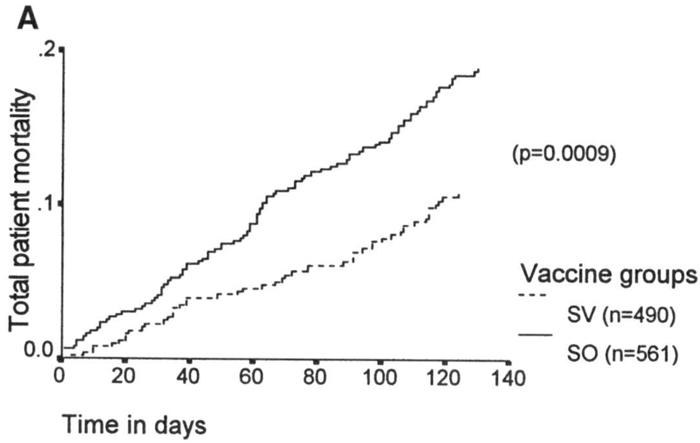

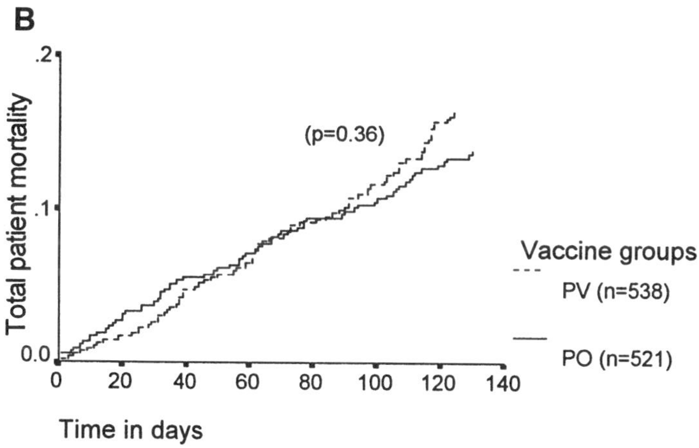

FIGURE 1.—Total patient mortality (proportion of all patients) in **A**, geriatric long-term care hospital sites where HCWs were offered influenza vaccine (SV) compared with sites where they were not offered vaccine (SO), and **B**, hospital sites where patients were routinely given vaccine (opt-out policy, PV) compared with sites where they were not routinely vaccinated (opt-in-policy, PO). Time course is from 31 October 1994 (time 0). (Courtesy of Potter J, Stott DJ, Roberts MA, et al: Influence vaccination of health care workers in long-term–care hospitals reduces the mortality of elderly patients. *J Infect Dis* 175:1–6, 1997. Copyright © 1997 The University of Chicago.)

jor problem is that the randomization was not patient randomization but randomization of institutions. Because of this, it is critical to understand the baseline mortality in the randomized institutions. This information was not provided.

Nevertheless, it is an intuitive finding that staff should be vaccinated, and most medical directors insist on this in nursing homes in the United States. I believe that we should be serious about vaccinating patients as well as staff. The medical director, attending physicians, and nursing director ought to set the standard by being the first to be vaccinated, and they should probably do so in front of the staff.

The herd immunity that occurs from vaccinating all patients (except those who have allergies or strong resistance to vaccination) has been demonstrated in the past, so the established bottom line in the United States is: vaccinate patients in long-term care institutions broadly, but also vaccinate all the staff starting with the medical director, director of nursing, and administrator.

I'd like to acknowledge the insightful help I received in analyzing this paper from two of my colleagues at Johns Hopkins, Donald W. Scott, M.D. and William B. Greenough, M.D.

J.R. Burton, M.D.

Increasing Influenza Immunization Among High-Risk Patients: Education or Financial Incentive?

Moran WP, Nelson K, Wofford JL, et al (Wake Forest Univ, Winston Salem, NC; Boston City Hosp)

Am J Med 101:612–620, 1996 2–9

Objective.—Because of the morbidity and mortality resulting from influenza, it is recommended that at-risk persons be vaccinated. Only about half of these individuals actually get vaccinated primarily because physician appointments are required in most cases. It has been suggested that standing orders be left to immunize at-risk individuals; that brochures be mailed that stress prevention of discomfort, not infecting others, and that include a physician's recommendation; or that financial incentives in the form of a lottery-type prize be provided to encourage immunization of older individuals. Information about these incentives were mailed to high-risk individuals to assess their effect in encouraging immunization.

Methods.—During the 1991–1992 influenza season, a brochure or lottery-type incentive or nothing was mailed to high-risk patients randomly allocated to receive either incentive, both incentives a week apart, or nothing. Postcard follow-up were mailed to 100 randomly selected individuals not documented as receiving an immunization to determine whether they were vaccinated at another site. Demographic variables were statistically analyzed to assess those characteristics predictive of getting an influenza vaccination.

Results.—A total of 797 patients (34% men), age 18–99, were included in the analysis. There were 397 in the brochure group, 397 in the incentive group, and 400 in the control group.

The brochure incentive interaction was significant (Table 3). Those immunized in the prior year were significantly more likely to seek immunization in the current year (OR = 4.21) and the likelihood of immunization increased with age. Associated costs were $0.54 per brochure and $0.75 per lottery-type incentive. Response rate to the postcards was low (25%).

TABLE 3.—Baseline Comparison of Covariates by Group

	All Patients (n = 797)			Patients with prior immunization history known (n = 328)		
	Odds ratio	95% CI	p value	Odds ratio	95% CI	p value
Educational brochure	2.29	1.45–3.61	0.0004	3.95	1.92–8.10	0.0002
Incentive	1.68	1.05–2.68	0.0308	1.59	0.769–3.28	0.2113
Educational brochure and incentive	1.41	0.88–2.27	0.1527	1.56	0.731–3.34	0.2460
Immunization in prior year	—	—	—	4.21	2.48–7.14	0.0001
Age	1.02	1.01–1.03	0.0003	—	—	—
Pulmonary disease	1.80	1.25–2.58	0.0015	—	—	—
Diabetes mellitus	1.73	1.09–2.74	0.0215	—	—	—
Alcoholism	—	—	—	0.395	0.151–1.03*	0.0405*

*Standard deviation.

(Reprinted by permission of the publisher from Moran WP, Nelson K, Wofford JL, et al: Increasing influenza immunization among high-risk patients: Education or financial incentive? *Am J Med* 101:612–620, Copyright 1996 by Excerpta Medica, Inc.)

Conclusion.—Brochures significantly increased influenza immunization by high-risk populations, lottery-type incentives were much less effective, and both together were not effective.

▶ This is a nice article on the value of a simple educational program to increase influenza vaccination among high-risk patients. In this study of patients using a community health center, there was a greater than twofold increase in immunization among those patients sent a simple educational cartoon about the importance of influenza vaccination. Such strategies make enormous sense and, I believe, should be widely used.

J.R. Burton, M.D.

A Comparison of Nursing Home–acquired Pneumonia Patients With Patients With Community-acquired Pneumonia and Nursing Home Patients Without Pneumonia

Marrie TJ, Blanchard W (Dalhousie Univ, Halifax, NS; Victoria Gen Hosp, Halifax, NS)

J Am Geriatr Soc 45:50–55, 1997 2–10

Objective.—Although the mortality rate of nursing home patients admitted for pneumonia is 40%, the proportion of deaths attributed to pneumonia vs. general ill health is not known. Mortality rates of patients with nursing home–acquired pneumonia (NHAP), patients with community-acquired pneumonia (CAP), and patients admitted to nursing homes for other reasons (NP) were compared.

Methods.—*Pneumonia* was defined as new opacity on chest radiograph and 2 or more signs, including cough, shortness of breath, fever, sputum production, or crackles on auscultation. Patients with NHAP were age- and sex-matched with 2 CAP and 2 NP patients. After discharge, patients

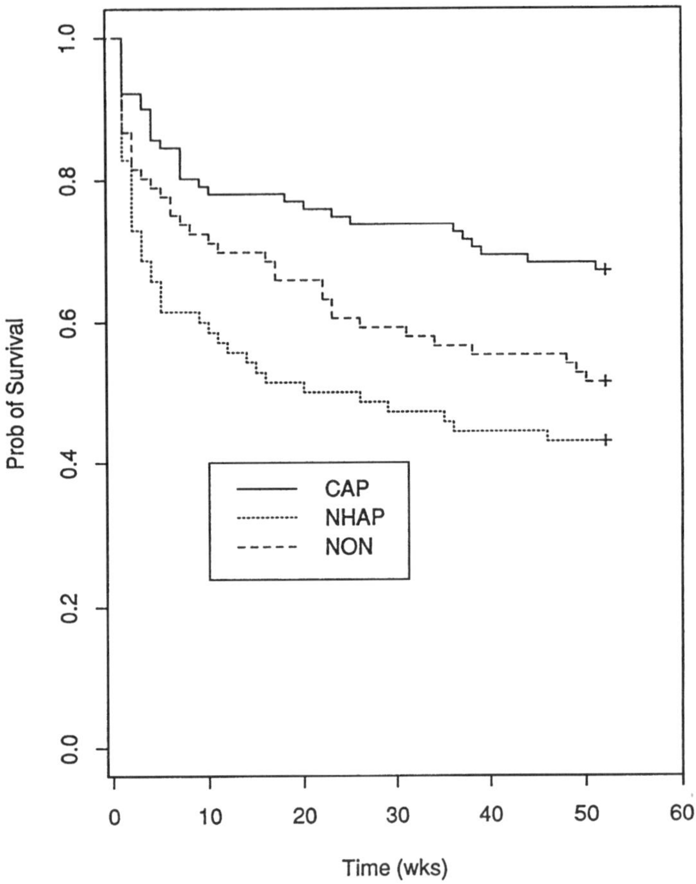

FIGURE 1.—Kaplan-Meirer (sic) plot of survival for patients with community-acquired pneumonia (CAP), nursing home acquired pneumonia (NHAP), and for patients from nursing homes admitted for conditions other than pneumonia (non). The survival rate for CAP patients is higher than that for NHAP patients ($p < 0.01$). (Courtesy of Marrie TJ, Blanchard W: A comparison of nursing home–acquired pneumonia patients with patients with community-acquired pneumonia and nursing home patients without pneumonia. *J Am Geriatr Soc* 45[1]:50–55, 1997.)

were contacted by telephone at 6, 12, 36, and 52 weeks. Survival was analyzed and compared statistically.

Results.—There were more females than males in the NP group, which was also older than the CAP group. In-hospital mortality was significantly higher for the NHAP group than for the CAP group but not for the NP group (32% vs. 14% vs. 23%, respectively). The NHAP group had the lowest number of self-sufficient patients (6%), the CAP group had the highest number taking corticosteroids (24%), and antibiotic use was similar among groups. Numbers of patients with no comorbidity was significantly different between groups with 32% in the CAP group, 8% in the NHAP group, and 5% in the NP group. NHAP patients were significantly more likely to be hypoxemic than CAP patients (68 vs. 44%), whereas significantly more CAP and NHAP patients than NP patients had positive blood cultures (85% vs. 85% vs. 31%), with CAP patients having predominantly *Streptococcus pneumonia* and NHAP patients having both *S. pneumonia* and aerobic gram-negative organisms that resembled the NP group more closely. Ventilatory support was required for 13% of CAP patients, 3% of NHAP patients, and 4% of NP patients. Pneumonia patients commonly had diarrhea caused by *Clostridium difficile*. Mortality was 58% for NHAP, 33% for CAP, and 50% for NP (Fig 1).

Conclusion.—The mortality rate for NHAP patients is significantly higher than for CAP patients and is primarily dependent on self-sufficiency and in-hospital complications rather than on group.

► This study shows the relative seriousness of pneumonia among patients admitted to hospital from nursing homes and from the community. It is no surprise that nursing home patients have a significantly higher mortality rate. The authors then compare nursing home patients admitted to hospital with pneumonia and with other causes. Mortality is predicted by two important factors: hospital complication rate and the level of self-sufficiency at the time of admission. The in-hospital mortality rate for patients with pneumonia admitted from nursing homes was 32%; this is significantly higher than the 14% rate among those admitted from the community but not significantly higher than the 23% rate for nursing home patients admitted for causes other than pneumonia.

J.R. Burton, M.D.

A Prediction Rule to Identify Low-risk Patients With Community-acquired Pneumonia

Fine MJ, Auble TE, Yealy DM, et al (Univ of Pittsburgh, Pittsburgh, Pa; Massachusetts Gen Hosp, Boston; Harvard Med School, Boston; et al)

N Engl J Med 336:243–250, 1997 2–11

Background.—About 4 million new cases of adult community-acquired pneumonia occur in the United States each year. Hospital admission rates vary from region to region, indicating that admission criteria may be inconsistent. Physicians tend to overestimate the risk of death, and patients at low risk are often hospitalized. Accurate, objective models for identifying low-risk patients with pneumonia may improve decisions about hospitalization.

Methods.—A prediction rule for patients with community-acquired pneumonia was derived from the analysis data from almost 14,200 adult inpatients. Patients were categorized into 5 classes on the basis of risk of 30-day hospital mortality. The prediction rule was validated with data from more than 38,000 inpatients and almost 2,300 additional inpatients and outpatients. In step 1 of the prediction rule, patients at low risk of death are identified on the basis of history and physical examination findings. In step 2, the remaining patients are classified on the basis of findings from step 1 plus laboratory and radiographic data (Table 2).

Results.—Mortality rates were similar in the 5 risk classes in the 3 patient cohorts (Table 3). Mortality was 0.1% to 0.4% in class I, 0.6% to 0.7% in class II, and 0.9% to 2.8% in class III. There were only 7 deaths among 1,575 patients in the 3 lowest risk classes from the group of almost 2,300 inpatients and outpatients; only 4 of the 7 deaths were pneumonia related. Risk class was significantly associated with risk of hospitalization

TABLE 2.—Point Scoring System for Step 2 of the Prediction Rule for Assignment to Risk Classes II, III, IV, and V

Characteristic	Points Assigned*
Demographic factor	
Age	
Men	Age (yr)
Women	Age (yr) − 10
Nursing home resident	+10
Coexisting illnesses†	
Neoplastic disease	+30
Liver disease	+20
Congestive heart failure	+10
Cerebrovascular disease	+10
Renal disease	+10
Physical-examination findings	
Altered mental status‡	+20
Respiratory rate ≥30/min	+20
Systolic blood pressure <90 mm Hg	+20
Temperature <35°C or ≥40°C	+15
Pulse ≥125/min	+10
Laboratory and radiographic findings	
Arterial pH <7.35	+30
Blood urea nitrogen ≥30 mg/dl (11 mmol/liter)	+20
Sodium <130 mmol/liter	+20
Glucose ≥250 mg/dl (14 mmol/liter)	+10
Hematocrit <30%	+10
Partial pressure of arterial oxygen <60 mm Hg§	+10
Pleural effusion	+10

*A total point score for a given patient is obtained by summing the patient's age in years (age minus 10 for women) and the points for each applicable characteristic. The points assigned to each predictor variable were based on coefficients obtained from the logistic-regression model used in step 2 of the prediction rule (see the Methods section of original article).

†Neoplastic disease is defined as any cancer except basal- or squamous-cell cancer of the skin that was active at the time of presentation or diagnosed within 1 year of presentation. Liver disease is defined as a clinical or histologic diagnosis of cirrhosis or another form of chronic liver disease, such as chronic active hepatitis. Congestive heart failure is defined as systolic or diastolic ventricular dysfunction documented by history, physical examination, and chest radiograph, echocardiogram, multiple gated acquisition scan, or left ventriculogram. Cerebrovascular disease is defined as a clinical diagnosis of stroke or transient ischemic attack or stroke documented by magnetic resonance imaging or computed tomography. Renal disease is defined as a history of chronic renal disease or abnormal blood urea nitrogen and creatinine concentrations documented in the medical record.

‡Altered mental status is defined as disorientation with respect to person, place, or time that is not known to be chronic, stupor, or coma.

§In the Pneumonia PORT cohort study, an oxygen saturation of less than 90% on pulse oximetry or intubation before admission was also considered abnormal.

TABLE 3.—Comparison of Risk-Class–Specific Mortality Rates in the Derivation and Validation Cohorts

Risk Class (no. of points)*	MedisGroups Derivation Cohort		MedisGroups Validation Cohort		Pneumonia PORT Validation Cohort					
					Inpatients		Outpatients		All patients	
	no. of patients	% who died	no. of patients	% who died	no. of patients	% who died	no. of patients	% who died	no. of patients	% who died
I	1,372	0.4	3,034	0.1	185	0.5	587	0.0	772	0.1
II (≤70)	2,412	0.7	5,778	0.6	233	0.9	244	0.4	477	0.6
III (71–90)	2,632	2.8	6,790	2.8	254	1.2	72	0.0	326	0.9
IV (91–130)	4,697	8.5	13,104	8.2	446	9.0	40	12.5	486	9.3
V (>130)	3,086	31.1	9,333	29.2	225	27.1	1	0.0	226	27.0
Total	14,199	10.2	38,039	10.6	1343	8.0	944	0.6	2287	5.2

Note: There were no statistically significant differences in overall mortality or mortality within risk class among patients in the MedisGroups derivation, MedisGroups validation, or overall Pneumonia PORT validation cohort. The P values for the comparisons of mortality across risk classes are as follows: class I, $P = 0.22$; class II, $P = 0.67$; class III, $P = 0.12$; class IV, $P = 0.69$; and class V, $P = 0.09$.

*Inclusion in risk class I was determined by the absence of all predictors identified in step 1 of the prediction rule. Inclusion in risk classes II, III, IV, and V was determined by a patient's total risk score, which was computed according to the scoring system shown in Table 2.

(Reprinted by permission of *The New England Journal of Medicine* from Fine MJ, Auble TE, Yealy DM, et al: A prediction rule to identify low-risk patients with community-acquired pneumonia. *N Engl J Med* 336:243–250.)

among outpatients and with use of intensive care and number of days admitted among inpatients.

Conclusions.—This prognostic model accurately identified patients with community-acquired pneumonia at low risk of death. This rule may help physicians make better decisions about hospitalizing patients with pneumonia. The predictor variables are well defined and may be evaluated at the initial examination, and patients can be assigned to the lowest risk class on the basis of information from the history and initial examination.

▶ Deciding which patients with community-acquired pneumonia should be admitted to the hospital requires considerable physician judgment.

Precious few data exist to guide the clinician in this decision. This study is important because it provides a theoretical framework with which to make the decision. It defines risk class for death within 30 days for patients with community-acquired pneumonia. The investigators predict risk by analysis of data in 3 cohorts totaling 53,581 patients with community-acquired pneumonia.

I believe this risk classification is valuable, but it remains to be seen whether physicians will use the method. A controlled study should be conducted next.

J.R. Burton, M.D.

Handwashing and Glove Use in a Long-term–Care Facility

Thompson BL, Dwyer DM, Ussery XT, et al (Ctrs for Disease Control and Prevention, Atlanta; Maryland Dept of Health and Mental Hygiene, Baltimore; Johns Hopkins Univ, Baltimore, et al)

Infect Control Hosp Epidemiol 18:97–103, 1997 2–12

Introduction.—In acute and long-term care facilities, universal precaution and body substance isolation guidelines have been accepted. The incidence of nosocomial disease, a major cause of morbidity and mortality in medical care settings, has been improved with these precautions. However, little is known of the effect of these precautions on nosocomial disease in long-term care facilities. The use of gloves and handwashing, the factors associated with infection-control practices, and the frequency of potential microbial transmission were determined in a long-term care facility.

Methods.—In a 266-bed, university-based long-term care facility, 230 staff-resident interactions were studied in which resident characteristics, type of activity, staff credentials, and movements of the staff members' hands were recorded. Appropriateness of glove use and handwashing was judged by using the long-term care facility's guidelines. Patients were divided into 2 wards. Ward A had 56 beds and a ventilator unit, and many residents had severe decubitus ulcers. Ward B had 60 residents, with no ventilator beds, and residents were not admitted for special care of decubitus ulcers.

TABLE 2.—Percentage of Interactions During Which the Facility's Guidelines Were Followed or in Which Potential Microbial Transmission Occurred, Wards A and B

	Percentage (Proportion)	
	Ward A	Ward B
Gloves used	82 (139/170)	100 (22/22)
Gloves changed	16 (21/132)	15 (3/20)
Hands always washed*	4 (7/189)	9 (2/22)
Hands washed before	27 (19/70)	67 (6/9)
Hands washed during	0 (0/162)	5 (1/20)
Hands washed after	63 (104/166)	83 (10/12)
PMT occurred	83 (144/173)	70 (14/20)

*Washed at every required instance during the interaction.
Abbreviation: PMT, potential microbial transmission.
(Courtesy of Thompson BL, Dwyer DM, Ussery XT, et al: Handwashing and glove use in a long-term–care facility. *Infect Control Hosp Epidemiol* 18:97–103, 1997.)

Results.—In 139 of 170 interactions (82%), gloves were worn. They were changed appropriately in 21 of 132 interactions (16%) (Table 2). Before an interaction, hands were washed appropriately in 27% of instances. They were washed during an interaction when needed in 0% of instances and in 63% after an interaction. In the care of residents with gastrostomy tubes, gloves were less likely to be used than in the care of other residents. Guidelines were followed more frequently during wound care than during other activities. In 152 of 193 evaluable interactions (82%), microbial transmission could have occurred. Potential microbial interactions occurred in 85% of interactions involving nursing assistants, in 83% of interactions involving Licensed Practical Nurses, and in 82% of interactions involving Registered Nurses.

Conclusion.—Glove use and handwashing were markedly deficient in this long-term care facility. Multivariate techniques were not used to control for confounding factors or to evaluate potential effect modifiers.

▶ This article from my own institution points out that we are simply not practicing what we preach. Nursing homes are ideal arenas for the spread of germs from one frail, vulnerable patient to another. Often infectious agents are transferred among patients by staff. The appropriate use of handwashing and gloves by staff can markedly reduce the spread of infection. In this operational study, 82% of the staff-patient interactions could have resulted in microbial transmission because of failure by staff to wash their hands or use gloves appropriately!

Perhaps we all should focus a bit on the obvious and work on these simple hygiene methods.

J.R. Burton, M.D.

Ethics and Advance Directives

The Illusion of End-of-life Resource Savings With Advance Directives

Teno J, for the SUPPORT Investigators (George Washington Univ, Washington, DC; et al)

J Am Geriatr Soc 45:513–518, 1997 2–13

Background.—There is increasing attention being focused on the high cost of medical care at the end of life. Almost 30% of the Medicare budget is spent on the 6% of recipients who die in a given year. Two recent studies reported a 35% and 68% decrease in hospitalization costs of terminally ill patients associated with documentation of advance directives in the medical record. Before enactment of the Patient Self-Determination Act, the authors reported no change in use of resources associated with advance directives among individuals who died in the hospital, but advance directives were rarely documented at that time.

Methods.—The association of resource use and documentation of advance directives by the third day of a serious illness was examined using data from the 2-year period before and after enactment of the Patient Self-Determination Act. There were 9,105 seriously ill patients enrolled in the Study to Understand Prognoses and Preferences for Outcomes and Risks of Treatments (SUPPORT). A nurse facilitated communication among patients, surrogates, and physicians about preferences for and outcomes of treatment and also documented advance directives in the medical record.

Results.—After enactment of the Patient Self-Determination Act and SUPPORT intervention, documentation of advance directives increased. However, no change in the use of hospital resources was seen among patients who died during their first hospital admission (Fig 1). Advance directives that were documented by the third day of serious illness were associated with a 23% decrease in resource use among control patients but not among patients receiving intervention, who had a higher rate of pre-existing, documented advance directives. Greater cost was associated with patients receiving intervention who had early documentation of advance directives than with patients without documented advance directives. The rate of documentation and the characteristics of patients with documented advance directives were different between control and patients who received intervention. Patients given intervention were more likely to have documented advance directives by the third day of illness, but control patients who were older, less wealthy, less educated, and more likely to prefer to forgo cardiopulmonary resuscitation and limit life-sustaining treatment had documented advance directives. These associations were not seen among patients receiving intervention.

Discussion.—These results show that the use of documented advance directives in the medical record does not necessarily decrease the use of hospital resources among adults who are seriously ill. Use of advance

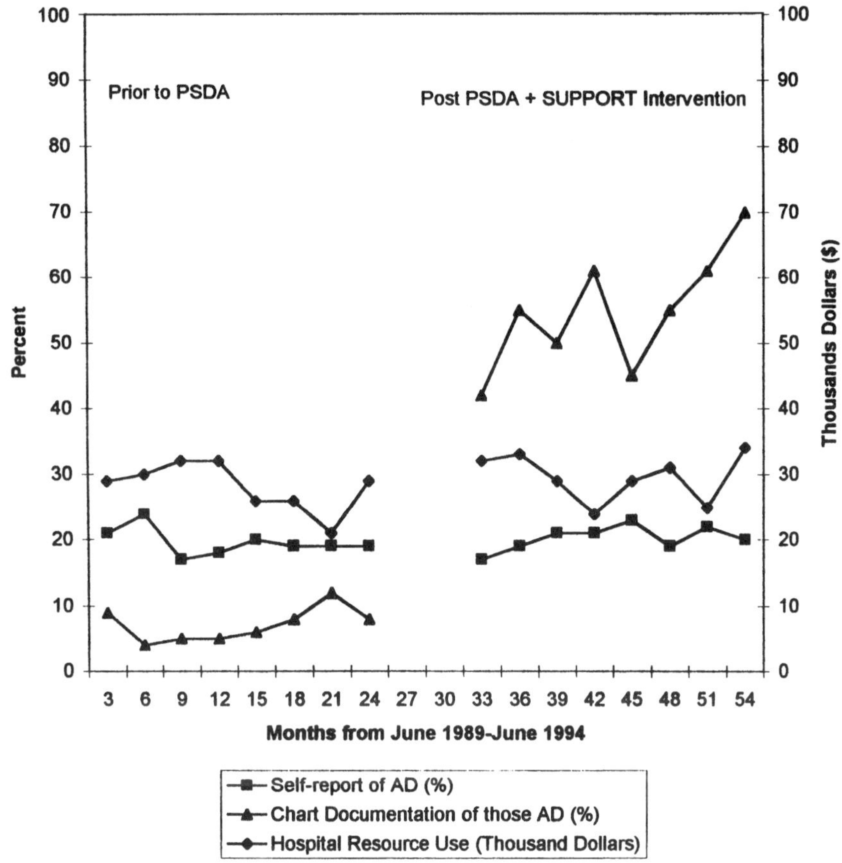

FIGURE 1.—Depicted are the association of the rates over time of self-reporting of advance directives (AD), documentation of those directives in the record by the third day, and hospital resource use among 680 intervention patients who died on the enrollment admission. *Abbreviations: PSDA*, Patient Self-Determination Act; *SUPPORT*, Study to Understand Prognoses and Preferences for Outcomes of Risks of Treatment. (Courtesy of Teno J, for the SUPPORT Investigators: The illusion of end-of-life resource savings with advance directives. *J Am Geriatr Soc* 45[4]:513–518, 1997.)

directives does not seem to increase communication between patients and physicians.

► It is commonly believed that the cost for care of patients with a terminal hospitalization would be considerably lessened in those with established advance directives. This study of the SUPPORT[1] group analyzes resource use based on the presence or absence of advance directives in the patient's record by the third day of hospitalization for a serious illness. The study spans the period of 2 years before and 2 years after the implementation of the Patient Self-Determination Act in 1992. Figure 1 shows no reduction in hospital resource use in spite of a significant increase in the documentation of advance directives in the medical record. The issue, as the authors point out, may not be simply to increase the number of patients with advance directives but rather to have physicians and other health care providers meaningfully discuss advance directives with the patients and then to appropriately respond to patient wishes.

Things are never as simple as they seem, but, clearly, nothing replaces both compassionate and thorough discussions by primary care clinicians about advance directives and the careful communication of patient wishes in the medical record and to other clinicians involved in the patient's care. This is particularly critical at the time of the hospitalization for a serious illness.

J.R. Burton, M.D.

Reference

1. The SUPPORT Investigators: A controlled trial to improve outcomes for seriously ill hospitalized adults: The study to understand prognoses and preferences for outcomes and risks of treatments (SUPPORT). *JAMA* 274:1591–1598, 1995.

Do Advance Directives Provide Instructions That Direct Care?

Teno JM, for the SUPPORT Investigators (George Washington Univ, Washington, DC; et al)

J Am Geriatr Soc 45:508–512, 1997 2–14

Background.—Although advance directives are intended to guide the medical treatment of seriously ill patients, it has been reported that these directives are not associated with improved decision making about resuscitation of seriously ill patients. There are 2 forms of advance directives: instructional directives stating decisions about future care and proxy directives naming a proxy decision maker. Living wills are the oldest advance directives. A standard living will states that there is a point at which the individual would prefer to die than continue living through artificial means, but they are generally not specific about which efforts to prolong life should cease and when. The content of documented advance directives was examined to determine whether they contained clear instructions to guide medical care.

Methods.—The Study to Understand Prognoses and Preferences for Outcomes and Risks of Treatments (SUPPORT) enrolled 4,804 patients with at least 1 of 9 serious illnesses after implementation of the Patient Self-Determination Act. A review of the advance directives from hospital medical records through 6 months follow-up or death noted content, date of completion, and whether they had been witnessed and notarized. The content of documents with instructions beyond the standard legal form was analyzed. Charts were reviewed for evidence of clinical decision making and use of life-sustaining treatment.

Results.—Only 688 documents from 569 patients showed advance directives placed in the medical record. About 66% were durable powers of attorney and 31% were standard living wills or other forms of written instructions. Only 90 documents had additional instructions beyond naming a proxy or stating preferences in a standard living will (Fig 1). Only 36 documents had specific instructions about use of life-sustaining treatment, and only 22 indicated that life-sustaining treatment should not be used in the patient's current medical condition. Some patients used terms like "no advanced life support" and "no cardiopulmonary resuscitation, no venti-

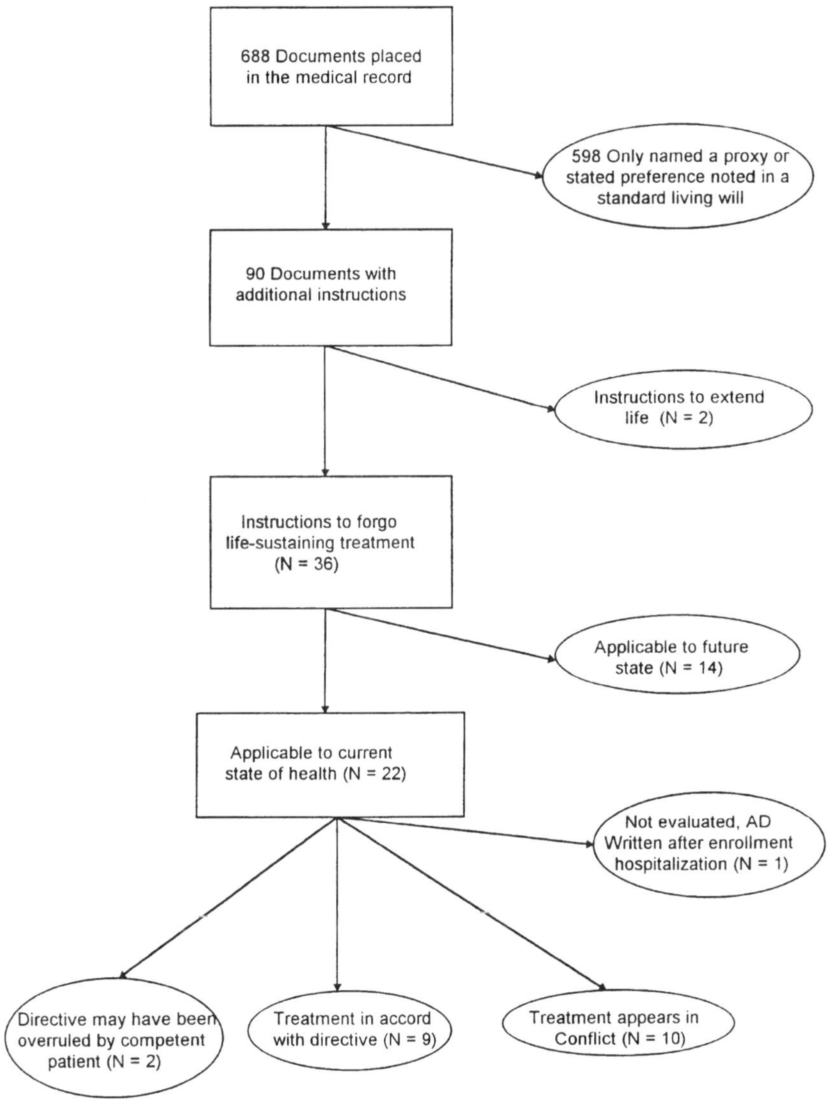

FIGURE 1.—Content of written advance directives (AD) placed in the medical record. (Courtesy of Teno JM, for the SUPPORT Investigators: Do advance directives provide instructions that direct care? *J Am Geriatr Soc* 45[4]:508–512, 1997.)

lators, no nasogastric G tubes." In 9 of these 22 patients, treatment was consistent with the patient's instructions, and 2 patients may have changed inconsistent instructions after discussion with hospital staff.

Discussion.—The naming of a health care proxy may provide valuable information to clinicians, but this outcome variable was not addressed in this study. In general, the advance directives examined did not provide specific instructions about medical treatment. Implementation of the Patient Self-Determination Act has not solved the problem of decision making for seriously ill individuals. This area of health care needs much improvement.

► Like the preceding article (Abstract 2–13), here are data derived from the SUPPORT work. This paper focuses on the written advance directives found in the patients' charts during hospitalization for serious illnesses and whether the documents provide clear instructions to direct care. Figure 1 shows that, of 688 documents that were placed in the medical record, only 36 had instructions to forgo life-sustaining treatment and, of those, only 22 were applicable to the current situation. What is remarkable is that in almost 50% of these 22 records, the treatment given to the patient was in conflict with what the investigators believed the content of the advance directive to be.

An article by the same group[1] accompanies this paper; in it, the authors further substantiate that advance directives did not substantially enhance physician–patient communications and did not enhance decision making about resuscitation.

Obviously, the federal legislation to require that all patients be asked about advance directives at the time of admission to a hospital (and other health care environments) is not fully working. Most individuals do not have clear advance directives, and, often, when they do, there is conflict between the care given and the recorded advance directive. Nevertheless, it is important to continue to try to understand more clearly what is accounting for these discrepancies so that patient wishes can be known and followed precisely.

J.R. Burton, M.D.

Reference

1. Teno J, Lynn J, Wenger N, et al: Advance directives for seriously ill hospitalized patients: Effectiveness with the Patient Self-Determination Act and the SUPPORT intervention 1995. *J Am Geriatr Soc* 45:500–507, 1997.

Continuity of Do-not Resuscitate Orders Between Hospital and Nursing Home Settings

Ghusn HF, Teasdale TA, Jordan D (Baylor College of Medicine, Houston; Houston Veterans Affairs Med Ctr)

J Am Geriatr Soc 45:465–469, 1997 2–15

Background.—In the United States, patients, their surrogates, and health care workers are involved in decisions about their health care, including consent to diagnostic tests and life-sustaining treatment such as cardiopulmonary resuscitation. Recent studies indicate that advance directives are often not presented to or followed by health care workers.

Methods.—A review was conducted of the hospital and nursing home records of 166 patients discharged from a veterans hospital to either a hospital-affiliated nursing home or a community nursing home. The hospital-affiliated nursing home received full medical records, but the community nursing homes received only hospital discharge summaries prepared by house staff.

Results.—The details of discussions of advance directives were documented in nursing home charts for 35% of patients (Fig 1). Of 43 patients in nursing homes with do-not-resuscitate orders, 81% had dementia, 35% had cerebrovascular accidents, 33% had cardiovascular diseases, 30% had chronic obstructive pulmonary disease, and 26% had cancer. Overall, 26% of patients discharged to nursing homes had do-not-resuscitate orders (Fig 2). Slightly more than 50% of patients with a hospital do-not-resuscitate order continued that status in the nursing home. Although twice as many patients with hospital do-not-resuscitate orders were discharged to community nursing homes as to the hospital-affiliated nursing

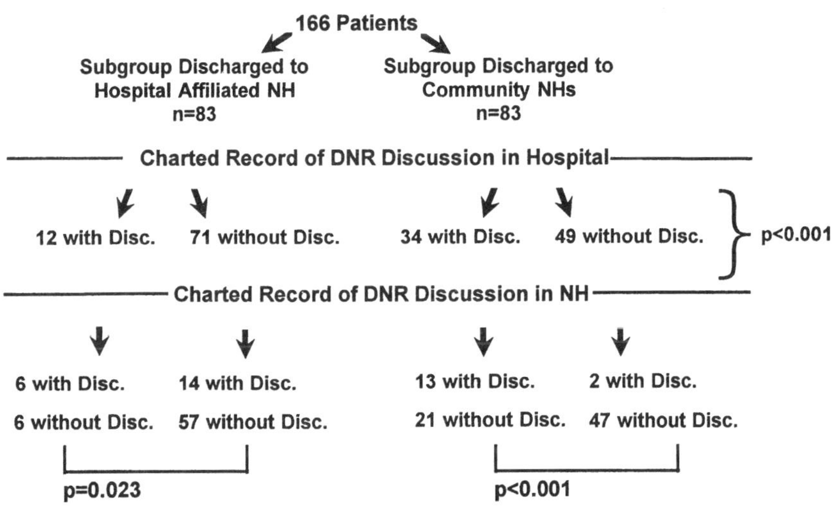

FIGURE 1.—Continuity of do-not-resuscitate (DNR) discussions (Disc) between hospital and nursing home (NH) settings. (Courtesy of Ghusn HF, Teasdale TA, Jordan D: Continuity of do-not resuscitate orders between hospital and nursing home settings. *J Am Geriatr Soc* 45[4]:465–469, 1997.)

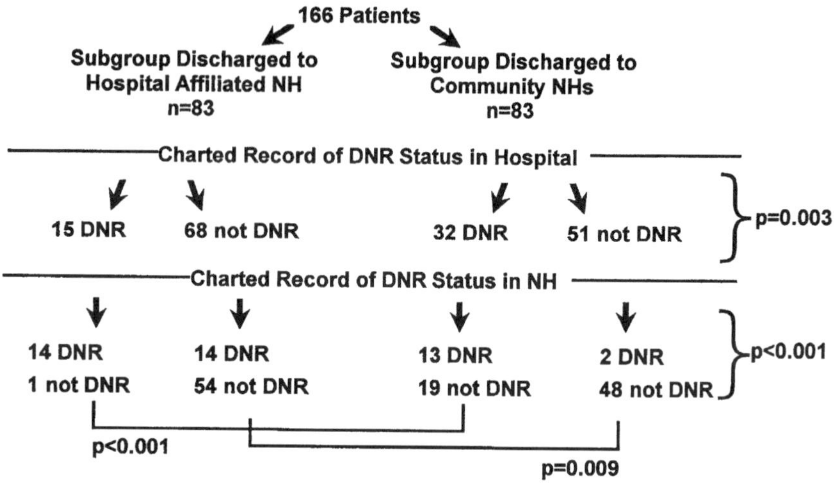

FIGURE 2.—Continuity of do-not-resuscitate (DNR) status between hospital and nursing home (NH) settings. (Courtesy of Ghusn HF, Teasdale TA, Jordan D: Continuity of do-not resuscitate orders between hospital and nursing home settings. *J Am Geriatr Soc* 45[4]:465–469, 1997.)

home, the continuity of do-not-resuscitate orders was greater between the hospital and hospital-affiliated nursing home. Specific communication of do-not-resuscitate orders to the nursing home by the hospital was associated with better continuity of those orders.

Discussion.—Discussions of advance directives are infrequent before hospitalized patients are discharged to a nursing home. Better continuity of advance directives was seen between this veterans hospital and its affiliated nursing home. There is a need for better communication between health care facilities about patients' health care wishes. Hospital discharge summaries should include a paragraph dedicated to advance directives even when none have been executed. Suggested information to be included in such paragraphs is shown in Table 2 of the original article.

▶ Did you ever wonder what happens to a patient's advance directives when the individual leaves the hospital and goes to a nursing home? Look at the figures: when going to a nursing home not closely affiliated with the short-term care hospital, there is a marked discrepancy when compared with patients transferred to a nursing home tightly affiliated with the hospital, in this case in the same building. We simply must work on communication of critical medical information such as advance directives, particularly as patients move from 1 unit to another within a facility or from 1 facility to another. Such transfers are increasingly common with the development of very short-term care and rehabilitation units and the increasingly rapid transfer of ill patients from hospitals to such units and to nursing homes; it is a phenomenon that parallels the seemingly ever-decreasing length of stay in short-term care hospitals.

J.R. Burton, M.D.

The Doctor's Role in Discussing Advance Preferences for End-of-life Care: Perceptions of Physicians Practicing in the VA

Markson L, Clark J, Glantz L, et al (Edith Nourse Rogers Mem Veterans Hosp, Bedford, Mass; Boston Univ)

J Am Geriatr Soc 45:399–406, 1997 2–16

Background.—Although in the United States individuals who are mentally competent have the legal right to make informed decisions about their health care, many individuals do not actually make decisions about life-sustaining treatment until after they have become ill and mentally incapacitated. Studies also indicate that proxy decision makers may not predict the patient's desires accurately. Advance directives are intended to enhance autonomy and facilitate end-of-life decisions about medical treatment. Laws such as the Patient Self-Determination Act require community health care centers to tell patients about their legal right to prepare advance directives. Many surveys report that physicians as well as patients believe that patients should discuss their preferences for medical treatment with their physicians and document their preferences.

Methods.—Data were collected from a national survey of physicians in VA medical centers. Questionnaires were sent to 1,050 physicians. The questionnaire contained 178 items covering the physicians' actual experiences discussing advance directives with patients and following those directives, obligations of their role in helping patients make advance decisions and in complying with those decisions, attitudes toward factors that help or hinder discussion of advance preferences with their patients, and opinions on the content and the format of advance directive forms.

Results.—The response rate was 67%. About 79% of respondents had discussed advance preferences with at least 1 patient in the previous year, and 19% had talked to more than 25 patients. Overall, 73% stated they had used a written directive to make decisions about treatment of at least 1 patient. Independent factors associated with discussing advance directives were younger age, board certification, less time spent in the outpatient setting, and personal experience with advance decision making. Of physicians who had discussed advance preferences with patients, 59% had often initiated the discussion, 55% usually had such discussions in inpatient settings, and 31% usually had such discussions in outpatient settings. About 82% believed that physicians should initiate discussions about advance preferences, 91% would try to persuade a patient to change a decision that was not well-informed, 88% would try to change a decision that was not medically reasonable, and 88% would try to change a decision that was not in the patient's best interest. Only 14% would try to change a decision that conflicted with their own moral beliefs. When asked about factors that would make it easier to discuss advance preferences with patients, 80% reported that they expected a discussion of advance preferences to make future decisions easier, and 76% believed that having such discussions was a professional responsibility (Fig 1). When asked about factors that would make it difficult to discuss advance preferences

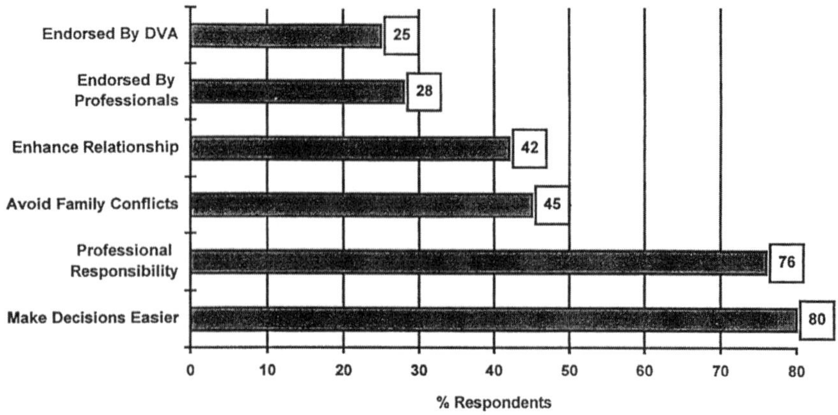

FIGURE 1.—Percentage of respondents who indicated that the factor would greatly increase discussions. *Abbreviation: DVA,* Department of Veterans Affairs. (Courtesy of Markson L, Clark J, Glantz L, et al: The doctor's role in discussing advance preferences for end-of-life care: Perceptions of physicians practicing in the VA. *J Am Geriatr Soc* 45[4]:399–406, 1997.)

with patients, 34% named discontinuity of care between inpatient and outpatient settings, 23% named pressure to see many patients in a given period of time, and 21% named scheduling policies as major factors (Fig 2).

Discussion.—These findings show that a large number of physicians in VA ambulatory and hospital centers discuss and carry out advance preferences about medical treatment of seriously ill patients. Most of the respondents in this survey believed that physicians should be involved in their patients' decision making about future treatment if they become seriously ill. Some have argued that physicians have never had a tradition of sharing information or decisions with their patients. This trend may be

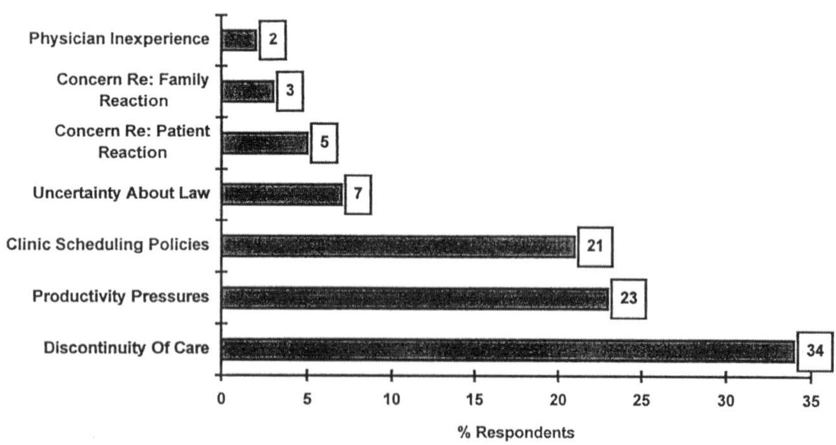

FIGURE 2.—Percentage of respondents who indicated that the factor would greatly decrease discussions. (Courtesy of Markson L, Clark J, Glantz L, et al: The doctor's role in discussing advance preferences for end-of-life care: Perceptions of physicians practicing in the VA. *J Am Geriatr Soc* 45[4]:399–406, 1997.)

shifting because of the greater availability of life-sustaining technology, physicians' serious moral concerns about the use of such treatment at the end of life, and a greater emphasis on death and dying in medical schools in the last 10 years.

▶ Here is even more new information on advance directives. In this study, the behavior of the VA health care system primary care physicians in their communications with patients about advance directives is analyzed. The results are derived from the responses of a national sample of 67% of 1,050 randomly selected physicians who were queried about these issues. This large and geographically diverse group adds great strength to the study. It is still limited, however, in being representative only of primary care physicians in the VA health care system.

This paper is helpful because it gets to the heart of the issue in establishing advance directives, namely, the dynamic of physician–patient communications. It describes areas of bias and physician apprehension. This paper and the others[1] on this subject all are efforts that are clearly needed on the local and national level to improve patients' use and understanding of advance directives and to improve health care systems' recognition of and adherence to developed advance directives.

J.R. Burton, M.D.

Reference

1. Teno J, Lynn J, Wenger N, et al: Advance directives for seriously ill hospitalized patients: Effectiveness with the Patient Self-Determination Act and the SUPPORT intervention 1995. *J Am Geriatr Soc* 45:500–507, 1997.

Nursing Home Issues

A Ten-Year Review of the Effect of OBRA-87 on Psychotropic Prescribing Practices in an Academic Nursing Home

Lantz MS, Giambanco V, Buchalter EN (Mount Sinai School of Medicine, New York)

Psychiatric Serv 47:951–955, 1996 2–17

Background.—The use of psychotropic medications in long-term care facilities has been controversial, with suggestions of overuse and misuse. The Omnibus Budget Reconciliation Act of 1987 (OBRA-1987) included provisions regulating psychotropic medication in long-term care facilities. The effects of OBRA-1987 on prescribing patterns were examined in a nursing home affiliated with a large medical school.

Methods.—The study was done in a 514-bed, nonprofit facility in New York City. The average age of facility residents was 87. There were 7 consulting psychiatrists attending the facility during the course of the study. Nursing staff turnover was low. Computerized pharmacy records for March 1984 through July 1994 were reviewed for prescription pat-

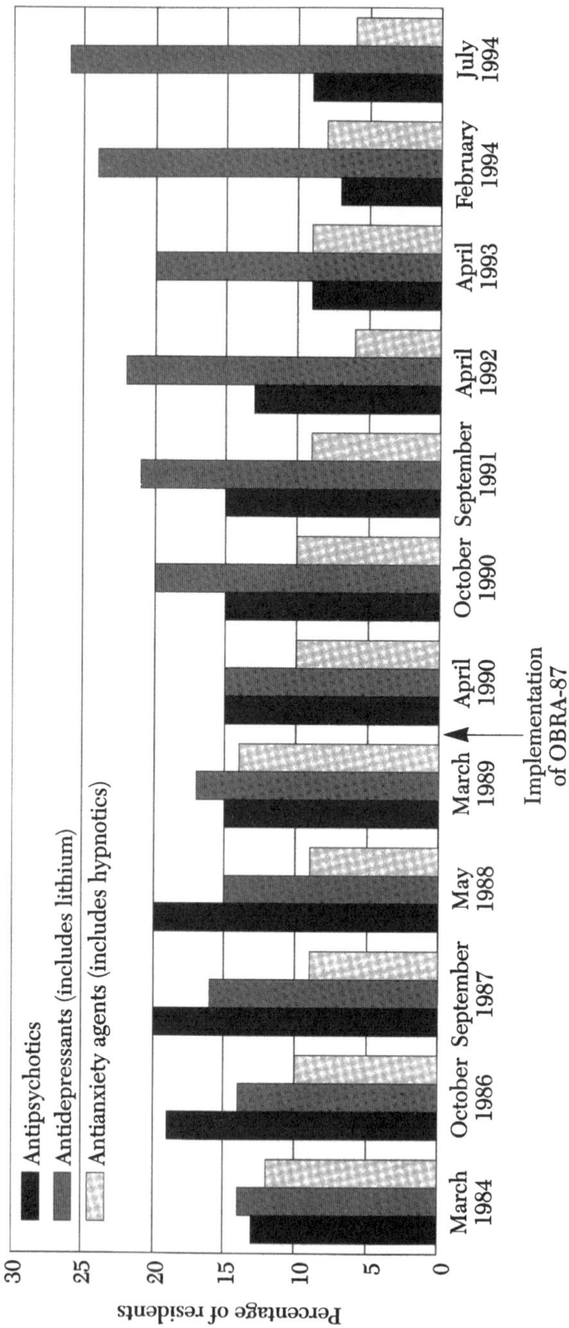

FIGURE 1.—Percentages of nursing home residents with prescriptions for 3 categories of psychotropic medication in selected months before and after implementation of the Omnibus Budget Reconciliation Act of 1987 (*OBRA-87*). (Courtesy of Lantz MS, Giambanco V, Buchalter EN: A ten-year review of the effect of OBRA-87 on psychotropic prescribing practices in an academic nursing home. *Psychiatric Serv* 47:951–955, 1996. Copyright 1996, the American Psychiatric Association. Reprinted by permission.)

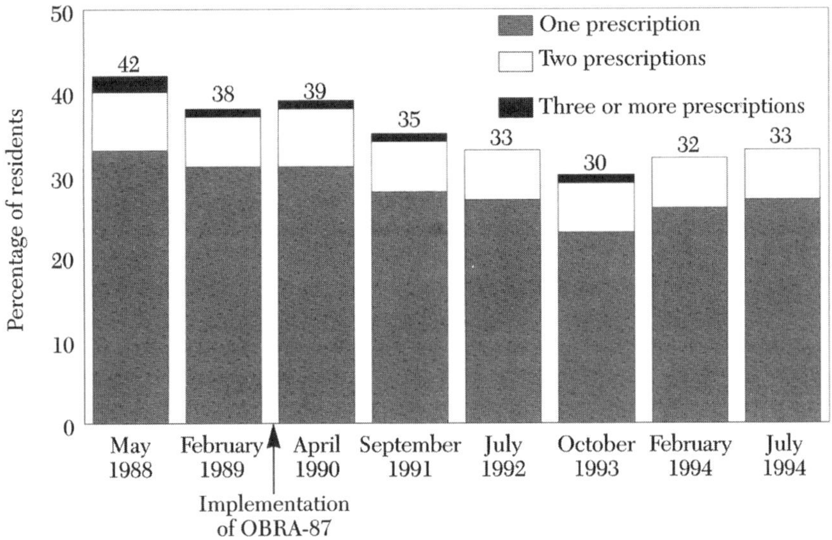

FIGURE 2.—Percentages of nursing home residents with 1, 2, or 3 or more concurrent prescriptions for psychotropic medication in selected months before and after implementation of the Omnibus Budget Reconciliation Act of 1987 (*OBRA-87*). The overall percentage of nursing home residents who received any psychotropic medication is shown above each *bar*. (Courtesy of Lantz MS, Giambanco V, Buchalter EN: A ten-year review of the effect of OBRA-87 on psychotropic prescribing practices in an Academic Nursing Home. *Psychiatric Serv* 47:951–955, 1996. Copyright 1996, the American Psychiatric Association. Reprinted by permission.)

terns of antipsychotic, anxiolytic and sedative-hypnotic, and antidepressant medications.

Results.—Before implementation of OBRA-1987, the percentage of facility residents who received antidepressants, anxiolytics and sedative-hypnotics, and antipsychotic medications was stable (Fig 1). After implementation of OBRA-1987, prescription of antidepressants increased significantly, whereas prescription of anxiolytic and sedative-hypnotics and antipsychotics was reduced (Fig 2). The total number of residents who received psychotropic medication decreased. There was a trend toward more prescription of the type of agents recommended for geriatric use, such as short-acting benzodiazepines and tertiary tricyclic antidepressants.

Conclusions.—Implementation of OBRA-1987 at a nonprofit residential geriatric facility appears to have served as an impetus for clinical review and a change in practice style to more closely reflect current understanding of optimal geriatric care.

▶ As a physician, I have always been embarrassed that it took federal regulation to improve the prescribing pattern of psychotropic drugs for patients in nursing homes, especially because the data about the benefit of OBRA-87 implemented October 1, 1990, have been overwhelmingly positive. This article presents the dramatic response, over a 10-year period, to the implementation of OBRA-87. The use of antipsychotic and anxiolytic drugs went down markedly, and the number of prescriptions per patient on average decreased significantly. Note, however, the significant increase in the prescription of antidepressants. This may be a positive outcome. Data do exist suggesting that depression is very common among nursing home patients, approaching 26%.[1] It may be that physicians are now recognizing depression among nursing home patients more commonly. It would be informative to know whether the changes in prescribing patterns in this study had a positive effect on patient outcomes and function, but such outcomes were not studied.

I believe that every nursing home and every physician prescribing in a nursing home should have easy access to the prescribing profile of the nursing home as well as his own prescribing profile. Only by reviewing prescribing patterns can a critical assessment of pharmacotherapy be possible. I believe such regular surveillance will significantly improve care.

One final point: I believe it is wise for the physician, at the monthly visit to a nursing home patient, to always review the patient's medications with an eye toward discontinuing what may no longer be needed and reducing dose wherever possible. Such decisions, in my view, require a careful review with the nursing staff if truly effective multidisciplinary care is to be practiced.

J.R. Burton, M.D.

Reference

1. Rovner BW, Kafonek S, Filipp L, et al: Prevalence of mental illness in a community nursing home. *Am J Psychiatry* 143:1446–1449, 1986.

Can Medicaid Long-term Care Expenditures for the Elderly Be Reduced?

Wiener JM (Urban Inst, Washington, DC)

Gerontologist 36:800–811, 1996 2–18

Introduction.—Several methods are proposed for reducing Medicaid expenditures, including the block grant approach of MediGrant (legislation passed by Congress in 1995 and vetoed by President Clinton), a per-beneficiary limit on the growth of expenditures (proposed by the Clinton administration), and a blend of these 2 proposals developed by the National Governors' Association. Each would dramatically reduce the rate of growth in Medicaid spending and affect long-term care for the elderly. However, it is not clear that large savings can be achieved by giving states greater flexibility while reducing federal Medicaid spending.

Strategies to Control Spending.—Three broad strategies might be used by states to control the growth of expenditures for the elderly who, together with the disabled, account for two thirds of Medicaid spending. More private resources might be brought into the long-term care system to offset Medicaid's expenditures; the delivery system could be reformed to provide care at lower cost; and reductions might be made in Medicaid eligibility, reimbursement, and service coverage.

Effects of Spending Control on Long-term Care.—Available research provides little evidence to suggest that large savings can be achieved without adversely affecting beneficiaries' eligibility, access to services, and quality of care. Few elderly can afford to purchase private long-term care insurance, and those who might afford it are unlikely to anticipate the need for this coverage. Transferring of assets by middle- and upper-class elderly is not as common as is often assumed, so legislation to prevent this practice would yield little in savings. Estate-recovery programs, which take from the estates of deceased Medicaid beneficiaries, have recouped only a small portion of nursing home expenditures. Similarly, research does not suggest that a solution to the problem of Medicaid spending will be found in other recommendations: integrating acute and long-term care services through managed care, expanding home- and community-based services, requiring family contributions, cutting reimbursement rates, reducing nursing home quality standards and enforcement, stopping construction of new nursing home beds, and reducing coverage for home- and community-based services.

Conclusions.—Because states already have substantial flexibility for coverage, reimbursement, and eligibility, they could lower long-term care spending. Yet large savings will not be obtained easily and painlessly, and substantial reductions are likely to adversely affect Medicaid beneficiaries. Medicaid pays only the costs that the elderly themselves cannot, and the system's payment rates are now much lower than those of Medicare and the private sector. From this perspective, the current method of Medicaid financing is a rather economical one.

▶ Dramatic changes in Medicaid are planned now and in the near future. These changes in essence amount to increasing state autonomy, with less federal support for the Medicaid program. Dr. Wiener, the author of this article, is considered by most as the leading authority on Medicaid financing in this country. This article presents a summary of his thinking and is, in particular, focused on the specific question of whether the Medicaid long-term care expenditure for the elderly can be reduced.

Dr. Wiener suggests that the existing data provide little evidence that savings will be found without several significant adverse outcomes. He believes that if savings are to be significant, then change in eligibility, access, or the quality of care delivered will result. In particular, long-term institutional health care is in for a tough time. I fear that those patients who are most vulnerable, the poor and the frail elderly, will suffer most with the proposed cost-saving changes.

J.R. Burton, M.D.

An Analysis of the Use of the Telephone in the Management of Patients in Skilled Nursing Facilities

Fowkes W, Christenson D, McKay D (Stanford Univ Med School, Calif; San Jose Hosp, Calif)

J Am Geriatr Soc 45:67–70, 1997 2–19

Introduction.—Most physician-directed medical care for patients in skilled nursing facilities (SNFs) is provided by telephone communication because of low reimbursement schedules for nursing home visits, time pressures, and practice priorities. Second to poor reimbursement, problems with communication are a great source of frustration for physicians caring for patients in SNFs. The impact of a voice mail system installed to manage the burden of communication between physician and SNFs was evaluated.

Methods.—Calls between physicians and SNFs with a standard answering service were evaluated for a period of 1 year. A voice mail system was then installed, and patients and staff in SNFs were encouraged to use voice mail rather than the answering service. Medical care providers, the staffs of 13 SNFs, and an average of 207 covered patients were monitored for 1 year. The total number of calls by patients and facilities, reasons for calls, outcome, and timing were evaluated. Comparisons were made between the standard answering service and voice mail.

Results.—Patients and staff of 13 SNFs made 10,264 calls regarding an average of 207 continuously covered patients receiving long-term care. This averaged about 50 calls per year per patient. Most calls were routine; only about 5% of calls were concerning acute illness (Table 2). A new treatment was started as a result of about one third of calls, but no new orders were issued in response to 23% of calls (Table 3). About 1 in 200 calls resulted in hospitalization. About 1 in 5 calls did not require a return call. Some facilities had significantly higher numbers of calls per patient per month, reflecting either a higher level of care provided or less frequent contact with providers on site (Table 1). A recent follow-up indicated that of 692 calls received in 1 month, 93% were received through voice mail.

TABLE 2.—Reason for Call

Reason	Percentage
Laboratory or X-ray report	18
New observation	17
Administrative	11
Medication or prescription request	9
New event	9
Status or parameter report	8
PT, OT, ST, podiatry, dental, equipment request	7
Acute illness	5

Note: Other categories each accounted for less than 3% of calls.
Abbreviations: PT, physical therapy; *OT*, occupational therapy; *ST*, speech therapy.
(Courtesy of Fowkes W, Christenson D, McKay D: An analysis of the use of the telephone in the management of patients in skilled nursing facilities. *J Am Geriatr Soc* 45[1]:67–70, 1996.)

TABLE 3.—Outcomes of Calls

Outcome	Percentage
Treatment or Prescription	32%
Nothing done	23%
Order a study, lab or x-ray	5%
PT, OT, ST, podiatry, dentistry	5%
Accept new patient	4%
Order observation or parameter	3%
Family contact	2%

Notes: The decision to see the patient was made in 2% of instances. Patients were transferred to the hospital in 0.5% of calls.

(Courtesy of Fowkes W, Christenson D, McKay D: An analysis of the use of the telephone in the management of patients in skilled nursing facilities. *J Am Geriatr Soc* 45[1]:67–70, 1996.)

Conclusion.—Communication between SNFs and physicians is driven by patient need and the Omnibus Reconciliation Act of 1987, which requires that any significant condition change be reported to the resident's physician. The voice mail system described can help relieve some of the significant communication burden of managing patients in SNFs.

▶ The value and characteristics of phone communications to physicians from skilled nursing facilities is reported in this study.

Over a period of 1 year, a group practice analyzed the phone calls related to an average nursing home practice population of 207 patients in 15 differernt nursing homes. After a year-long survey, a voice mail system was installed and the impact of this on the efficiency of the care of nursing home patients was increased.

On average, there were 50 calls per patient per year. These data are summarized in the table. Only 0.05% of calls were felt to be urgent, for 2% of calls the physician decided to visit the patient, and for 0.5% of calls the

TABLE 1.—Facilities and Calls

Facility	Average Census (%)*	Number of Calls (%)†	Calls/Patient‡
1.	53 (25)	2682 (26)	50.6
2.	38 (18)	1591 (16)	41.9
3.	37 (18)	1169 (11)	31.6
4.	30 (15)	1954 (18)	65.1
5.	11 (5)	759 (7)	69.0
6.	11 (5)	762 (7)	69.3
Total	108 (100%)	8917 (100%)	Average 49.5

Note: Facilities with 10 or more covered patients.

*Average number of patients covered at the facility with the percent of the total to the nearest percentage point.

†Total number of telephone calls received from the facility during a 12-month period, with the percentage of the total to the nearest percentage point.

‡Calls for each facility divided by its average census. The difference in rates between six facilities is significant at p 0.001 by chi-square.

(Courtesy of Fowkes W, Christenson D, McKay D: An analysis of the use of the telephone in the management of patients in skilled nursing facilities. *J Am Geriatr Soc* 45[1]:67–70, 1996.)

physician decided to transfer the patient to the hospital or the emergency department.

After the introduction of a voice mail system, 93% of calls were handled by the system, and of those, about 20% did not require a return call.

This kind of study I find very valuable for planning programs and managing a clinical practice.

J.R. Burton, M.D.

Frailty and Hospitalization of Long-term Stay Nursing Home Residents

Fried TR, Mor V (Yale Univ, New Haven, Conn; Brown Univ, Providence, RI)

J Am Geriatr Soc 45:265–269, 1997 2–20

Introduction.—Most agree that the rate of hospitalization of nursing home residents should be reduced because nursing home residents are at substantial risk of iatrogenic complications, hospitalization is expensive, and transfers can be emotionally traumatic for families and residents. For the most frail of nursing home residents, for those with severe functional status and cognitive impairments, the benefit-burden ratio of hospitalization is likely to be the lowest. The relationship between frailty and risk of hospitalization was examined in long-term–stay nursing home residents.

Methods.—One hundred three nursing homes had 3,782 residents who had had no transitions out of the nursing home during the first 6 months of their stays. Residents were 65 or older. The analysis was focused on determining whether residents were hospitalized and for what reason. Residents were also assessed for functional status and its association with hospitalization.

Results.—During the second 6 months of their hospital stays, 931 residents (25%) were hospitalized at least once. Hospitalization was associated with severe functional impairment, worsening performance of activities of daily life, presence of a decubitus ulcer, presence of a feeding tube, primary diagnosis of congestive heart failure, and primary diagnosis of respiratory disease. A lower rate of hospitalization was not associated with advance directives.

Conclusions.—The residents most likely to be hospitalized are the physically frail patients. No association was found between lower rates of hospitalization and "do-not-hospitalize" orders, suggesting that barriers exist to providing acute care in nursing homes. Certain patients may be targeted successfully for reduction in hospitalization rates, such as those with recent functional decline and primary diagnosis of congestive heart failure and respiratory disease.

▶ Understanding the reasons for the widely prevalent practice of transferring patients from the nursing home to an acute hospital is important. I believe there is an excess number of such transfers. Certainly the transfer rate varies among institutions.[1] Acute care hospitals can be very stressful environments for frail older persons, especially those admitted from nursing homes. Responding to an acute problem in a nursing home patient in the nursing home itself whenever possible, in my view, is so much better for the patient than transfer to the acute care hospital.

This study was designed to quantify the transfer of nursing home patients to acute care hospitals. Nursing home patients who had not been transferred were analyzed during their second 6 months in a long-term care facility. Twenty-five percent of this large cohort were transferred in the second 6 months. In fact, even "do-not-hospitalize" advance directives did not modify this high rate of transfer.

I believe there is great room for improvement here. One important requirement of improving the care of nursing home patients who become acutely ill is to have physicians based full-time in the nursing home. This can easily be done if nursing homes expand their focus beyond long-term institutional care and become comprehensive geriatric centers by adding services such as outpatient facilities and day care.[2]

J.R. Burton, M.D.

References

1. Teresi JR, Holmes D, Bloom HG, et al: Factors differentiating hospital transfers from long-term care facilities with high and low transfer rates. *Gerontologist* 31:795–806, 1991.
2. Burton JR: The evolution of nursing homes into comprehensive geriatrics center: A perspective. *J Am Geriat Soc* 42:794–796, 1994.

General Surgical Care in the Nursing Home Patient: Results of a Dedicated Geriatric Surgery Consult Service

Zenilman ME, Bender JS, Magnuson TH, et al (Johns Hopkins Bayview Med Ctr, Baltimore, Md)

J Am Coll Surg 183:361–370, 1996 2–21

Background.—As the population ages, an increasing proportion of elderly people will require nursing home admission. The number of nursing home surgical patients will increase as well. There have been no scientific

TABLE 4.—Consult Diagnoses for the Geriatric Surgery Consult Service

Diagnosis	*Percent*
Maintenance	32.5
Abdominal or rectal disease	27.7
Peripheral vascular disease	16
Breast disease	10.6
Hernia	4.6
Hemodialysis access	1.2
Total	92.6*

Note: Maintenance-decubitus care, care related to long-term IV lines, and care related to enterostomy and enteral tubes.

*The other 7.4% of patients had lymphadenopathy, trauma (fall), hyperparathyroidism, or a gynecologic diagnosis.

(Courtesy of Zenilman ME, Bender JS, Magnuson TH, et al: General surgical care in the nursing home patient: Results of a dedicated geriatric surgery consult service. *J Am Coll Surg* 183:361–370, 1996. By permission of the *Journal of the American College of Surgeons*.)

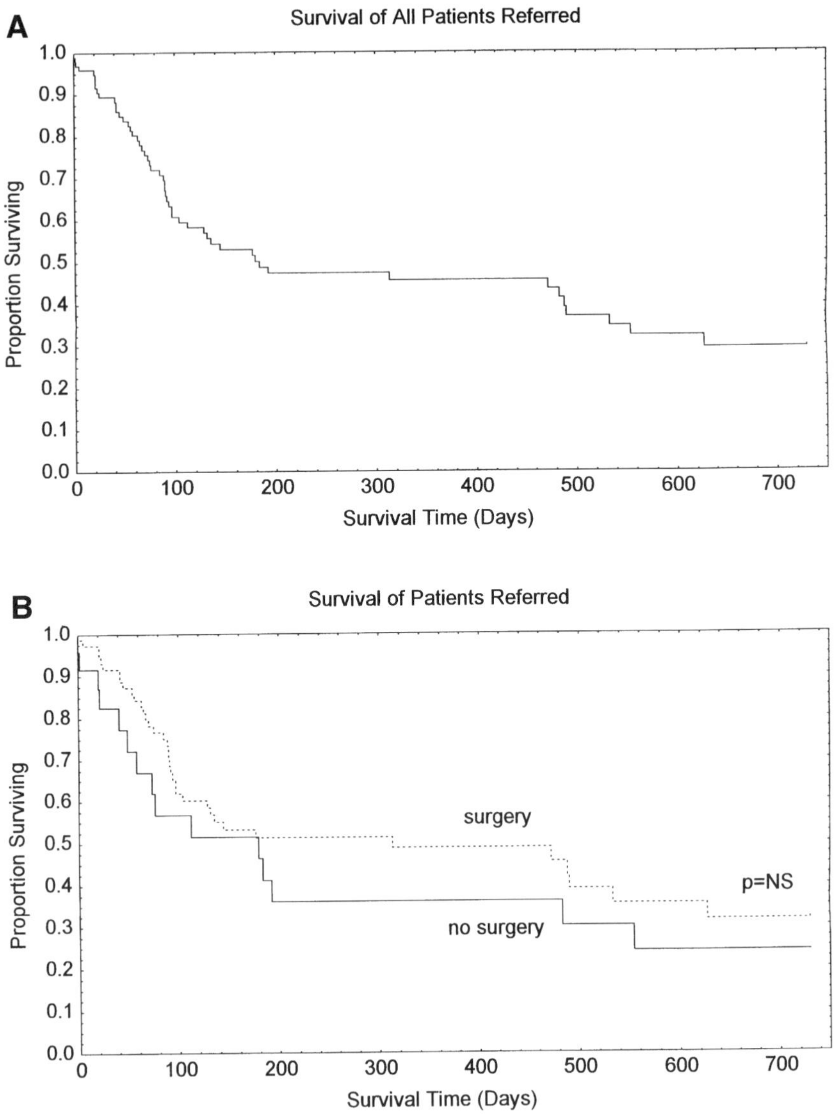

FIGURE 2.—A, overall survival of patients referred to the geriatric surgery consult service. B, comparison of survival between those who did and did not need surgical intervention. There was no statistical difference. *Abbreviation: NS*, not significant. (Courtesy of Zenilman ME, Bender JS, Magnuson TH, et al: General surgical care in the nursing home patient: Results of a dedicated geriatric surgery consult service. *J Am Coll Surg* 183:361–370, 1996. By permission of the *Journal of the American College of Surgeons*.)

studies of surgery in nursing home patients. A follow-up study of patients seen on a geriatric surgery consult service (GSCS) was reported.

Patients.—The GSCS saw all patients at a long-term care facility who required surgical consultation. One hundred fifty-three such patients were seen over a 20-month period. The major reason for admission to the long-term care facility was CNS dysfunction resulting from dementia or stroke. One hundred seventeen of the patients actually underwent 1 or more surgical procedures. Of the 168 procedures performed, 79 were done at the bedside and 89 were done in the operating room. About one third of the referrals were for maintenance care, such as treatment related to decubitus ulcers, stoma, and enteral tubes (Table 4). However, 55% were for common abdominal, breast, and vascular surgical problems.

Outcomes.—In the 30 days after surgery, the mortality rate was 8.5%. The complication rate was 9% overall and 18% for patients undergoing major abdominal or vascular surgery. The actuarial survival was 46% at 1 year and 35% at 18 months (Fig 2). Factors associated with reduced survival were a history of coronary artery disease, a diagnosis of dementia, and age older than 70 years. However, survival was unaffected by the need for a surgical procedure, major vs. minor surgery, sex, comorbidity, or resuscitative status.

Conclusion.—Experience on the authors' GSCS shows poor survival for long-term care patients referred for surgical evaluations. However, undergoing surgery per se does not reduce overall survival. Although surgical care in the elderly nursing home population is generally not curative, neither is it futile. Decisions regarding surgery should take into consideration quality of life, patient dignity, and relief of suffering.

▶ This study, from my own institution, is the first to document the activities of a GSCS. The service was designed to provide geriatrically focused care for nursing home residents. The results, based on a 29-month experience, show that appropriate surgery does not increase the mortality rate among nursing home residents, as shown in the figure. The common problems encountered by the surgeons are catagorized in the table. I am sure that other institutions have developed similar GSCSs, and I think these are extremely valuable. Such a service is able to develop continuity among surgeons and generalists and can build expertise among the surgeons in evaluating and treating frail elderly nursing home patients. Although not discussed in this paper, 1 of the greatest advantages of this service, in my opinion, is that the surgeons see the patients in the nursing home. This practice has, I believe, markedly improved the quality of the consultation and the management recommendations.

J.R. Burton, M.D.

Percutaneous Feeding Tube Changes in Long-term–Care Facility Patients

Graham S, Sim G, Laughren R, et al (Univ of Manitoba, Canada)
Infect Control Hosp Epidemiol 17:732–736, 1996 2–22

Introduction.—Percutaneous tubes placed directly into the stomach or jejunum are frequently used to provide nutritional support to patients in long-term–care facilities. Changing the feeding tube may be uncomfortable for the patient, but prolonged use of a tube increases the occurrence of complications. A prospective, randomized study compared patient outcomes when tubes were changed routinely each month or only when clinically necessary (PRN).

Methods.—The nonblinded, crossover study was conducted at a 416-bed long-term–care facility. Twenty-six patients were enrolled in the study and initially assigned to either routine monthly tubing changes or to PRN changes. After 6 months, they were crossed over to the alternate frequency of tubing changes for an additional 6 months. During the study period, patients were monitored for clinical status, antimicrobial therapy, and feeding tube changes. Temperatures were taken every 12 hours during the 48 hours after tube re-insertion.

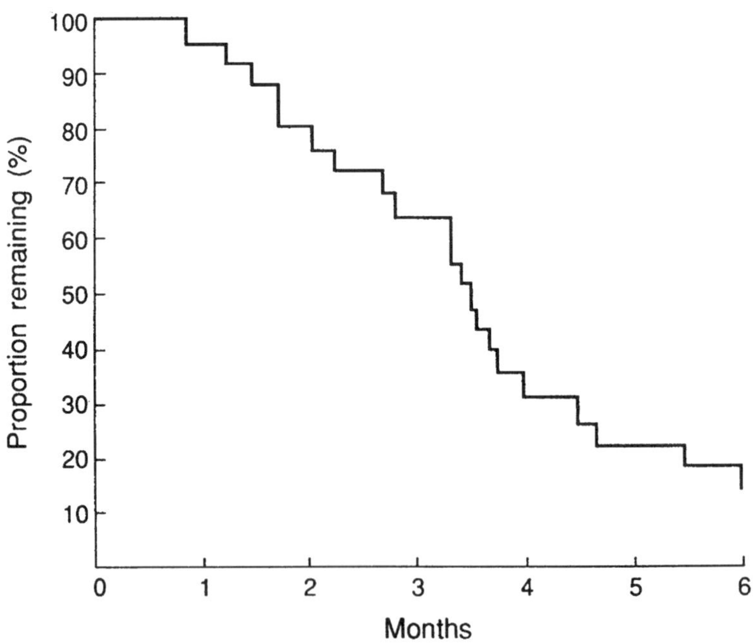

FIGURE.—Survival curve of feeding tubes inserted during as-necessary (*prn*) tube change interval. The *curve* displays the proportion of feeding tubes that had been inserted at onset of the prn observation period and that remained in situ without having been changed at a given time from insertion. (Courtesy of Graham S, Sim G, Laughren R, et al: Percutaneous feeding tube changes in long-term–care facility patients. *Infect Control Hosp Epidemiol* 17:732–736, 1996.)

Results.—Fifteen of the 26 patients had severe brain injury but few associated illnesses; 11 patients had a variety of illnesses and multiple co-morbidities. Twelve of 24 assessable patients were randomly assigned initially to PRN changes. The monthly change periods differed from the PRN change periods only in frequency of tube changes. Tube changes were 2.9 times more frequent with monthly changes than with PRN changes. The frequency of stomal site infections, antibiotic courses, fever episodes, and episodes of emesis was similar for the 2 tube-change protocols. In both protocols, the feeding tubes were significantly more likely to fall out and require replacement within 24 hours of previous tube replacement. The half-life of feeding tubes in the prn period (Figure) was approximately 104 days.

Conclusion.—In these patients who were receiving long-term nutritional support via percutaneous feeding tubes, changing the tube monthly on a routine basis offered no advantages over changing the tube only when required because of malfunction or displacement.

▶ Should a percutaneous feeding tube be changed routinely? This study of 26 individuals was prospective, randomized, and crossed over. Although the study was small, the design of the study leads the authors with confidence to answer the question "No." The average tube lasts about 100 days.

J.R. Burton, M.D.

Falls

The Modified Gait Abnormality Rating Scale for Recognizing the Risk of Recurrent Falls in Community-dwelling Elderly Adults

VanSwearingen JM, Paschal KA, Bonino P, et al (Univ of Pittsburgh, Pa; Creighton Univ, Omaha, Neb)

Phys Ther 76:994–1002, 1996 2–23

Background.—For older adults living in the community, mobility is important for independence, and loss of independence often accompanies a fall. This implies that identifying the older individual at risk for falling is an important objective of geriatric assessment. Gait changes have been related to a history of falls among frail older adults. A videotaped system for rating qualitative abnormalities of gait that may identify those at increased risk for falling has been developed, the Gait Abnormality Rating Scale (GARS-M). The reliability and validity of the GARS-M was studied in distinguishing between community-dwelling, frail older individuals with a history of falls and those without a history of falls.

Methods.—The study participants were 52 veterans referred to the Geriatric Evaluation and Management program for evaluation from December 1991 to December 1993. Their average age was 75. Each participant or caregiver reported the number of falls over the past year. There were no significant differences in age, height, or weight between those with a history of falls and those without such a history. A standard camcorder was used to record the participant walking at a self-selected pace on the tile surface of the out patient clinic hallway. Participants walked past the camcorder, turned around and walked back, for a total of 152 m. Videotapes were replayed with slow-motion and stop-action capability. Three physical therapists determined the GARS-M score.

Results.—The scores obtained by the 3 raters indicated moderate to substantial interrater reliability. Concurrent validity was shown for the relation between GARS-M scores and stride length, as well as GARS-M scores and walking speed. The average GARS-M score distinguished between frail older individuals with a history of falls and those without a history of falls.

Conclusions.—The GARS-M score is a valid and reliable measure that may be useful in predicting the risk of falling in frail, community-dwelling older adults. The GARS-M score may be useful in determining when intervention is necessary to reduce the risk of falling in an older, frail individual.

▶ The analysis of gait in frail elderly individuals in an office setting is increasingly important as a measure of the risk of falling. The old practice of watching a patient walk into the office and perhaps back and forth 15–20 ft in the hall is not terribly reliable. These authors have shown interobserver reliability and validity of gait analysis using a camcorder and then reviewing that video at slow motion. Such gait analyses should increasingly become a part of the assessment of older individuals. The technique appears to be useful, reliable, and relatively easy to accomplish. The recording of gait and the development of a normal rating scale has been established for a number of years.[1] That article should be reviewed by those interested in establishing such a program in their own assessment clinic.

J.R. Burton, M.D.

Reference

1. Wolfson L, Wipple R, Amerman P, et al: Gait assessment in the elderly: The Gait Abnormality Rating Scale and its relationship to falls. *J Gerontol* 45:M12–M19, 1990.

Falls Presenting to the Accident and Emergency Department: Types of Presentation and Risk Factor Profile

Davies AJ, Kenny RA (Royal Victoria Infirmary, Newcastle Upon Tyne, England)

Age Ageing 25:362–366, 1996 2–24

Objective.—The incidence of falls in the elderly is estimated to be 28% to 35% for those over 65 and more than 40% for those over age 75. The mental and physical consequences of falls can be devastating. Results of a study characterizing falls and risk factors in elderly U.K. patients who came to 1 inner-city emergency department are presented.

Methods.—Between August and September 1994, 188 elderly fallers (141 women), 44% over age 65, in the Royal Victoria Infirmary emergency department were screened for cognitive impairment. Those who were not deemed impaired and able to describe their falls were included in the study. In addition to a complete physical examination and history, visual impairment, gait and balance abnormalities, depression, medication problems, orthostatic hypotension, carotid sinus hypersensitivity, vasovagal hypersensitivity, arrhythmia, and positional vertigo were assessed.

Results.—Most fallers (92%) came to the emergency department between midnight and 8 PM. Of the 30% who were hospitalized, 48% had no significant soft-tissue or bony injuries, but 29 had long bone fractures, 17 had other fractures, and 18 required stitches. Of 26 patients (21 women) participating in additional studies, 18 had unexplained or recurrent falls and 9 had unexplained loss of consciousness. Risk factors were identified in 23. Although all were cognitively and physically normal, they had an average of 3 risk factors including vision problems (23%), gait abnormalities (19%), depression (31%), 4 or more medications (27%), culprit medications (39%), and benign postural vertigo (8%). Twenty patients had abnormal cardiovascular findings, and 7 patients had loss of consciousness (LOC) and amnesia for LOC.

Conclusion.—Although falls are relatively common in the elderly, they are explained in only one third of cases. Modifiable risk factors identified in this study include cardiovascular indications, depression, and culprit medications.

► I like this paper because it represents an "in the trenches" experience and evaluation of patients who have fallen. It provides an emergency department focus which is a typical place where many patients are initially seen after a serious fall. A group of 200 patients with falls was accumulated over just less than a month. An emergency department assessment resulted in approximately one third of patients with either unexplained falls or recurrent falls. Subsequently, a group of 26 of these individuals was fully investigated. Almost all of these patients had risk factors for falls that included medications, gait abnormalities, or carotid sinus hypersensitivity. The study points out the value of a targeted, multidimensional, relatively easily performed assessment for patients with unexplained or recurrent falls. The data in this paper could be used by individuals interested in targeting patients for appropriate evaluation who have had falls and who present to emergency departments. Over one third of the patients who presented with falls were admitted to the hospital. It is possible that with the appropriate initial evaluation as outlined in this paper some of these admissions might have been prevented. The basic evaluation of patients who have fallen with no obvious immediate explanation and who were not cognitively impaired was relatively simple. It included a focused history and physical examination, simple laboratory tests, a basic neurologic screen, standard visual and auditory measurements, and a measurement of gait and balance. Orthostatic blood pressure, a carotid sinus massage, and head-up tilt test were performed in all patients. Selectively, other more invasive studies such as EEG,

CT, or Holter monitoring were performed. The assessment is relatively simple if targeted.

J.R. Burton, M.D.

Outcomes and Costs After Hip Fracture and Stroke: A Comparison of Rehabilitation Settings

Kramer AM, Steiner JF, Schlenker RE, et al (Univ of Colorado, Denver)
JAMA 277:396–404, 1997 2–25

Introduction.—For older persons, functional losses after acute events have devastating consequences. The ability to walk is lost by up to 60% of those with hip fractures, and up to 75% lose their ability to perform activities of daily living. Moderate functional impairment affects up to 40% of stroke survivors. There has been a rapid growth in the number of rehabilitation facilities. The most common disabling conditions in older patients are still not known. The effectiveness and cost of rehabilitation for patients with hip fracture and with stroke was studied in rehabilitation facilities, subacute skilled-nursing facilities, and traditional skilled-nursing facilities.

Methods.—The study comprised 485 stroke survivors and 518 patients with hip fracture in 17 states. At 6 months the patients were evaluated to compare community residence, Medicare costs, recovery to premorbid levels in 5 activities of daily living, and the numbers of physician and therapy visits. Adjustments in outcome were made for mobility impairments, sensory deficits, depression, cognition, admission function, comorbid illness, caregiver availability, and premorbid residence and function.

Results.—Rehabilitation hospital patients were more likely to have caregivers and better cognitive and physical function on admission. No difference was detected between hip fracture patients admitted to rehabilitation hospitals and those admitted to nursing homes in the number of activities of daily living recovered to premorbid level or in returning to the community. Stroke patients, however, were more likely to recover activities of daily living and to return to the community if they were admitted to rehabilitation hospitals rather than nursing homes. Traditional nursing home patients with stroke were less likely to return to the community than were subacute nursing home patients. For patients with hip fracture, there was no difference in return to the community among traditional or subacute nursing home patients. Medicare costs were greater for rehabilitation hospital patients than those for subacute nursing home patients. Costs for traditional nursing home patients were less than those for subacute nursing home patients.

Conclusions.—Outcomes were enhanced for stroke patients treated in rehabilitation hospitals but not for hip-fracture patients. Despite comparable functional outcomes, subacute nursing homes were more effective than traditional nursing homes in returning patients with stroke to the community.

▶ What are the outcomes and cost differences among older patients admitted to a variety of rehabilitation settings? There are important data in this study. This article, to my knowledge, is the first substantive report using a large national dataset. It uses a case-mix adjustment scheme to account for the different levels of dysfunction and comorbidity of patients admitted to rehabilitation facilities. The results show that stroke patients have better outcomes but higher costs after admission to a rehabilitation facility compared with a subacute or traditional skilled nursing facility. Also, outcomes were better, with higher costs, in subacute than in traditional skilled-nursing facilities. However, there was no difference among treatment sites in functional outcomes in patients with hip fracture.

Certainly such data are critical for health policy decisions, especially in light of the enormous increase in recent years in subacute and rehabilitation beds in the United States.

J.R. Burton, M.D.

▶ This outcomes study involved a stratified, random sample of rehabilitation facilities and 2 kinds of skilled nursing facilities, standard and so-called "subacute" units. A random sample of patients with hip fracture and stroke were studied. This kind of study is important because of the variety of facilities to which physicians try to direct their patients within the limitations of their community and health insurance plans. Increasing numbers of subacute units are under development within nursing home facilities and in the hospital systems. As we work toward more integrated care for the elderly, watching the evolution of these subacute units at the interface between acute care and chronic care will be critical.

What is interesting in this study is the somewhat better outcome obtained for stroke patients in the rehabilitation facilities. These are more expensive in general and will likely be limited by changes in Medicare reimbursement, whereas subacute units may grow. The lessons learned from this study can assist those developing rehabilitation programs. The authors conclude that comprehensive rehabilitation, including recreational therapy, psychological services, physical occupational, and speech therapy provided better outcomes. Thus, attention to the psychosocial factors is critical to successful community reintegration.

P.J. Whitehouse, M.D., Ph.D.

Physical Restraints

Facility and Area Variation Affecting the Use of Physical Restraints in Nursing Homes

Phillips CD, Hawes C, Mor V, et al (Research Triangle Inst, Research Triangle Park, NC; Brown Univ, Providence, RI; Univ of Michigan, Ann Arbor; et al)
Med Care 34:1149–1162, 1996 2–26

Introduction.—The use of physical restraints in nursing homes has a long history and a serious potential for abuse. Although efforts have been

TABLE 4.—Area Differences in Restraint Use

Areas	% Restrained	*P*
Oakland, CA	50.1	<0.01
Hartford, CT	41.3	>0.05*
Des Moines, IA	41.1	>0.05*
Baltimore, MD	34.4	>0.05*
Minneapolis, MN	31.5	>0.05*
Cleveland, OH	40.6	>0.05*
Portland, OR	51.5	<0.01
Nashville, TN	34.7	>0.05*
Dallas, TX	21.8	<0.01
Newport News, VA	46.4	<0.01

*Not significant.

(Courtesy of Phillips CD, Hawes C, Mor V, et al: Facility and area variation affecting the use of physical restraints in nursing homes. *Med Care* 34:1149–1162, 1996.)

made to reduce the use of mechanical restraints, the prevalence remains high in some areas. To determine the influence of individual, facility, and area indicators on the likelihood of restraint use, data collected from more than 250 nursing homes in 10 different areas were analyzed.

Methods.—The elderly nursing home residents included in this study lived in Medicare- or Medicaid-certified facilities in 42 counties in 10 states. States selected varied considerably in Medicaid payment levels and reimbursement schemes, nurse staffing, and geographic regions. A stratified, random sample of residents was selected within each facility; 8 residents were usually included, 6 who had been in the facility for more than 90 days and 2 who had 30–90 days of residency. Resident data were collected in 1990 by research nurses using the Minimum Data Set for Nursing Home Resident Assessment and Care Screening. Facility data were gathered by telephone interviews with staff.

Results.—The study sample of 2,127 nursing home residents was predominantly female (78%); 46% were older than 84 and 45% had dementia. Approximately two thirds required assistance in 4–5 activities of daily living. After controlling for the residents' physical and cognitive function, both facility characteristics and location (Table 4) had a significant impact on restraint practices. Overall, more than one third of residents in the sample were restrained, and only 1 of the 10 geographic areas had a rate significantly lower than the other areas. Facilities with low nurse staffing were more likely to use restraints, and physical restraints tended to be used more often for residents difficult to control and for those in greatest need of assistance.

Conclusions.—Nursing homes vary considerably in their use of physical restraints for residents. As noted in previous studies, residents whose physical and cognitive function was considerably impaired were more likely to be restrained than those with less need of assistance. After controlling for these factors, however, the level of nurse staffing and geographic area had a significant impact on restraint policies.

► Although there has been a significant reduction in the use of mechanical restraints in nursing homes in the United States in recent years, there is still room for improvement. The reduction of restraints in this country, in part, was because of the implementation of the Omnibus Budget Reconciliation Act in 1990.

This study analyzed restraint use within nursing homes in different geographic areas of the United States. The overall rate of restraint use was approximately 33%. The sample size was 2,127 patients, a very large study group, which heightens the value of these data. The remarkable finding in this study is the variability of greater than twofold of restraint use in various regions of the country. Restraint use varied from a low of 21% to a high of 50%. It seems not so much that the patient population is different in the various homes but rather that the homes themselves have a different attitude, a different nursing staff-to-patient ratio, or both. For example, facilities that had a nursing staff-to-patient ratio that was higher than the median used half the number of restraints than those facilities with nursing staff-to-patient ratios below the median.

I think we can do better in the reduction of mechanical restraints in this country. It does, however, take a major faculty initiative and requires adequate nursing.

J.R. Burton, M.D.

Physical Restraints in Geriatric Care in Sweden: Prevalence and Patient Characteristics

Karlsson S, Bucht G, Eriksson S, et al (Umeå Univ, Sweden)
J Am Geriatr Soc 44:1348–1354, 1996 2–27

Objective.—Geriatric patients with dementia or delirium frequently are physically restrained for safety reasons. Some have argued that restraints are overused. Results of a study of the prevalence of physical restraints in various geriatric care settings and of characteristics of patients restrained are given.

Methods.—A 1-week point prevalence study involved 1,325 patients (64% female), average age 82, performed in northern Sweden in 8 nursing homes, 15 old people's homes, a somatic geriatric clinic, and a psychogeriatric clinic with a total of 1,403 beds. Patients were assessed with the Multi-Dimensional Dementia Assessment Scale (MDDAS).

Results.—There were 312 patients (24%) restrained (Fig 1). Dependent patients, older patients, cognitively impaired patients, patients with impaired speech, and patients with impaired walking ability were significantly more likely to be restrained. Most restrained patients (94%) were cognitively impaired. Restrained patients were significantly more likely to be given 1 or more psychoactive drugs. Restrained patients imposed significantly higher physical and psychologic workloads on staff than unrestrained patients. Patients who yelled and shouted continuously, were aggressive or threatening to other patients and staff, refused to get dressed

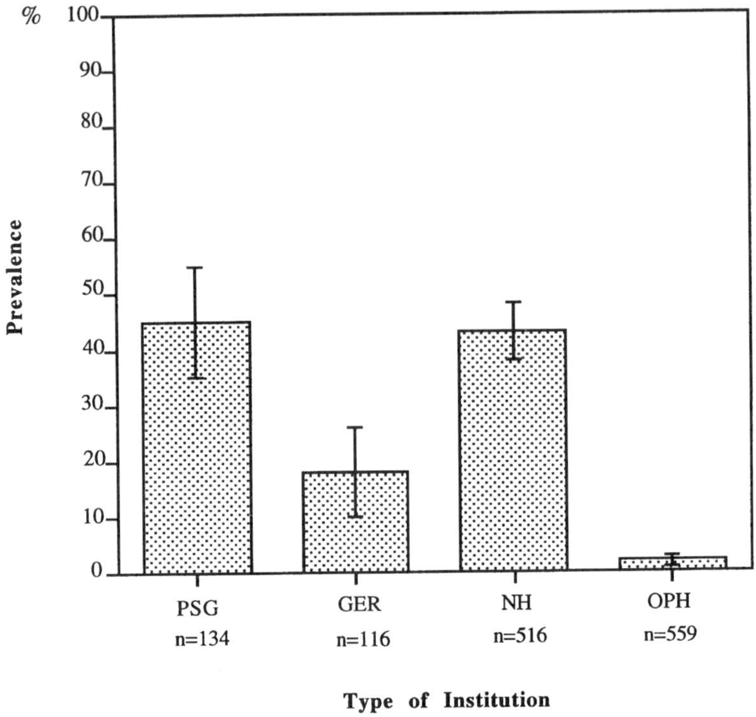

FIGURE 1.—Prevalence (% and 95% CI) of physical restraints in institutions investigated. *Abbreviations: PSG*, psychogeriatric clinic; *GER*, somatic geriatric clinic; *NH*, nursing home; *OPH*, old people's home. (Courtesy of Karlsson S, Bucht G, Eriksson S, et al: *J Am Geriatr* 44[11]:1348–1354, 1996.)

or undressed, were disturbed or restless, or exhibited anxiety were significantly more likely to be restrained.

Conclusion.—Swedish geriatric patients are frequently physically restrained, particularly if they are cognitively or physically impaired.

▶ For years it has been widely touted that Sweden was a model of care with respect to the elderly and particularly in the use of mechanical restraints. This large study, however, questions that belief. Overall the restraint use in Sweden was slightly less in various settings than in the United States (see Abstract 2–26), but there is still a profound problem in Sweden, and this is especially so in geropsychiatric institutes and in nursing homes. In this study, there was a 24% use of restraints among the 1,325 residents evaluated over a 1-week period. The use of restraints was remarkably high, 45% and 43%, in patients in geropsychogeriatric programs and in nursing homes, respectively. Sweden has a different system of health care, so comparisons are hard, but this study points out that the use of restraints is a multinational problem.

J.R. Burton, M.D.

Effects of a Restraint Reduction Intervention and OBRA '87 Regulations on Psychoactive Drug Use in Nursing Homes

Siegler EL, Capezuti E, Maislin G, et al (New York Univ; Univ of Pennsylvania, Philadelphia)

J Am Geriatr Soc 45:791–796, 1997 2–28

Background.—In nursing homes, behavioral problems historically have been treated with physical and "chemical" restraints, such as psychoactive medications. A previous study in 3 Philadelphia nursing homes showed that staff education and expert consultation can lead to a significant decline in the number of restraints used. These authors expanded those previous findings to determine whether a reduction in the use of physical restraints had an effect on the use of psychoactive medications.

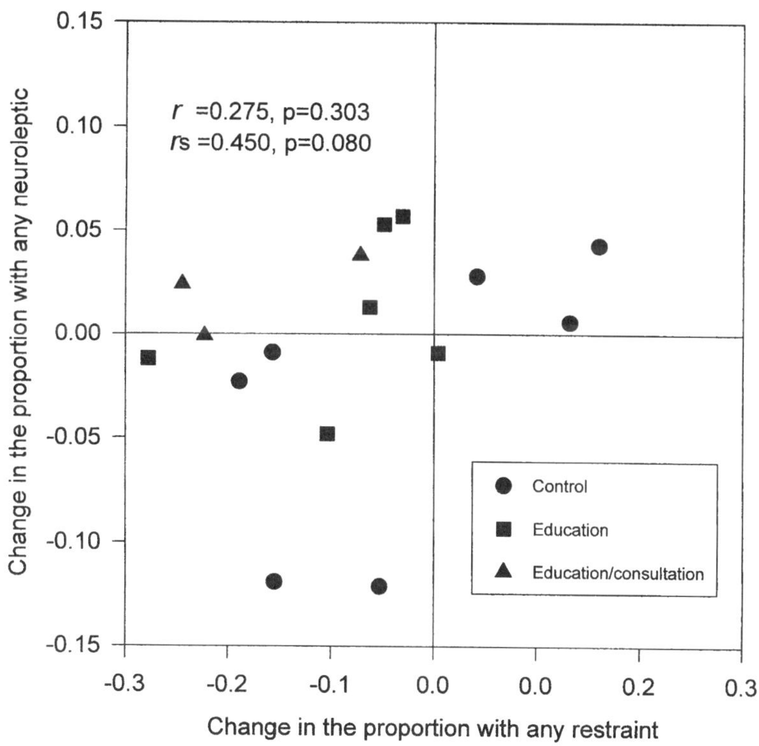

FIGURE 1.—This figure is based on the proportion of residents using neuroleptic drugs and restraints on each ward (n = 16) and is a plot of the change in the proportions between baseline and end. In the upper left quadrant are points representing those wards in which neuroleptic drug use increased and restraint use decreased. In the lower left quadrant are those wards in which neuroleptic drug and restraint use decreased. In the upper right quadrant are those wards in which neuroleptic drug and restraint use increased, and in the lower right quadrant is the ward in which neuroleptic drug use decreased and restraint use increased. (Courtesy of Siegler EL, Capezuti E, Maislin G, et al: Effects of a restraint reduction intervention and OBRA '87 regulations on psychoactive drug use in nursing homes. *J Am Geriatr Soc* 45[7]:791–796, 1997.)

Methods.—Three nursing homes were studied (446 residents in 16 wards): a control site, a site that received staff education about restraint use, and a site that received education coupled with expert consultation. Data on the use of neuroleptics, benzodiazepines, and antidepressants were evaluated to see whether drug use changed over time. Evaluations were based on measurements taken after the Omnibus Budget Reconciliation Act (OBRA) mandates of 1987 (T1), immediately after the educational intervention (T2), and 3 (T3) and 6 (T4) months after the intervention.

Findings.—Neuroleptic medications were used at T1 in 19%, 14%, and 18% of the control, education, and education plus consultation sites, respectively. After 6 months (T4), only the control site had a significant decrease in neuroleptic drug use (11%, 16%, and 19% for the 3 sites, respectively). Benzodiazepine use, however, declined significantly from T1 to T4 in all 3 sites (from 33% to 27% in the control site, from 37% to 27% in the education site, and from 22% to 18% in the education plus consultation site). Antidepressant use varied greatly and nonlinearly, but in general, it was low. In each ward, the use of neuroleptic drugs and physical restraints seemed to either decrease or increase together (Fig 1).

Conclusions.—Using fewer restraints did not cause an increase in the use of psychoactive drugs. In fact, in many wards the use of benzodiazepines and physical restraints decreased in tandem. Although the effects of the OBRA 1987 mandate were not uniform (especially with regard to antidepressant use), each of the 3 sites did show reductions in the use of physical and/or chemical restraints over time.

▶ This important study has had an additional impact on the reduction of mechanical restraints among nursing home patients. This is a secondary analysis focused on psychoactive drug use associated with a program of restraint reduction that resulted from the OBRA 1987 regulations. The original paper focused on the effectiveness of an educational program and a nursing consultation service in mechanical restraint reduction.[1]

This study shows that an effective program of restraint reduction is not associated with an increased use of psychotrophic drugs. I believe both of these articles are of critical importance to those who work in long-term care facilities and are further evidence that care among the elderly in nursing homes can be accomplished without the use of extensive mechanical restraints or neuroleptic medication. Also, I believe that mechanical restraints violate individual dignity and often lead to agitation and deteriorating mental and physical functioning. I am delighted that programs such as the one in this report have been so successful in reducing the use of mechanical restraints. Also, the fear that many have that reducing mechanical restraints would lead to increased use of psychoactive drugs is not borne out. It does not appear that patients were suffering more from delusions or hallucinations, which are target symptoms that might be improved by the use of neuroleptic drugs. All in all, this is good news and important for medical directors and directors of nursing in long-term care facilities. They should be familiar with and review it with the staff in their institutions.

J.R. Burton, M.D.

Reference

1. Evans LK, Stumpf NE, Allen-Taylor SL, et al: A clinical trial to reduce restraints in nursing homes. *J Am Geriatr Soc* 45:675–681, 1997.

Deaths Caused by Bedrails

Parker K, Miles SH (St Paul Ramsey Med Ctr, Minn; Univ of Minnesota, Minneapolis)

J Am Geriatr Soc 45:797–802, 1997 2–29

Objective.—Even though bedrails are heavily used in hospitals and nursing homes, and federal law requires a physician's order before bedrail restraints can be used in nursing homes, the risks and benefits of their use have not been studied. Deaths caused by bedrails have not been reviewed in the literature. Information is presented on adult deaths and injuries caused by bedrails. The information is taken from the Death Certificate File, Reported Incidents File, and National Injury Information Clearinghouse Accident Investigations File of the U.S. Consumer Product Safety Commission. The data in these files show how bedrails cause death and why manufacturers and regulators should devise standards and promote research to improve design of bed systems.

Methods.—Information on individuals older than 18 who were killed or injured between 1966 and 1996 on adult-size beds, mattresses, and bedrails while they were in bed were included.

Results.—There were 74 deaths—51 women, 21 men, and 2 of unreported sex. There were 51 (69%) deaths of individuals older than 70 and 26 (35%) deaths of individuals ages 81–90. Deaths were caused by asphyxiation between the bedrail and the side of the mattress in 52 cases (Fig 1),insertion of the head between widely spaced vertical bars in the bedrails in 13 cases, sliding on the back or abdomen through the slot between the head and foot rails, jamming the head and neck into a hyperflexed or hyperextended position on the floor, or sliding the legs first through the slot until the neck was caught against the rail. Bedrails are most often appropriate for sedated or somnolent patients or for patients receiving life-sustaining treatment. Key dimensions of beds, rails, and mattresses should be standardized and spaces between vertical bars should be narrowed to avoid entrapment of patients' heads. Design recommendations are included.

Conclusion.—Deaths caused by bedrails are more common than was previously suspected. These deaths are preventable. Standards for beds, rails, and mattresses need to be developed. Bedrails should not be used indiscriminately, and their use should be restricted only to those patients who require them.

▶ Bedrails are widely used in nursing homes and acute care hospitals. Generally, bedrails are considered safe, even though they are a mechanical restraint. I am unaware of any reports in the literature concerning their effectiveness or safety. I selected this article because it makes the point

A

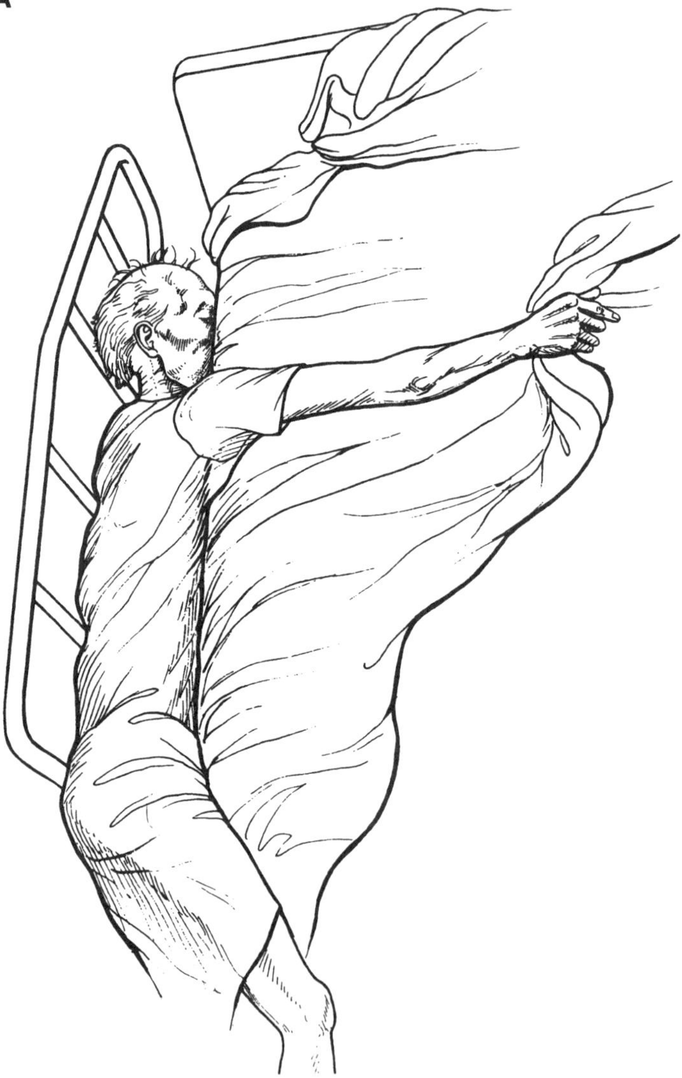

(Continued)

FIGURE 1 (cont.)

B

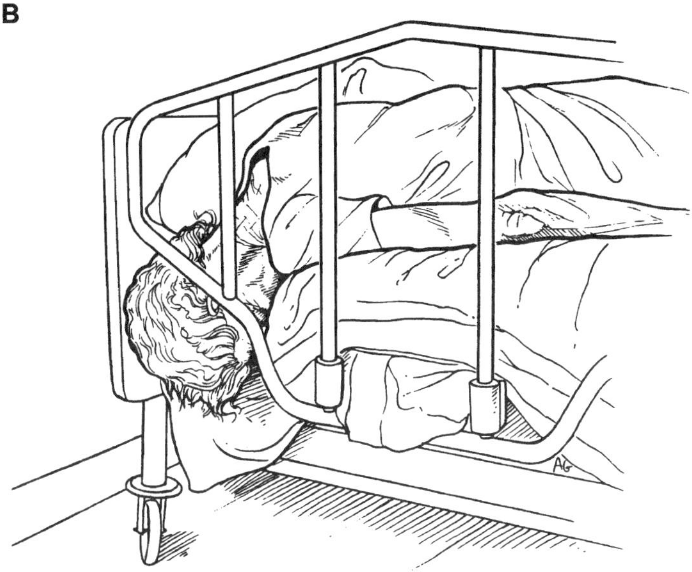

FIGURE 1.—Bed, rail, and mattress entrapment. (Courtesy of Parker K, Miles SH: Deaths caused by bedrails. *J Am Geriatr Soc* 45[7]:797–802, 1997. Copyright by Williams & Wikins 1997.)

that bedrails may cause death. The authors identified 54 deaths from their review of the U.S. Consumer Product Safety Commission files. Nearly all the deaths were of older individuals. Of these deaths, 77% occurred by entrapment of the patient between the bedrail and the mattress, as shown in Fig 1. A few patients were trapped between the rails, and others slipped out of the bed and became entrapped in the rail. The authors suggest improvements that might be applied to bedrail construction.

Over the years, I have selected many articles on the ill effects of mechanical restraints. We must develop alternative ways to reduce falls.

J.R. Burton, M.D.

Pressure Sores

Hospital-acquired Pressure Ulcers and Risk of Death

Thomas DR, Goode PS, Tarquine PH, et al (Univ of Alabama, Birmingham)
J Am Geriatr Soc 44:1435–1440, 1996 2–30

Introduction.—Pressure ulcers appear to be associated with increased mortality, but it is uncertain whether the ulcers cause death directly or tend to occur in frail patients with greater disease severity. A prospective study of 286 patients assessed the impact of in-hospital pressure ulcer development on mortality.

Methods.—The study setting was a tertiary, acute care, urban teaching hospital. Participants were drawn from patients 55 years or older who were admitted from December 1988 through June 1991. Those eligible had no pressure ulcers at entry and were expected to be alive, in the hospital, and confined to a bed or chair for at least 5 days. Baseline

TABLE 4.—Factors at Hospital Discharge Associated With Increased 1-Year Mortality

Variable	Risk Ratio	95% Confidence Limits	*P* Value
When total incident complications are known			
MD Assessment of Life Expectancy <5 Years	2.3	1.9, 2.8	<.001
Any weight loss	2.3	1.5, 3.3	<.001
Total Incident Complications Score	1.3	1.2, 1.5	<.001
When discharge bed-bound status is known			
MD Assessment of Life Expectancy <5 Years	2.2	1.8, 2.6	<.001
Any weight loss	2.2	1.5, 3.2	<.001
Confined to bed or chair at discharge	1.9	1.2, 3.1	.01
Total Incident Complications Score	1.3	1.2, 1.5	<.001

(Courtesy of Thomas DR, Goode PS, Tarquine PH, et al: Hospital-acquired pressure ulcers and risk of death. *J Am Geriatr Soc* 44[12]:1435–1440, 1996.)

demographic, medical, functional, and nutritional data were gathered for each patient. Also recorded were estimates of disease severity and life expectancy and the acute physiology score of APACHE II. Vital status was determined at 3, 6, 9, and 12 months after hospital discharge.

Results.—Patients included in the analyses had a mean age of 73.7; 60.8% were women and 58.4% were white. Their severe functional impairment was reflected in the mean Activity of Daily Living Score (0.3) and mean Norton Score (12.7). In-hospital stage 2 or greater pressure ulcers developed in 37 patients, for a cumulative incidence of 12.9%. Four patients had stage 3 and 33 had stage 2 ulcers. Forty (14.0%) of the patients died before discharge and 77 (26.9%) died during the year after discharge. Of those with pressure ulcers, 24.3% died in the hospital and 46.4% died after hospital discharge; corresponding death rates for those without pressure ulcers were 12.4% and 29.4%, respectively. After adjusting for other predictors of mortality at hospital admission, however, the development of pressure ulcers was not independently associated with decreased survival. Predictors of mortality at admission in multivariate analysis were weight loss in the 6 months before admission, physician estimate of life expectancy, and the Co-morbidity Damage Index. Also determined were factors at discharge associated with increased 1-year mortality (Table 4).

Conclusion.—In these older, severely ill patients, the development of pressure ulcers (predominantly stage 2) during acute hospitalization was not associated with reduced 1-year survival after adjustment for other relevant variables.

► Pressure sores are predictors of death within 1 year of their development. Just why this is so is uncertain. This study addresses this uncertainty with reference to hospitalized patients. In this study, 13% of 286 patients had pressure sores in the hospital. Of this group, however, only about 10% were stage 3 or 4. Ninety percent of these pressure sores were stage 2. Stage 1 ulcers were not considered.

The new information derived from this study is that pressure sores are not an independent predictor of death after adjusting for nutrition, functional status, other global measures of severity of disease, and noninfectious complications occurring in the hospital. There was no intervention in this study, so it is not known whether targeting patients with nutritional and rehabilitation strategies and focusing on decreasing hospital complications will actually change outcomes.

I suggest that those interested in the subject read the editorial accompanying the original article.[1] The editorial is by Dr. Graney, the deputy editor of the *Journal of the American Geriatrics Society.* Dr. Graney questions whether multivariant analysis, the analytic technique used in Dr. Thomas' article, can establish or rule out causality. He suggests that the relation between pressure sores and mortality may derive from their relation to other factors.

J.R. Burton, M.D.

Reference

1. Graney MJ: Can multivariant analysis rule out causality? *J Amer Geriatr Soc* 44:1476, 1996.

Predictors of Pressure Ulcer Healing Among Long-term Care Residents
Berlowitz DR, Brandeis GH, Anderson J, et al (Bedford VA Hosp, Mass)
J Am Geriatr Soc 45:30–34, 1997 2–31

Introduction.—In residents of long-term care facilities, pressure ulcers commonly develop. These can be very difficult to treat. Clinical practice guidelines for the management of these ulcers are now available. However, there are few data on the characteristics associated with healing of pressure ulcers. This information is needed for use in evaluation of health services, as well as for clinical reasons. A large population of long-term care residents in Veterans Administration (VA) facilities was studied to gain insight into the healing of pressure ulcers.

Methods.—The data base used for the study included information on the stage of the largest pressure ulcer present at the time of evaluation. Other information included ability to perform activities of daily living. The analysis included all residents of VA long-term care facilities who had a stage 2 or greater pressure ulcer as of April 1993. Ulcer outcomes were assessed in October of the same year. Predictors of healing were evaluated by analysis of variance and chi-square tests.

Results.—Of nearly 20,000 residents included in the data base, 1,529 (8%) had a pressure ulcer in April 1993. Eight hundred nineteen of these

TABLE 3.—Results of Logistic Regression Modeling Identifying Factors Independently Associated With Pressure Ulcer Healing

Characteristic	Odds Ratio	(95% CI)
Age (≥75 years)	1.5	(1.1, 2.0)
Rehabilitation services (per no. received)	1.3	(1.1, 1.6)
Immobility	0.3	(0.1, 0.5)
Incontinence	0.7	(0.4, 1.0)
Stage 2 ulcer (compared with stage 4)	5.2	(3.5, 7.7)
Stage 3 ulcer (compared with stage 4)	1.5	(1.0, 2.3)

Note: Model c statistic = 0.74.

(Courtesy of Berlowitz DR, Brandeis GH, Anderson J, et al: Predictors of pressure ulcer healing among long-term care residents. *J Am Geriatr Soc* 45[1]:30–34, 1997.)

patients were still institutionalized in October. The pressure ulcers healed in 54% of patients. The rate of freedom from pressure ulcers at 6 months was 72% for stage 2 ulcers, 45% for stage 3 ulcers, and 31% for stage 4 ulcers. Healing was more likely in residents older than 75 years and in residents admitted within the previous month. Residents who were not receiving rehabilitation therapies, who had multiple sclerosis or quadriplegia, were receiving oxygen therapy, or were dependent in any of the activities of daily living were less likely to have ulcer healing. Factors independently associated with ulcer healing were smaller ulcer size, patient age over 75, and receiving rehabilitation services. Factors independently associated with ulcer nonhealing were immobility and incontinence (Table 3).

Conclusion.—The findings regarding factors associated with healing and nonhealing of pressure ulcers among residents of long-term care facilities will allow targeted therapy of patients with risk factors for poor healing. They will also be useful in assessing the facility's performance in treating ulcers. This VA experience with healing of pressure ulcers is similar to that reported by a national chain of nursing homes.

▶ Predicting the healing of pressure sores has great significance for clinicians and administrative staff of nursing homes. These data are, therefore, important. They represent a large national population of VA Medical Center patients with pressure sores who could be followed for at least 6 months. At the end of this period, most stage 2 ulcers had healed, but only 45% and 31% of stage 3 and 4 ulcers, respectively, had healed. The factors associated with ulcer healing are summarized in the table. More such data are desperately needed.

Quite impressive are 2 facts: sores are extremely slow to heal and they are not necessarily a predictor of increased mortality; rather they may be just another sign of severe illness. A companion paper based on this large data set reports on the effect of pressure sores on survival. This abstract (2–32) follows.

J.R. Burton, M.D.

Effect of Pressure Ulcers on the Survival of Long-term Care Residents
Berlowitz DR, Brandeis GH, Anderson J, et al (Edith Nourse Rogers Mem Veterans Hosp, Bedford, Mass)
J Gerontol 52A:M106–M110, 1997 2–32

Objective.—For long-term care residents, pressure ulcers carry significant morbidity and mortality. Through infection leading to bacteremia, pressure ulcers could cause death. However, their independent effects on survival are unclear. This study analyzed the impact of pressure ulcers on survival among residents of Veterans Administration (VA) long-term care facilities.

Methods.—Data on 19,981 long-term care residents were obtained from VA data bases. These included information on pressure ulcer status, among many other characteristics. The main outcome was survival over a 6-month period between standard evaluations. Potential predictors of survival included demographic variables; age, dependency, and other risk factors for survival; and other factors with a clinically plausible impact on survival.

Results.—Thirteen percent of evaluable residents died during the 6-month follow-up period. The mortality rate was 26% in residents with a pressure ulcer vs. 12% in those without, for a relative risk of 2.37. Risk of death was similar for residents with superficial vs. deeper pressure ulcers, which are more likely to become infected. After adjustment for other

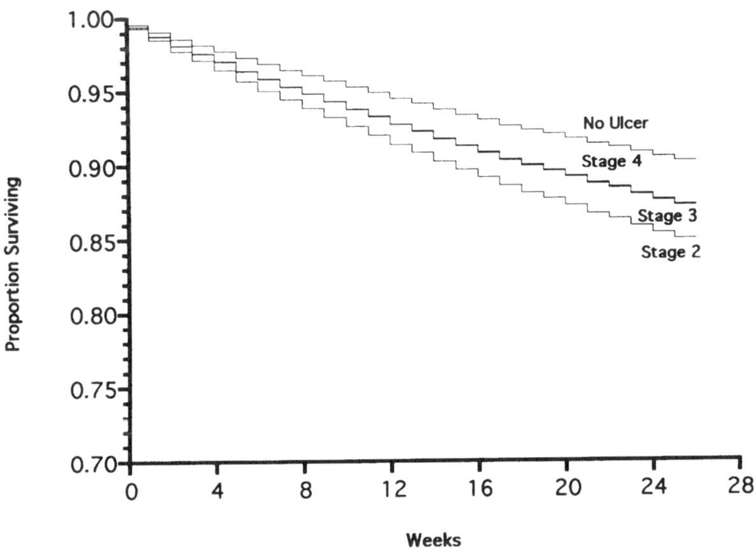

FIGURE 2.—Proportional hazards estimates of the proportion of patients surviving, by weeks from baseline, for the no–pressure ulcer and the ulcer stage 2, 3, and 4 subject groups, after adjustment for other factors. (Courtesy of Berlowitz DR, Brandeis GH, Anderson J, et al: Effect of pressure ulcers on the survival of long-term care residents. *J Gerontol* 52A:M106–M110. Copyright 1997, The Gerontological Society of America.)

factors, the relative risk of death associated with pressure ulcers declined to 1.45 (Fig 2).

Conclusion.—Long-term care residents with pressure ulcers were at significantly increased risk of death during 6 months of follow-up. However, most of the excess mortality was related to associated factors, such as frailty and diseases. The presence of a pressure ulcer may reflect clinical factors, other than risk of serious infection, that are not included in the authors' model. The findings suggest that decisions about pressure ulcer treatment in the long-term care setting should take into consideration the patient's overall medical condition.

▶ Pressure sores have long been considered a risk factor for death. However, this large VA Medical Center national study in which patient survival data are available for a 6-month period showed that the increased risk is mainly the result of associated factors such as the underlying disease and frailty.

J.R. Burton, M.D.

Managed Care

Predictive Validity of the P_{ra} Instrument Among Older Recipients of Managed Care

Pacala JT, Boult C, Reed RL, et al (Univ of Minnesota, Minneapolis; Value Health Sciences, Santa Monica, Calif)

J Am Geriatr Soc 45:614–617, 1997 2–33

Background.—Two strategies can improve the cost-effectiveness of medical care: (1) identifying individuals who are at the greatest risk for critical medical events and (2) providing them with special care to improve their health and reduce their need for expensive medical services. The P_{ra}

APPENDIX.—Questions That Solicit Data for Computing P_{ra}

1. In general would you say your health is: [excellent; very good; good; fair; poor].
2. In the previous 12 months, have you stayed overnight as a patient in a hospital? [not at all; one time; two or three times; more than three times.]
3. In the previous 12 months, how many times did you visit a physician or clinic? [not at all; one time; two or three times; four to six times; more than six times.]
4. In the previous 12 months, did you have diabetes? [yes; no.]
5. Have you ever had: Coronary heart disease? [yes; no.] Angina pectoris? [yes; no.] A myocardial infarction? [yes; no.] Any other heart attack? [yes; no.]
6. Your sex? [male; female.]
7. Is there a friend, relative or neighbor who would take care of you for a few days, if necessary? [yes; no.]
8. Your date of birth? [month ; day ; year .]

(Courtesy of Pacala JT, Boult C, Reel RL, et al. Predictive validity of the P_{ra} instrument among older recipients of managed care. *J Am Geriatr Soc* 45[5]:614–617, 1997.)

TABLE 1.—Predictive Validity of P_{ra} in a Managed Care Population

Outcome	Mean Resource Use by P_{ra} Risk Level: Low Risk (n = 5086)	High Risk (n = 1716)	High/Low Ratio
Claims ($/member/yr)	960	2,637	2.7
Hospital admissions (#/member/yr)	.110	.270	2.5
Emergency room visits (#/member/yr)	.089	.180	2.0
Nursing home admissions (#/member/yr)	.020	.072	3.6
Home visits (#/member/yr)	.069	.240	3.5

(Courtesy of Pacala JT, Boult C, Reel RL, et al. Predictive validity of the P_{ra} instrument among older recipients of managed care. *J Am Geriatr Soc* 45[5]:614–617, 1997.)

(probability of repeat admission) screening instrument, which consists of 8 questions (Appendix) to evaluate a patient's probability of repeated admission to the hospital, was developed for the fee-for-service environment. It proved to be both reliable and practical. Whether this formula would continue to be reliable and practical in the managed care environment is the focus of this report.

Methods.—Enrollees in a Medicare TEFRA risk plan, who were at least 65 years old and who completed and returned a 4-page standardized health inventory were eligible. Responses to the questionnaire were sufficient to calculate the P_{ra} score in 6,802 participants. Research subjects were divided into high-risk (highest quartile) and low-risk (other three quartiles) groups on the basis of their P_{ra} score. The ratio of service use among high-risk subjects to that of low-risk subjects in the year after the survey was taken as the predictive value of the P_{ra} score.

Findings.—High-risk subjects used significantly more health resources than low-risk subjects (Table 1), as measured by the P_{ra} risk level.

Conclusions.—The P_{ra} instrument accurately identified older people in a managed care setting who used significantly more health resources in the year after the survey was taken than their lower risk peers did. Such individuals can be identified and provided with special interventions to minimize the effects of disease and the costs of treatment.

► Risk adjusters are increasingly important in clinical medicine for targeting populations that may require special attention. This is especially so for the elderly. This simple 8-question instrument seems to predict reliably those patients who may require increased clinical services. Basically, the instrument uses age, sex, certain diseases, and the number of health care encounters in the previous 12 months. This risk adjuster requires specific data collection which cannot be derived from the usual existing data sets. Existing risk-adjusting instruments are available that use existing data sets and are, therefore, theoretically similar. For example, claims data are a reliable source of information, and several sophisticated systems of risk adjustment using the codes for services given and diagnoses for these services have been developed. Adjustments are made based on claims data from the previous year. To set up and maintain claims-based risk adjustors, computer programming resources are needed. Such resources are usually reserved for large-scale adjusting, such as the payment adjusting done by a state or the Health Care Financing Administration. Increasingly, health care providers will need to be familiar with these risk-adjusting instruments.

J.R. Burton, M.D.

Post-Hospital Sub-Acute Care: An Example of a Managed Care Model

von Sternberg T, Hepburn K, Cibuzar P, et al (Univ of Minnesota, Minneapolis)

J Am Geriatr Soc 45:87–91, 1997 2–34

Objective.—Economics are encouraging timely hospital discharge of geriatric patients, providing for subacute care in alternative facilities, including units on separate hospital floors, acute rehabilitation units, and geriatric rehabilitation hospitals. Type of care, therapeutic goals, cost reduction, length of stay, and discharge arrangements need to be considered. A staff model nonprofit HMO in Bloomington, Minnesota, with 21,000 geriatric patients enrolled under a TEFRA contract reports its experience with the transitional care centers (TCC).

Methods.—The staffing mix permits care of patients with acute needs. The institution has a high nurse-patient ratio (1 to 9), can admit around the clock, offers physical and occupational therapy 6 days a week, and can provide TPN and IV therapy, heparin therapy, and IV hydration. The clinical team consists of a board-certified geriatrician, a GNP worker, and nursing, therapy, and social worker staff. Admission occurs directly or by transfer from an acute care facility. About 80% of patients are hospital transfers, one third of whom are orthopedic, one third deconditioned, and one third postsurgical patients. Patients receive care as dictated by a discharge summary of the patient's laboratory data from the last 3 days. Advance directive status is determined on admission by the team, which meets weekly to discuss patient status and goals. Patients are seen several times weekly by the geriatrician and the GNP, who update the patient's primary care physician. The patient is discharged when the individual can no longer benefit from the sub-acute care provided.

Outcomes.—Frail, disabled patients can be cared for successfully, as the 2-year program has shown, when compared with other nursing home units (Table 1). The average length of stay, monitored for 1 year, was 14.3 days. Social workers obtained patient information at 3 and 6 months after discharge. Primary care physicians and patients were satisfied with patient care and team communication. The program was cost effective, using 0.75 full-time equivalent (FTE) of a GNP and 0.2 FTE of a geriatrician.

Conclusion.—The TCC provided quality care of geriatric patients that satisfied patients and primary care physicians at a cost that was 38%

TABLE 1.—Summary Table Comparing TCC Units With Non-contract Facilities Accepting Patients for Post-hospital Care and Rehabilitation

	Transitional Care Facilities	Non-contract Facilities
Average length of stay	14.3	20.5
Per diem costs (including therapies)	$185	$280–$300
Re-hospitalization rate per 100 admits	0.06	0.05
Re-hospitalization rate for infections (urosepsis, pneumonia) per 100 admits	0.03	0.06

(Courtesy of von Sternberg T, Hepburn K, Cibuzar P, et al: Post-hospital sub-acute care: An example of a managed care model. *J Am Geriatr Soc* 45[1]:87–91, 1997.)

below that of noncontracted nursing homes. Rehospitalization rates were comparable with other geriatric settings.

▶ New systems of care are a part of the shifting paradigm of health care in the United States. This study reviewed an experience with a sub-acute care program in a managed care system. The results are favorable. There were significant cost savings, and, more important, there was an excellent level of satisfaction among referring primary care physicians and among patients who used the transitional care units. Also in these units, there did not appear to be any unusually high level of transfer of patients back to acute care hospitals. There was a critical role for a team, consisting of a geriatrician and a geriatric nurse practitioner, in the management of these patients, and it provided a highly functional multidisciplinary core for these patients.

J.R. Burton, M.D.

Alzheimer's Disease

Predicting Time to Nursing Home Care and Death in Individuals With Alzheimer Disease

Stern Y, Tang M-X, Albert MS, et al (Columbia Univ, New York; Harvard Med School, Boston; Johns Hopkins Univ, Baltimore Md)
JAMA 277:806–812, 1997 2–35

Background.—Patients with Alzheimer's disease (AD) and their families commonly ask how long it will be until the patient needs nursing home admission or dies. These questions cannot be answered on the basis of empirical data. This study sought to use clinical features to predict such important outcomes in individual patients with AD.

Methods.—The study included 236 patients who met the National Institute of Neurological and Communicative Disorders and Stroke–Alzheimer's Disease and Related Disorders Association criteria for probable AD. The patients were 140 women and 96 men with a mean age of 73. Their mean duration of AD was about 4 years. All had mild dementia at baseline, with a modified Mini-Mental State Examination (mMMS) score of 30 or higher, and had not taken neuroleptic medications for at least 1 month. Patients with substance abuse, schizophrenia, major affective disorder, previous electroconvulsive therapy, or evidence of stroke were excluded. The potential predictors evaluated included duration of illness, age at onset, extrapyramidal signs, psychosis, and cognition. Starting in the sixth year of the study, apolipoprotein E genotype was considered as well. Outcomes evaluated were nursing home placement or its equivalent and death.

Results.—Although 28% of patients had abnormal medical findings at baseline, none of these were believed to be contributing to dementia. Sixty-nine percent of patients reached the point of needing nursing home care during the maximum follow-up of 7 years. Forty-two percent of patients died. Mortality was lower for women, patients with longer duration of illness, and higher mMMS scores; it was higher for patients with extrapyramidal signs. Prediction algorithms based on Cox proportional hazard models were used to generate survival curves for time to either of the study outcomes. When predictor variables from a validation cohort of 105 patients were entered into the algorithms, predicted survival fell within the 95% confidence bands of the actual survival curves.

Conclusions.—Prediction algorithms for time to nursing home admission or death in patients with AD represent an initial step toward providing specific prognoses for individual patients with AD. The approach could be useful in the design and interpretation of clinical trials by providing an expected time course to be compared with the patient's actual course.

▶ Clinicians need to be able to educate patients and their caregivers as precisely as possible regarding the natural history of a disease. This is especially so in common, chronic neurologic conditions such as AD, in which medical care resource utilization and family caregiver burden may eventually be substantial. However, such data have been lacking for AD, and clinicians have been forced to discuss the course of this disease in only the broadest of terms.

This study is important in that it aims to refine the predictability of the course of AD. Prediction algorithms were developed for 2 outcomes: the equivalent of nursing home placement and death. To develop the models, initial clinical data from 236 patients seen early in their disease at 3 AD research centers were analyzed. Clearly, these predictive models are just a start in this process, and larger numbers of patients and a broader experience will be necessary before such models will be widely used. Nevertheless, this paper describes an early approach, and it holds promise for what is to come.

J.R. Burton, M.D.

▶ This is an important study that is methodologically sophisticated and provides information of utility to both clinicians and researchers. Two convenient samples were followed. Predictors of nursing home placement include younger age at onset, greater cognitive impairment, shorter duration of illness, and the presence of psychotic and extrapyramidal symptoms. These findings support a growing body of knowledge suggesting that nursing home placement is not necessitated by any 1 factor but rather by a combination of cognitive and non-cognitive symptoms. The finding that shorter duration and poor mMMS score predict placement supports the contention that disease severity is a primary predictor. This is also likely to be true for the presence of extrapyramidal symptoms.

The finding that psychotic symptoms present at onset predict placements raises the possibility that treating the patients might delay or prevent placement. There is no data to support this hypothesis in the literature to my knowledge.

It is also of note that the predictors of death are similar to those for placement. This similarity supports the contention that factors intrinsic to the disease play a major role in both rate of progression and mortality. However, this study does not rule out the possibility that at least 1 apolipoprotein (APO) $\epsilon 4$ allele also increased the risk of both placement and death (since the confidence intervals for each of these includes 1). Thus, the finding could be due to chance. While this would be compatible with the hypothesis that these individuals were more likely to have Alzheimer's disease, the autopsy data suggest that the authors were diagnostically accurate whatever the APO ϵ status. The authors did not include APO ϵ status in the prediction algorithms. Thus, the relationship between their capacity to predict in relationship to the other variables is not known.

Clinicians will need to be cautious in applying these findings since there can be a danger in going from group data to individual patients. Nevertheless, this does provide some guidance to clinicians in predicting prognosis. Since many family members and patients benefit from prognostic data, the findings can serve as a general guide. From a research perspective, these findings might guide studies aimed at delaying nursing home placement. Conversely, they could be used to develop criteria supporting placement. Used either as a guide to placement or treatment intervention, studies should be approached with caution since nursing home care benefits many individuals.

P.V. Rabins, M.D., M.P.H.

Long-term Tacrine (Cognex) Treatment: Effects on Nursing Home Placement and Mortality

Knopman D, and the Tacrine Study Group (Univ of Minnesota, Minneapolis; et al)

Neurology 47:166–177, 1996 2–36

Background.—Tacrine, a cholinesterase inhibitor, has been shown to have clinically significant effects on cognition and function in patients with Alzheimer's disease (AD) who have taken this drug as part of 12- to 30-week randomized, placebo-controlled trials. The long-term effect of tacrine on this group has not been investigated. To determine the effect of

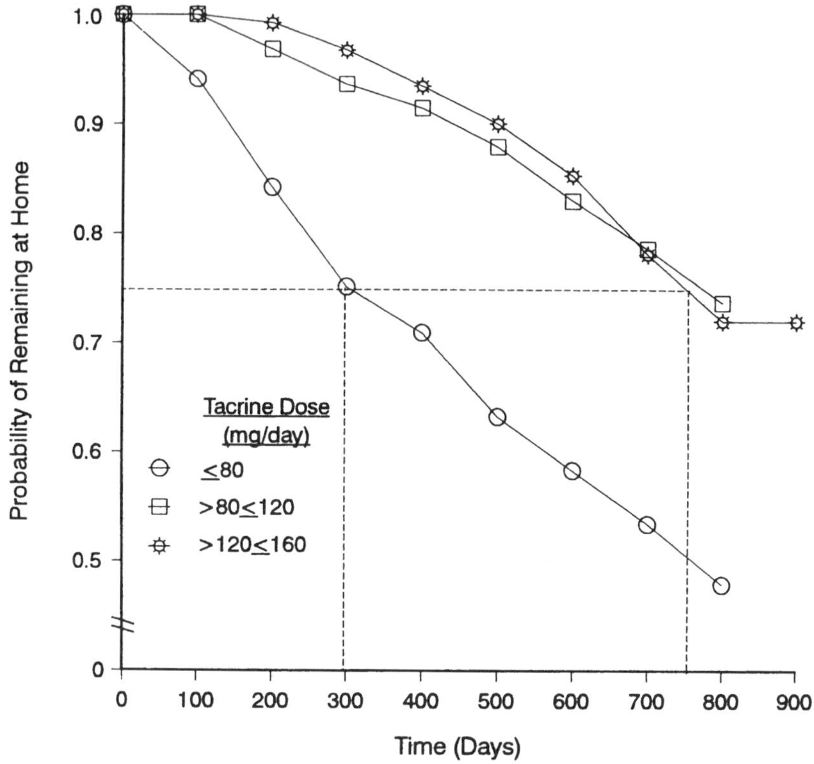

Effective Sample Size

	0	100	200	300	400	500	600	700	800	900
≤80	102	95	83	72	64	52	36	20	7	0
>80≤120	96	95	89	85	80	71	57	32	8	0
>120≤160	122	122	121	118	110	95	72	38	12	2

FIGURE 2.—Probability of remaining at home according to final daily tacrine dose for patients who continued to receive tacrine up to or within 60 days of nursing home placement or death, for whom exact date of nursing home placement was available. Effective sample sizes at each interval are given below the graph. (Courtesy of Knopman D, and the Tacrine Study Group: Long-term tacrine [Cognex] treatment: Effects on nursing home placement and mortality. *Neurology* 47:166–177, 1996. Copyright American Academy of Neurology. Used with permission of Lippincott-Raven.)

long-term tacrine treatment on nursing home placement and mortality in this population, a group of patients with AD who were involved in a 30-week trial of tacrine was followed up for 2 years.

Methods.—A 30-week randomized, double-blind, placebo-controlled, parallel-group clinical trial of tacrine was conducted at 33 American medical centers. Participants in this study were healthy men and women at least 50 with a diagnosis of probable AD. Disease severity was mild to moderate based on a Mini-Mental State Examination. Caregivers ensured compliance with the medical regimen. Patients who completed this study were eligible to receive long-term, open-label tacrine treatment. The initial dose was 40 mg/day, which could be increased every 4 weeks to a maximum dose of 160 mg/day.

Results.—Patients who continued to take tacrine for the full 2-year period and who received doses greater than 80 mg/day were significantly less likely to have entered a nursing home at 2-year follow-up than those taking lower doses or those who discontinued the medication (Fig 2). There was also a trend toward lower mortality among patients receiving more than 120 mg/day of tacrine.

Conclusions.—Patients with AD who received long-term, high-dose tacrine treatment had a significantly lower risk of nursing home placement and a trend toward lower mortality. More research is needed to prospectively replicate and expand the findings of this study in the AD population.

▶ This is an interesting study of the benefit of tacrine. It is a follow-up of a 30-week randomized, controlled trial of high doses of tacrine in patients with AD.[1] What was reported here was an additional minimum of 2 years of follow-up. The outcomes of nursing home placement and death were analyzed using logistic regression.

The results are significant. The patients who continued to receive tacrine and were receiving doses greater than 80 mg/day or greater than 120 mg/day were less likely to enter a nursing home than patients receiving lower doses. A tendency toward lower mortality for patients receiving greater than 120 mg/day was noted. These are the kinds of outcome data that we must have.

J.R. Burton, M.D.

Reference

1. Knapp MJ, Knopman DS, Solomon PR, et al: A 30-week randomized controlled trial of high-dose tacrine in patients with Alzheimer's disease. *JAMA* 217:985–991, 194.

Miscellaneous

Do Drug Costs Affect Physicians' Prescription Decisions?

Hart J, Salman H, Bergman M, et al (Tel Aviv Univ, Israel)

J Intern Med 241:415–420, 1997 2–37

Background.—In this era of increasing demands to control health care costs, controlling the costs of drug therapy figures prominently. Would physicians' prescription practices differ if they knew the cost of the drugs they were prescribing? Two patient simulations were used to address this question.

Methods.—Two patient simulations—one with mild urinary tract infection (UTI), and another with severe UTI—were presented to 30 family physicians from outpatient clinics and 30 physicians from a hospital department of internal medicine. Physicians read a case history in which the symptoms of the UTI were described, and 6 or 7 possible drug therapies were listed. Physicians were interviewed twice, first without knowing the cost of the drugs (phase 1) and then 2 months later with the cost of the

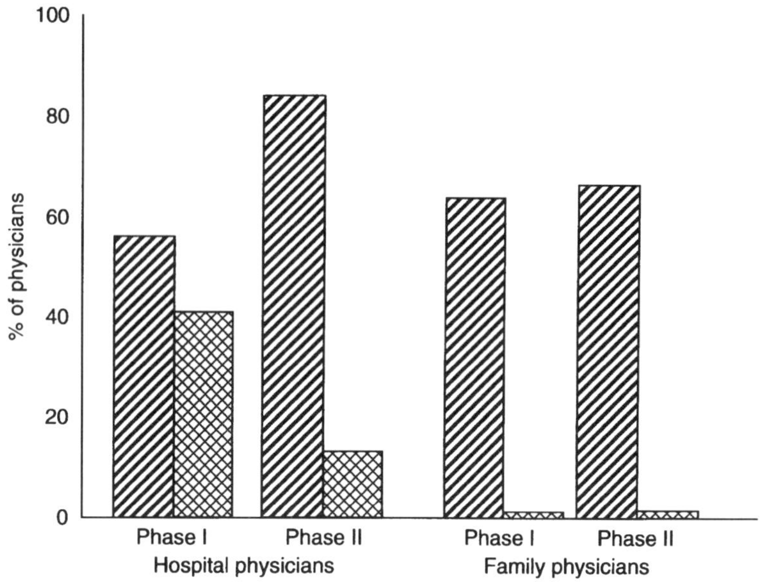

FIGURE 1.—Preferences in drug prescription for patient 1 (mild form of UTI) by the hospital and family physicians in both phases of the study, both without and with an awareness of the drug costs. *Diagonal hatches*, TMP-SMZ; *crosshatches*, quinolone. (Courtesy of Hart J, Salman H, Bergman M, et al.: Do drug costs affect physicians' prescription decisions? *J Intern Med* 241:415–420, 1997. Published by Blackwell Science Ltd.)

drugs supplied (phase 2). Physicians were not informed that the second interview would take place. Thus, it was assumed that they would not remember the drug they had assigned during the first phase.

Findings.—For the patient with mild UTI, 60% of family physicians chose trimethoprim and sulfamethoxazole (TMP–SMZ) regardless of whether they knew the cost of the drugs or not (Fig 1). Hospital physicians, however, changed their prescribing pattern significantly when the cost of the drugs was known (Fig 1). For the patient with severe UTI, 74% of family physicians chose gentamicin, regardless of whether they knew the costs of the drugs or not (Fig 2). Again, hospital physicians changed their prescribing pattern significantly when the cost of the drugs was known (Fig 2). For the family physicians, years of practice did not correlate with their choice of drugs. For the hospital physicians, those with fewer years of practice prescribed expensive drugs significantly more often during phase 1 of both simulations.

Conclusions.—The physician's knowledge of a drug's cost can significantly affect his or her prescription patterns. At the authors' institution, it is estimated that prescribing less costly drugs in these 2 patient simulations would result in a monthly savings of $34,000.

► How sensitive are physicians to drug costs when selecting an agent to prescribe for a patient? Probably not as sensitive as they should be. For this

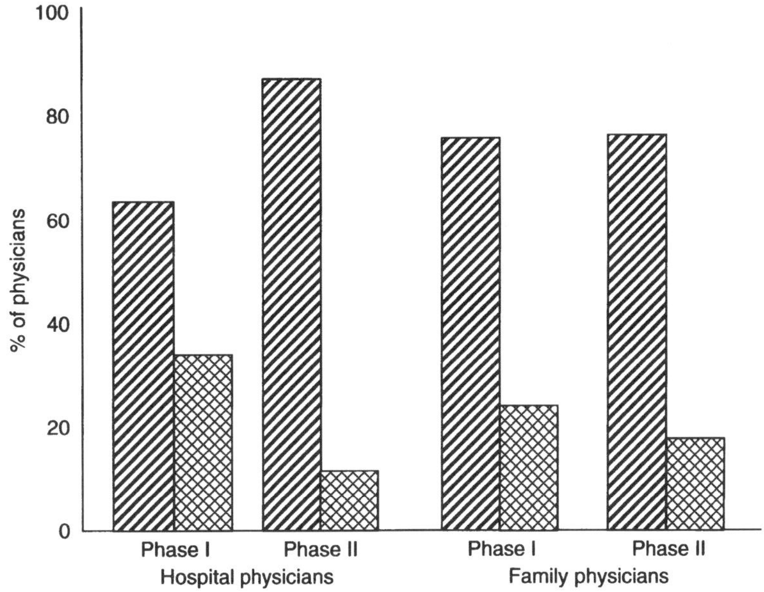

FIGURE 2.—Evaluation of preferences in drug prescription for patient 2 (severe form of UTI) by hospital and family physicians in both phases of the study, both without and with an awareness of the drug costs. *Diagonal hatches*, gentamicin; *crosshatches*, cephalosporin. (Courtesy of Hart J, Salman H, Bergman M, et al: Do drug costs affect physicians' prescription decisions? *J Intern Med* 241:415–420, 1997. Published by Blackwell Science Ltd.)

reason, this small study is valuable. Although it was done in Israel, I believe the results are applicable to the United States.

Two patient simulations were presented to family physicians based in clinics and internal medicine physicians based in community hospitals. The simulated patients had either simple or complex urinary tract infections, cases in which many equally effective drugs are available for treatment. The physicians served as their own controls, and drug costs were available only at the second phase of the simulation.

The awareness of cost definitely affected the selection of the drug in the study among hospital physicians but not among family physicians, who for the most part, had already selected lower-cost drugs. This study shows that substantial savings were incurred when the physician was aware of the cost of the drugs.

Frankly, I think it would be a great advance if commonly used books and other references used by physicians when prescribing had information about drug costs. Overall cost-savings to patients, insurers, and hospitals would be enormous, with likely no loss in benefit.

J.R. Burton, M.D.

Faithful Patients: The Effect of Long-term Physician-Patient Relationships on the Costs and Use of Health Care by Older Americans

Weiss LJ, Blustein J (Columbia College, New York)

Am J Public Health 86:1742–1747, 1996 2–38

Objective.—It is believed that the duration of the physician-patient relationship has a positive effect on patient well-being and costs, although these positive effects have not been quantitated. With the advent of managed care, many of these relationships have been severed. One survey found that 41% of patients switched physicians when joining an HMO. From publicly available data, the benefits of long-standing doctor-patient Medicare fee-for-service relationships were quantitated.

Methods.—Enrollees from 107 sampling units in the U.S. Medicare program were surveyed. The response rate was 83.3% or 12,677 patients

TABLE 2.—Health Care Use, Health Behaviors, and Health Care Costs of All Subjects and Those in Poor Health by the Duration of their Tie to a Usual Source of Care

Outcome Measure	Duration of Tie to Usual Source of Care, y <1	1–3	3–5	5–10	10+
Had influenza vaccine previous winter, %					
All subjects	38.5	40.6	46.0	44.7	47.2*
Subjects in poor health	37.2	46.1	44.5	46.0	48.2
Had a mammogram during the previous year, % of females					
All subjects	37.6	37.8	39.2	39.5	37.7
Subjects in poor health	32.1	28.4	32.0	32.0	29.6
Smoke now, % of ever smoked					
All subjects	27.0	27.9	27.5	23.7	25.6
Subjects in poor health	28.3	27.4	33.0	23.1	26.6
Obese, %					
All subjects	16.3	16.9	17.2	18.1	16.1
Subjects in poor health	22.6	25.1	16.6	26.5	22.6
Used emergency room during the previous year, %					
All subjects	16.1	13.1	12.1	11.6	11.9
Subjects in poor health	23.0	22.1	26.4	22.5	21.5
Any hospital admissions, %					
All subjects	21.3	17.3	19.3	18.6	15.1*
Subjects in poor health	46.4	36.8	41.0	36.2	33.1
Mean Part A reimbursement, $					
All subjects	2140	1847	1686	1713	1223**
Subjects in poor health	5180	4424	5910	4793	3374
Mean Part B reimbursement, $					
All subjects	1458	1307	1254	1317	1018**
Subjects in poor health	2703	2889	3044	2852	2044
Mean no. office visits					
All subjects	6.12	6.09	5.76	5.89	5.59**
Subjects in poor health	8.59	8.89	8.05	9.95	7.75

*$P < .05$ (chi-square analysis of the overall association between this outcome measure and the duration of tie to usual source of care).

**$P < .05$ (ANOVA examining the overall association between this outcome measure and the duration of tie to usual source of care).

(Courtesy of Weiss LJ, Blustein J: Faithful patients: The effect of long-term physician-patient relationships on the costs and use of health care by older Americans. *Am J Public Health* 86:1742–1747.

of whom 8,068 with specific physician ties were included. Usual provider and duration of tie, health care use, healthy behaviors, cost of care, and sociodemographic and health status measures were recorded. The magnitude and variability effects of the duration of the relationship on each outcome was subjected to multivariate analysis.

Results.—Approximately 55% of the respondents had relationships of 5 or more years with their doctors, and about 35% had relationships lasting 10 years or longer. Duration of the physician-patient relationship was associated with receiving an influenza vaccine the previous winter, hospitalization, part A reimbursement, the number of office visits, and part B reimbursements (Table 2). The usual source of care was listed as the doctor's office by 78.7% of patients. Of the 251 patients who had been seeing their physician for less than 1 year, 81.8% said they had been seeing another physician previously. Most said they changed because of changes affecting accessibility.

Conclusion.—In this study, relatively healthy older Americans in fee-for-service organizations did not tend to change physicians. The fact that individuals were free to switch providers at any time and the lack of ability to quantify many of the benefits of a long-term physician-patient relationship were limitations of this study. Lasting physician-patient relationships are important even in the era of managed care.

▶ This important study was designed to quantify the benefits of long-standing physician-patient relationships under the fee-for-service system within Medicare. The study was based on a cluster sampling of just over 100 sampling units with a net sample available for analysis of just over 8,000 individuals. It is remarkable to note that approximately 55% of individuals had seen a single physician for over 5 years and just over a third for over 10 years. Quiet reassuring is the finding that both part A and part B Medicare expenditures were lower for those individuals who had been with a physician for 10 years or longer. Also, hospitalization rates were lower for this group than for the group of patients who did not have a long-term relationship with a physician. This survey does not allow one to analyze the reasons for these differences, but future studies will be focused on that question. The data fit with the bias that most of us have that first class long-lasting primary care is the best form of health care, and this is especially important for frail elderly individuals who are the most vulnerable users of the health care system.

J.R. Burton, M.D.

Courier Robot Keeps Hospital Staff 'On the Job'

Deery J III (Abington Mem Hosp, Pa)

J Healthcare Qual 19:22–23, 1997 2–39

Objective.—Because of budget considerations and staff shortages—particularly in nutrition and supply, processing, and distribution (SPD) workers—Abington Memorial Hospital decided to investigate using a materials-transport robot. The trackless, self-guided courier robot is designed to transport materials, can travel anywhere in a building once programmed, and does not require modifications to existing buildings.

Installing the Robot.—The process took a few weeks and consisted of installing an infrared interface at the emergency room and elevator doors. Communication was via radio transceivers. Programming took a few days and consisted of installing a hospital map with "rules of the road": for example, staying away from walls and avoiding certain areas.

Using the Robot.—The nutrition and SPD departments share the robot, which functions mainly in the pickup and delivery mode between programmed stations and homebase. The robot times out for 2 minutes at each station and continues to the next stop if not serviced. The robot also has a 1-way mode used at 6 PM.

Communication.—The person at each station removes or deposits the load and pushes a button to dispatch the robot. A red button stops the robot in an emergency. The robot vocalizes its needs with a list of preprogrammed messages and instructs individuals at each station what they are to load or unload or to remove obstacles.

Control System.—The robot uses the service elevator only when its control system determines the need. The system allows persons on the elevator to stop on floors as they wish but ignores outside buttons when the robot is on board. The controller sends the elevator to the robot's floor.

Evaluating the Robot.—The costs are $5 per hour to rent the robot and $1 per hour to rent the elevator interface. The robot is dependable and reliable, is consistent in its travel time, and goes where it is sent by the most direct route.

▶ Well, what next? Here is a "case report" of a courier robot used in a general hospital. The robot was able to distribute late meal trays, other food items, and non-nutritional supplies throughout the hospital at a very low hourly cost. Be on the look out: high-tech medicine is now moving to courier robots!

J.R. Burton, M.D.

3 Geriatric Psychiatry

Introduction

Depression

Advances in understanding major depression in the elderly have come from several fronts this year. The importance of depression as a source of distress and in association with medical illness is clear. In a well-designed outcome study from a large HMO in the Seattle area, Unützer et al. (Abstract 3–1) demonstrate that the higher medical costs associated with depression (50% higher in their study) are independent of the costs of chronic medical illness. Since only 1% of total expenditures were for mental health services, these data provide one of the stronger supports for the need for earlier recognition and better treatment of depression as a source of cost savings as well as a source of morbidity relief.

The relationship between grief and major depression has intrigued clinicians since Freud, and a group from the University of Pittsburgh has developed important data suggesting that these two conditions are distinct (Abstract 3–4). The replication study reported by Prigerson et al. demonstrates that complicated bereavement meeting criteria for major depression is symptomatically distinct. This has important implications for treatment. The etiology of major depression remains unknown, but several papers reviewed this year strengthened the long-held belief that central nervous system vascular disease may be one cause. Alexopoulos et al. (Abstract 3–5) from Cornell-Westchester have codified these suggestions into a specific hypothesis and demonstrate neuropsychological data supporting it. Krishnan et al. (Abstract 3–6) and Lesser et al. (Abstract 3–8) tested these hypotheses on MRI and demonstrated that later onset cases are more likely to have evidence of vascular brain disease. A study by Greenwald et al. (Abstract 3–10) suggests that this association between vascular disease and depression might also presage the development of Alzheimer's disease.

It is surprising that major depression is often not listed as a risk factor for suicidal ideation. The study by Callahan et al. (Abstract 3–11) demonstrates that approximately 1% of individuals in primary care have suicidal ideation, but there is a five-fold increase among individuals with major depression. Whether improved recognition will lead to suicide prevention is an important question that has not been demonstrated. In this study of 300 individuals, none died of suicide. Therefore, it is likely that a very large number of subjects would need to be studied to determine effectiveness of any prevention strategy. The link between suicidal ideation and major depression is also confirmed in a study by Chiu et al. from Hong Kong (Abstract 3–12). Although suicide rates and methods vary greatly according to culture, perhaps the association between depression and suicide holds across many cultures.

A paper with important potential by Schneider et al. (Abstract 3–15) reports that estrogen replacement therapy and fluoxetine had a greater benefit in improving mood than either did alone. This is a retrospective finding and not too much should be made of it until it is replicated in prospective trials. It is a plausible finding because it has long been known that estrogens relate to mood. This could be an important finding particularly for the women who fail to improve under standard antidepressant medication therapy.

Dementia

The etiology of Alzheimer's disease (AD) is still unknown, but several issues have become clear. First and foremost, it is not a single disease but rather a syndrome with many etiologies. Much of the focus has been on molecular genetics since three genes (amyloid precursor protein on chromosome 21, presenilin 1 on chromosome 14 and presenilin 2 on chromosome 1) cause an autosomal dominant form of AD, linkage to chromosome 12 has been identified in late onset cases, a gene dosage effect operates in Down's syndrome, and apoliproprotein genotype influences age of onset. A majority of researchers have focused on the amyloid protein as the likely site of commonalities in etiology. Robert Terry, one of the pioneers in studying basic pathobiology of AD, suggests an alternative hypothesis based on cytoskeletal abnormalities as the initiating event (Abstract 3–16). The intense competition in this field is likely to lead to a more rapid discovery of causes; an open-mindedness about potential etiologies and pathways should likewise be beneficial. Levy et al. (Abstract 3–18) demonstrate that many of the non-cognitive symptoms of AD vary over time but are often persistent and recurrent. These symptoms remain a focus of treatment, and better understandings of their pathogenesis and therapy are urgently needed.

Among other forms of dementia, Lewy-body dementia has received a great deal of attention in recent years. The study of Klatka et al. (Abstract 3–20) confirms that depression, delusions, and hallucinations are common in diffuse Lewy-body disease and supports the use of these symptoms in making the proper diagnosis.

Several other articles that are reviewed this year address other clinically relevant issues. An article from Sweden and Finland (Abstract 3–21) demonstrates that elderly individuals dying in automobile accidents are highly likely to have the neuropathological and genetic markers of AD. A study from Australia (Abstract 3–22) shows the difficulty in early recognition again demonstrated by the poor reliability of screening instruments. The complexities of informing patients with dementia about the diagnosis and of obtaining informed consent from persons with dementia are reviewed in 2 articles from Great Britain (Abstracts 3–24 and 3–25). In a study from the Stanford VA Hospital (Abstract 3–26), Zeiss et al. demonstrate that sexually inappropriate behavior is infrequent in persons with dementia but can be reliably identified. A study of cognitive processing in persons with Parkinson's disease (Abstract 3–27) demonstrates that incentive learning can be impaired when other forms are not. Such findings increase our knowledge of the biology of memory but also have clinical implications since impaired learning of this type is sometimes misinterpreted as a purposeful attempt at frustrating the care provider.

MISCELLANEOUS

A variety of other studies in this chapter reflect advances in knowledge. Perhaps most important is the study in Mittelman et al. (Abstract 3–28) demonstrating that a 2-month weekly structured intervention with caregivers can delay the placement of persons with AD in nursing homes by an average of 9 months. A collection of case reports from Duke (Abstract 3–29) demonstrates that anorexia nervosa can start in elderly individuals. Other common conditions, such as major depression and many physical illnesses, must obviously be ruled out before this diagnosis is made, however. Finally, an intriguing report by Cooper (Abstract 3–30) demonstrates that learning disabilities can be identified in the elderly. It will be important to determine whether these conditions are treatable.

Peter V. Rabins, M.D., M.P.H.

Depression

Depressive Symptoms and the Cost of Health Services in HMO Patients Aged 65 Years and Older: A 4-Year Prospective Study

Unützer J, Patrick DL, Simon G, et al (Univ of Washington, Seattle; Group Health Cooperative of Puget Sound, Seattle)

JAMA 277:1618–1623, 1997 3–1

Background.—Many elderly patients have symptoms of depression. The frequency of depressive symptoms (clinical or subthreshold) in elderly patients and whether such symptoms are associated with higher health care costs were investigated.

Methods.—Subjects were 2,558 HMO enrollees older than 65. They were divided into 2 groups: the control group received usual care from their primary care physician, whereas the treatment group also received preventive measures, including visits with a health promotion nurse and health promotion classes for specific health risks. Surveys and interviews performed 3 times during the 4-year study evaluated the patient's level of depression according to the Center for Epidemiological Studies Depression (CED-S) scale. Pharmacy data gave information about the number of medical conditions, and the HMO database tracked the cost of health services. Confounding variables such as age, sex, and severity of medical illness were controlled for by statistical analysis.

Findings.—On the basis of CED-S scores, 27% of patients showed symptoms of depression at at least 1 of the 3 follow-up points. No significant relationship existed between depressive symptoms and chronic medical illness. Total health care costs increased proportionally with time at all levels of medical illness. Patients with depression used significantly more medical services than controls. The costs associated with these services increased 1.9% for each grade increase in the CES-D score. Factors significantly associated with higher costs were a higher CES-D score, a higher chronic disease score, and age (higher for patients older than 70 years).

Conclusions.—These extensive data from an HMO show that patients with depression have health care costs about 50% higher than patients without such symptoms. Both depression and chronic medical illness were associated with greater health care costs, yet these 2 variables did not show a significant interaction. Mental health services accounted for only about 1% of the total costs, consistent with other reports in the literature. It is suggested that a greater focus on the treatment of depression might be cost-effective in the long run.

► This important prospective study confirms what several retrospective and cross-sectional studies have demonstrated: elderly individuals with depressive symptoms utilize more health care resources than other individuals. In this study, potential confounding variables such as severity of co-existing medical illness, age, and sex are controlled for, further strengthening the finding. The information presented illustrates that for all levels of chronic disease, the higher the number of depressive symptoms, the greater the health care expenditures. These higher costs are not accounted for by use of any formal mental health services. This suggests that there is a potential for cost savings if depressive symptoms are adequately treated. As the authors point out, this is a hypothesis that would need to be tested before it could be stated with any degree of certainty, but the data here clearly support the need for such studies.

The authors are also correct in noting that many of these individuals are seen in primary care and interventions focused on improving identification and treatment of patients in primary care would be of particular interest.

It should be noted that the instrument used in this study, the CES-D, is a measure of depressive symptoms rather than depressive disorder. The vast majority of patients had symptom scores below the threshold of 15, at which a diagnosable disorder is likely. Thus, many of these individuals had so-called subsyndromal depression. Whether different strategies need to be used for individuals with different levels of symptoms is unknown and whether the distinction between subsyndromal and syndromal depression has utility cannot be stated from this study. The finding of a continuum of expense with increasing score would suggest that the categorical model of syndromic and subsyndromic might not have clinical utility. This is another area of importance to both clinicians and researchers.

P.V. Rabins, M.D., M.P.H.

Effectiveness of a Psychosocial Intervention, Interpersonal Counseling, for Subdysthymic Depression in Medically Ill Elderly
Mossey JM, Knott KA, Higgins M, et al (Hahnemann Univ, Philadelphia)
J Gerontol 51A:M172–M178, 1996 3–2

Background.—Subdysthymic depression occurs in up to half of hospitalized elderly patients. This is depression that can be detected by self-report depression scales but does not meet diagnostic criteria for major depression or dysthymia. Subdysthymic depression has been linked to physical and social disability, delayed recovery, and excessive use of health services. However, there is little information about these depressive symptoms or how they should be treated. Interpersonal counseling (IPC)—a form of short-term psychotherapy—was assessed as a treatment for subdysthymic depression in hospitalized elderly.

Methods.—The study included 76 hospitalized patients, age 60 or older, with subdysthymic depression. All had a Geriatric Depression Scale score of more than 10 but did not meet DSM-III-R criteria for major depression or dysthymia. They were randomly assigned to IPC or usual care (UC). The IPC group received individual counseling from a psychiatric clinical nurse specialist after hospital discharge. This was an interactive process focusing on "here and now" problems. The patients received up to 10 IPC sessions of up to 60 minutes in length. The 2 groups were compared at baseline and at 3, 6, and 12 months. The main outcomes measures were GDS scores, health ratings, and measures of physical and social functioning.

Results.—The 3-month assessment showed greater improvement in all variables for the IPC group, though the difference was not significant. By 6 months, the IPC group had a significant advantage: 61% had GDS scores of 10 or less, compared with 35% of the UC group (Table 3). The benefit of IPC was confirmed by multivariate analysis. Although this treatment had a significant positive effect on self-rated health, there was no significant improvement in physical or social functioning.

Conclusions.—Interpersonal counseling appears to be a useful treatment for medically ill elderly patients with subdysthymic depression. It effectively achieves short-term reduction of depressive symptoms with an

TABLE 3.—Proportion of Individuals in the IPC and UC Groups With GDS Scores Less Than 11 at 3 Months and 6 Months

	3 Months	6 Months
Interpersonal Counseling	46.7%	60.6%*
Usual Care	36.8	35.1

(Courtesy of Mossey JM, Knott KA, Higgins M, et al: Effectiveness of a psychosocial intervention, interpersonal counseling, for subdysthymic depression in medically ill elderly. *J Gerontol* 51A:M172–M178. Copyright 1996 the Gerontological Society of America.)

accompanying improvement in self-rated health. The authors recommend IPC for subdysthymic hospitalized elderly patients.

▶ The effectiveness of psychotherapy/counseling for the elderly remains a question in many practitioners' minds. This is a well-designed study demonstrating that a form of short-term psychotherapy, interpersonal counseling (IPC), is effective in a group of older subjects who had depressive symptoms but did not meet DSM-IV criteria for major depression or dysthymia. Because these subjects were ascertained from inpatient medical, surgical, orthopedic, and neurologic services, the findings are clearly relevant to the many patients with emotional distress treated in the primary care setting. However, this does not mean that the results are applicable only to individuals with medical illness, because we do not know the reason that these individuals were admitted to those services. Thus, this study confirms the efficacy of counseling intervention in individuals with comorbid medical and depressive symptomatology.

The authors note that more than 75% of individuals screened for the study did not have an elevated score on the Geriatric Depression Scale (GDS) (11 or higher). Thus, a substantial majority of individuals admitted to inpatient medical and surgical services do not suffer from depression. Why some individuals develop symptoms while others do not remains a mystery. The demonstration that the medically ill with depressive symptoms can be helped by short-term counseling is an important one that deserves wide notice.

P.V. Rabins, M.D., M.P.H.

Randomised Controlled Trial of Effect of Intervention by Psychogeriatric Team on Depression in Frail Elderly People at Home

Banerjee S, Shamash K, Macdonald AJD, et al (Inst of Psychiatry, London; St Thomas's Hosps, London)

BMJ 313:1058–1061, 1996 3–3

Objective.—Home care enables the disabled elderly to be maintained in their own households. Unfortunately, the prevalence of depression in these patients is estimated to range from 26% to 44%. Results of a randomized controlled trial of intervention by a psychogeriatric team in southeast London are presented.

Methods.—A multidisciplinary team, consisting of community psychiatric nurses, occupational therapists, senior and junior medical staff, a social worker, and a psychologist, evaluated 69 depressed home care patients (12 male), 65 or older, and randomly allocated them to intervention (n = 33) or to the control group (n = 36) which received medical care only. Six months later, the patients were interviewed by a blinded observer. Recovery from depression was based on the AGECAT rating system. Results were compared statistically.

Results.—At follow up 4 patients in the intervention group and 3 in the control group had died. At baseline 3 control patients and 4 intervention patients were receiving antidepressant drugs. At follow-up 5 control patients and 20 intervention patients were taking antidepressant drugs. During the study 2 control patients were referred to the psychiatric team. Three intervention patients and 1 control patient were admitted to a psychiatric facility. Nineteen intervention patients and 9 control patients recovered. Use of antidepressant drugs did not produce a significant treatment effect. Increasingly severe depression and first episode of depression were predictive of a worse outcome at 6 months.

Conclusion.—Only one fourth of the control group recovered in 6 months, indicating that the natural course of this disease is grim. The poor prognosis after a first episode of depression is probably the result of a combination of factors including many irreversible physical or social factors that limit recovery. Additional investigations need to be conducted to determine the degree to which these depressed patients can be managed and the cost associated with that management.

► The pressure to show the effectiveness of all medical treatment is mounting. This important study from Great Britain documents better effectiveness of psychiatric treatment of depression in community-residing older individuals compared with standard care—that is, the care provided by a general practitioner. Individuals in the psychiatric treatment group were 2½ times more likely to recover than those in the control group. This is not only a statistically significant difference but a clinically meaningful difference.

The study has many strengths. It identified individuals residing in the community by using standardized epidemiologic screening methodology and carefully diagnosed and used research criteria to carefully diagnose them. One of the strengths of the study is that it describes the types of treatments provided on this individualized basis. Rather than relying on a single protocol for treatment, treatment plans were those devised by a care team. Thus, the study has the strength of examining a standard psychiatric team's use of pharmacotherapy, social therapy, and psychotherapy, depending on the needs of the particular individual.

The study makes the important point that spontaneous remission rates were infrequent, with only 25% of the control group recovering in 6 months. The authors also emphasize that therapeutic nihilism is inappropriate because 58% of the intervention group recovered.

The authors do not note one major limitation of this study: Although it is described as a comparison of care by a psychiatric team to standard care, the physicians of the patients in the control group were not notified that they were depressed. Thus, this is really a study that compares individuals referred to a psychiatric team for treatment of depression to individuals in general practice whose doctor may be unaware that they are depressed. The general practitioners were notified that their patient was a control in the study and that this should not affect the patient's management. This is an important study because it shows the effectiveness of treating major depression in community residing individuals as opposed to self-selected and highly unrepresentative samples that are usually included in treatment trials. The need to educate the public and primary care physicians about the treatability of major depression should remain a high priority.

P.V. Rabins, M.D., M.P.H.

Complicated Grief as a Disorder Distinct From Bereavement-Related Depression and Anxiety: A Replication Study

Prigerson HG, Bierhals AJ, Kasl SV, et al (Univ of Pittsburgh, Pa; Yale Univ, New Haven, Conn)

Am J Psychiatry 153:1484–1486, 1996 3–4

Introduction.—Recent findings indicate that symptoms of complicated grief are distinct from those of bereavement-related depression and anxiety in older adults. The symptoms of bereavement-related depression lessen over time, but the symptoms of complicated grief persist despite the passage of time and treatment with tricyclic antidepressants. One-hundred fifty individuals were interviewed 6 months after their deceased spouses' hospital admission to determine whether symptoms of complicated grief

TABLE 1.—Factor Loadings for Complicated Grief, Depression, and Anxiety of Bereaved Spouses at 6-Month Assessment (N = 135)*

Symptom	Loading on Factor 1 (Complicated Grief)†	Loading on Factor 2 (Depression)†	Loading on Factor 3 (Anxiety)†
Blues last week	0.07	**0.66**	−0.16
Depressed last week	0.10	**0.71**	−0.31
Everything an effort last week	0.13	**0.57**	−0.16
Happy last week	0.03	**−0.70**	0.15
Enjoyed life last week	−0.04	**−0.65**	0.17
Restlessness	−0.00	−0.14	**0.51**
Anxiousness	−0.18	−0.22	**0.52**
Nervousness	−0.13	−0.22	**0.81**
Fear of abandonment	−0.17	−0.30	**0.46**
Worried	0.04	−0.09	**0.54**
Yearns for spouse as before illness	**0.62**	0.21	0.02
Is preoccupied with thoughts of spouse	**0.68**	0.26	−0.10
Needs to call spouse's name	**0.73**	0.07	−0.27
Is drawn to associations with spouse	**0.71**	0.15	−0.12
Has mental images of spouse	**0.82**	−0.02	−0.08
Hears things associated with spouse	**0.80**	−0.10	−0.09
Feels spouse's presence	**0.82**	−0.02	−0.08
Dreams of spouse	**0.69**	−0.04	−0.06
Is unable to accept spouse's illness/death	**0.68**	0.17	−0.12
Has pain in same area as spouse	**0.77**	−0.03	0.02
Feels just like spouse	**0.50**	0.23	0.12

*Fifteen of the 150 cases were deleted because of missing data.
†Highest loadings are in bold underline.

(Courtesy of Prigerson HG, Bierhals AJ, Kasl SV, et al: Complicated grief as a disorder distinct from bereavement-related depression and anxiety: A replication study. *Am J Psychiatry* 153:1484–1486.

constitute a unique form of emotional distress distinct from the symptoms of bereavement-related depression and anxiety.

Methods.—In 150 individuals whose spouses died within 6 months of hospitalization, intensive face-to-face interviews were conducted upon spouses' hospital admission and 6 weeks, 6 months, 13 months, and 25 months after hospitalization. Rating scales were used to measure complicated grief, depression, and anxiety.

Results.—There were 3 distinct symptom dimensions: complicated grief, bereavement-related depression, and bereavement-related anxiety (Table 1). Symptoms of complicated grief predicted different mental and physical health outcomes from symptoms of bereavement-related depression and anxiety.

Conclusions.—Symptoms of complicated grief formed a distinctly different dimension from bereavement-related emotional distress. Findings suggest that the symptoms of complicated grief form a distinct clinical entity.

▶ In one of his best known and most widely cited papers, *Mourning and Melancholia*, Sigmund Freud suggested that grief and depression are intimately related. While he could not find parallels for every symptom of major depression (he particularly noted early morning awakening and guilt), he laid the groundwork for the formulation of Abraham that depression is grief and anger "turned inward."

This study confirms earlier findings by this group that major depression which develops in the context of grief has different symptomatology than grief. It adds further evidence to the suggestion that major depression, grief, and anxiety are different conditions. Table 1 shows the distinctions among the 3 factors and the relative independence of the 3 factors. These factors have face validity as well as statistical validity.

Of course Freud's formulation could still be correct—it is still possible that grief develops into major depression in some individuals and that the latter is just a more severe form of the former. However, the fact that the 3 factors in this study were identified in the same individuals does not support this interpretation. In addition, it should be noted that complicated grief and uncomplicated grief have significant overlap. This finding along with other work by this group showing that some symptoms respond to tricyclic antidepressants[1] also suggests that grief is a universal syndrome, whereas major depression is confined to some individuals.

P.V. Rabins, M.D., M.P.H.

Reference

1. Pasternak RE, Reynolds C, Schlernitzauer MA, et al: Open-trial nortriptyline therapy of bereavement-related depression in late life. *J Clin Psychiatry* 52:307–310, 1991.

Clinically Defined Vascular Depression

Alexopoulos GS, Meyers BS, Young RC, et al (Cornell Univ, New York; Cornell Inst of Geriatric Psychiatry, White Plains, NY)

Am J Psychiatry 154:562–565, 1997 3–5

Introduction.—There is a growing body of evidence to suggest that many patients with late-onset depression have neurologic brain disorders. Depression has been linked to damage of the basal ganglia and their connections to prefrontal structures. This type of damage can also cause a frontal lobe syndrome consisting of retardation, lack of insight, and impaired executive function. These types of signs and symptoms might therefore be expected in patients with vascular depression. The clinical findings of depressed elderly patients with and without risk factors for vascular depression were compared.

Methods.—The study included 65 consecutive elderly patients meeting the Research Diagnostic Criteria for major depression. Thirty-three had

TABLE 1.—Demographic and Clinical Characteristics of Elderly Patients With Vascular and Nonvascular Depression

	Patients With Vascular Depression (N=33)			Patients With Nonvascular Depression (N=32)		
Variable	N	Mean	SD	N	Mean	SD
Age (years)*	33	74.4	5.9	32	71.5	6.7
Disability (Multilevel Assessment Instrument score)	33	4.0	0.9	32	4.8	0.5
Dementia Rating Scale						
Total score	32	130.4	10.1	32	138.1	4.9
Fluency (words from C, F, or W in 1 minute [21])	32	35.9	10.9	32	41.1	9.6
Visual retention (recognition of Benton visual stimulus cards from a matrix of four cards)	29	6.2	2.1	26	7.8	1.9
Verbal memory (d' from 14-item Mattis-Kovner scale [22])	31	2.4	1.0	32	2.7	0.7
Comprehension (tokens of two shapes, two sizes, and five colors [20])	30	13.7	3.1	28	15.0	1.3
Visual naming (identification of 30 line drawings [21])	33	48.2	8.8	32	52.3	6.5
Construction: drawing clock (% abnormal)	33	36.3	27.6	32	15.6	20.5
Construction: copying Bender-Gestalt hexagon (% abnormal)	33	33.3	27.1	32	12.5	20.0
17-item Hamilton Depression Rating Scale						
Total score	33	25.96	6.76	32	27.00	5.95
Retardation	33	0.79	1.10	32	0.34	0.70
Agitation	33	0.12	0.33	32	0.41	0.61
Guilt feelings	33	1.03	0.92	32	1.50	0.72
Lack of insight	33	0.42	0.61	32	0.19	0.47

Note: The ratio of women to men in the group with vascular depression was 2.3:1, and in the group with nonvascular depression it was 1.5:1 ($\chi^2 = 0.75$, $df = 1$, n.s.).

*$t = 1.88$, $df = 63$, $P < 0.07$.

Abbreviation: n.s., nonsignificant

risk factors for vascular depression, as indicated by a vascular score of 1–4 on the Cumulative Illness Rating Scale—Geriatrics. The other 32 patients had no such risk factors. The clinical presentations of the 2 groups were compared, including cognitive deficits, disability, and depressive symptoms.

Results.—Cognitive impairment and disability were greater for the patients with vascular depression. This group also had increased retardation and reduced agitation, along with impairments in fluency and naming. Guilt feelings were relatively lower and lack of insight greater in the patients with vascular depression.

Conclusions.—This study demonstrates a distinct clinical profile associated with vascular depression in the elderly (Table 1). The symptoms identified are similar to those expected with damage to the striato-pallido-thalamo-cortical pathway and other areas. Vascular depression may prove to be a distinct syndrome that requires a different treatment approach. If so, then identification of its clinical profile could be important to treatment decision making.

▶ This study uses an operational definition of "vascular depression" and demonstrates that individuals meeting the criteria are more cognitively and functionally impaired than subjects with Alzheimer's disease. This offers some validation for the concept of vascular depression that George Alexopoulos has been championing. The development of specific criteria that rely on the Cumulative Illness Rating Scale-Geriatrics is a strength of this paper and an advancement in this field. The clear definition employed here should allow validation by other methods such as treatment response, neuroimaging, and long-term prognosis. The authors are right to point out that the study does not establish vascular dementia as the cause of the impairment. Their suggestion that vascular damage to pathways linking basal ganglia to frontal lobes might lead to both cognitive and mood impairment is an important hypothesis which deserves attention and further study.

P.V. Rabins, M.D., M.P.H.

MRI-defined Vascular Depression

Krishnan KRR, Hays JC, Blazer DG (Duke Univ, Durham, NC)
Am J Psychiatry 154:497–501, 1997 3–6

Background.—Risk factors for late-life onset of depression are not well understood. Genetic factors appear to be less important in this type of depression, whereas structural brain changes, especially vascular or ischemic changes, seem to be more important. The term "vascular depression" has been used to describe depression related to multiple infarcts in the brain. The clinical and demographic features of vascular depression were reported.

Methods.—Eighty-nine depressed patients were classified as having vascular (32 patients) or nonvascular (57 patients) depression based on brain

MR images. All patients were enrolled at the National Institute of Mental Health Clinical Research Center for the Study of Depression in Later Life.

Findings.—In bivariate analyses and a fully adjusted logistic regression model, patients with vascular depression were more likely to be older, to have a late age at onset, and to have a nonpsychotic subtype of depression compared with patients with nonvascular depression. Patients with vascular depression less often had a family history of mental illness. Anhedonia and functional disability were somewhat more common in patients with vascular depression.

Conclusion.—A better understanding of the profile of patients with vascular depression is needed. Such understanding is likely to result in better treatments for such patients.

▶ Forty years ago, Martin Roth[1] suggested that some cases of late onset dementia were likely to have a vascular cause. Similar suggestions were made even earlier by Kraepelin. This is 1 of the first modern studies to look at this issue and to use modern neuroimaging methods. Krishnan and colleagues used MRI to identify a group of individuals with major depression and significant brain vascular disease. They found that individuals thus defined as having "vascular depression" were older, were more like to have nonpsychotic depression, were less likely to have a family history of depression, and were more likely to be functionally disabled.

Several lines of evidence suggest linkages between depression and brain vascular disease. Robert Robinson[2] has demonstrated that frontal stroke has a high likelihood of inducing major depression. Some studies suggest that late-life onset depressives have more brain white matter disease changes on MRI than earlier-onset patients, although this has not always been replicated. As cited in this paper, Fujikawa and colleagues[3] found silent strokes in a number of older individuals with major depression.

Just how "late onset" depressions should be defined is controversial. In this study, vascular disease risk factors were risk factors for onset of depression after age 40 but not when the cutoff was set at 45 or 50 years. This would be a young age to choose if ones interest is the elderly. It is not clear whether this cutoff point was chosen a priori. However, in the logistic regression, age older than 59 was also associated with a higher prevalence of vascular depression.

Major depression is multifactorial. Genetic factors, life events, systemic disease, and drugs such as reserpine and steroids can induce major depressive disorder. The idea that atherosclerosis is linked to many psychiatric disorders of aging is not new, and this hypothesis had been discredited. Clearly, the hypothesis deserves a new and more careful look.

P.V. Rabins, M.D., M.P.H.

References

1. Roth MR, Kay DWK: Affective disorders arising in the senium: II. Physical disability as an etiologic factor. *J Ment Sci* 102:141–150, 1956.

2. Robinson RG, Kubos KL, Starr KL, et al: Mood disorders in stroke patients. *Brain* 107:81–93, 1984.
3. Fujikawa T, Tamawaki S, Touhouda Y: Incidence of silent cerebral infarction in patients with major depression. *Stroke* 24:1631–1634, 1993.

MRI Signal Hyperintensities in Geriatric Depression

Greenwald BS, Kramer-Ginsberg E, Krishnan KRR, et al (Long Island Jewish Med Ctr, Glen Oaks, NY; Albert Einstein College of Medicine, Bronx, NY; Duke Univ, Durham, NC)

Am J Psychiatry 153:1212–1215, 1996 3–7

Introduction.—Previous reports have described magnetic resonance imaging (MRI) signal intensities in the brains of elderly people, including healthy subjects and those with dementia. Some of these studies have suggested that more severe and more frequent hyperintensities are related to geriatric depression—particularly late-onset depression—but the specificity and significance of these changes remains uncertain. The meaning and associations of MRI signal hyperintensities in the elderly were studied.

Methods.—MRI brain scans were obtained in 2 groups of elderly people: 48 with DSM-III-R depression and 39 controls. The 2 groups were demographically similar. Two established rating systems were used to compare periventricular and subcortical signal hyperintensities in these groups. The analysis sought to determine whether the signal hyperintensities could distinguish between depressed and nondepressed elderly people and whether they could be linked to any clinical variables.

Results.—The depressed group had significantly more severe hyperintensity ratings in the subcortical gray matter than their nondepressed counterparts. This was the only significant difference on comparison of the MRI scans; there was no difference in periventricular or deep white matter hyperintensities. There was no difference in subcortical gray matter hyperintensities for subjects with similar current ages and cerebrovascular disease risk who had early- vs. late-onset depression.

Conclusions.—The subcortical gray matter hyperintensities are more severe in elderly people with depression than in nondepressed elderly controls. The results add weight to the theory the basal ganglia is involved in depression and geriatric depression. However, the previously reported link between late-onset depression and MRI hyperintensities is more likely related to cerebrovascular disease risk and age.

► An association between depression in the elderly and white matter hyperintensities on MRI scans has been widely reported. This study, from Long Island Jewish Medical Center and Duke University, confirms that older patients with depression have more severe hyperintensities in the subcortical gray matter. More important, however, the study found that when age and cerebrovascular risk factors are controlled for, cerebrovascular disease may be explanatory. Thus, these results suggest that cerebrovascular disease may cause both white matter hyperintensities and increase the likelihood of depression. This confirms a hypothesis stated 40 years ago by Martin Roth and David Kay.[1]

The authors also replicate the finding that hyperintensities involving basal ganglia may be particularly important in inducing depression. Given the high rates of mood disorder in patients with Parkinson's disease and Huntington's disease, 2 diseases in which the basal ganglia are involved, this finding supports the importance of the subcortical structures in development of mood disorder. A relationship between white matter hyperintensities and hypertension is well established, but hypertension does not explain all hyperintensities and remain undiscovered. Therefore, the possibility that white matter hyperintensities result from brain vascular disease and that the vascular disease triggers late-life onset depression remains plausible.

P.V. Rabins, M.D., M.P.H.

Reference

1. Roth MR, Kay DWK: Affective disorder arising in the senium: II. Physical disability as an aetiological factor. *J Men Sci* 102:141–150, 1956.

Cognition and White Matter Hyperintensities in Older Depressed Patients

Lesser IM, Boone KB, Mehringer CM, et al (Harbor-UCLA Med Ctr, Torrance, Calif)

Am J Psychiatry 153:1280–1287, 1996 3–8

Background.—The magnetic resonance imaging (MRI) finding of subcortical white matter hyperintensities has been linked to various psychiatric disorders in the elderly, particularly depression. Reports disagree as to the relation between white matter hyperintensities and cognitive function as well as about the cognitive function of elderly patients with major depression. The link between white matter hyperintensities and cognitive function was evaluated in older adults with depression.

Methods.—Three groups of adults over 50 were studied: 60 patients with current depression in whom depression first developed after age 50; 35 patients with depression in whom depression first developed before age 35; and 165 controls without psychiatric illness. All subjects underwent MRI with measurement of the area of white matter hyperintensity, and neuropsychologic tests.

Results.—The area of white matter hyperintensity was greater in patients with late-onset depression than in either of the other 2 groups. Cognitive scores were lower in the depressed patients than in the controls, including the domains of nonverbal intelligence, nonverbal memory, constructional ability, executive ability, and information processing speed. Mainly the patients with late-onset depression had cognitive abnormalities. Patients with large areas of white matter hyperintensity had significantly reduced executive skills, although most of these scores did not reach the level of significant impairment.

Conclusions.—Elderly patients with late-onset depression are more likely to have large areas of white matter hyperintensity than either non-depressed controls or elderly patients with early-onset depression. Patients with both types of depression have mild reductions in certain cognitive skills associated with the right hemisphere. In addition, those with late-onset depression have reduced information processing speed and executive functions. Executive function is significantly reduced in patients with large areas of white matter hyperintensity.

▶ This study explores the relation between white matter changes on MRI and cognitive performance in older individuals with depression. This has proven to be a complicated issue because studies among "normal" older individuals have only inconsistently found relations between the extent of white matter change and cognitive performance. The authors' finding that cognitive impairment was greatest in individuals with late-onset depression and that white matter was more involved in late-onset cases raises the question of whether the white matter lesions and the late-onset depression are both caused by the same factors becomes important. As reviewed above, Greenwald et al. (Abstract 3–7) also present data supporting this relation.

These studies raise the possibility that the prevention of cerebrovascular disease by earlier recognition and treatment of hypertension, diabetes, and hyperlipidemia might diminish the incidence of late-life depression is a distinct possibility. Such efforts must begin earlier in life. An important study by Skoog and co-workers[1] from Scandinavia demonstrates that blood pressure measured in early and mid-adulthood predicts the development of dementia. Other studies by this group[2] further support the link between mid-life hypertension and the development of late-life dementia. A link between mid-life hypertension and depression is not demonstrated by these studies, but the possibility that mid-life cerebrovascular disease leads to the development of both depression and dementia in late life remains.

P.V. Rabins, M.D., M.P.H.

References

1. Skoog I, Lernfelt B, Landahl S, et al: A 15-year longitudinal study of blood pressure and dementia. *Lancet* 347:1141–1145, 1996.
2. Skoog I, Palmertz B, Andreasson LA: The prevalence of white-matter lesions on computed tomography of the brain in demented and nondemented 85-year-olds. *J Geriatr Psychiatry Neurol* 7:169–175, 1994.

Longitudinal Analysis of the Association Between Depressive Symptomatology and Cognitive Deterioration

Dufouil C, Fuhrer R, Dartigues J-F, et al (INSERM U360, Paris; INSERM U330, Bordeaux, France)

Am J Epidemiol 144:634–641, 1996 3–9

Purpose.—It has long been suggested that there is a link between depression and dementia in the elderly. However, the nature of this association is undetermined; it is unknown which comes first, depressive symptoms or cognitive impairment. This longitudinal study assessed the risk of cognitive deterioration in elderly people with a high level of depressive symptoms.

Methods.—The prospective study included a community-based cohort of 1,600 noninstitutionalized elderly. They were assessed at baseline and at 3 years' follow-up. The assessment included the Mini-Mental State Examination (MMSE), with cognitive deterioration defined as a decline of at least 5 points between the 2 assessments. Depressive symptoms were evaluated on the Center for Epidemiologic Studies Depression (CES-D) Scale.

Results.—Level of depressive symptoms was significantly associated with cognitive function at both study time points. Subjects with a high level of depressive symptoms were at increased risk of cognitive impairment (odds ratio 2.6). However, a high level of depressive symptoms did not predict cognitive deterioration at follow up (relative risk 0.8). This was so even after sensitivity analysis was carried out because of the high proportion of nonresponders at follow-up. Subjects receiving psychotropic medications did appear to have a higher rate of cognitive deterioration.

Conclusions.—This longitudinal study indicates that the link between depressive symptoms and poor cognitive functioning is cross-sectional in nature. Although the results could be affected by selection bias, any effect in which high depressive symptoms led to cognitive deterioration would be weak. Epidemiologic studies of cognitive function should adjust for concomitant depressive symptoms.

► The frequent co-occurrence of cognitive impairment and depressive symptoms in the elderly remains a clinical challenge and unexplained. Among the explanations for this higher than expected co-occurrence are the hypotheses that dementing illnesses such as Alzheimer's disease may present first with depressive symptoms and only later manifest as major depression, that prior major depression may predispose to the development of cognitive disorder, and that a third factor, such as cerebrovascular disease, causes both depression and a dementing illness to develop.[1]

Contrary to what would be predicted if depression were a common precursor or predisposition to dementia, this study did not find that high levels of depressive symptomatology predict the development of dementia at 3 years. The authors suggest that other studies which have found a relationship between cognitive impairment and depressive symptomatology are cross-sectional in nature. Although the authors discuss several limitations to the study, including differential attrition rates over 3 years in individuals with cognitive disorder, depressive symptoms, or neither, they attempt to control for attrition. Another possible limitation is the 3-year length of the follow-up. Although some studies (including one by this reviewer) have not found that individuals with both cognitive and depressive symptoms have a higher likelihood of developing dementia within 2 years, Alexopoulous[2] has found at 5 years of follow-up that in many individuals with co-existing depressive and cognitive symptoms dementia had developed. Therefore, this study cannot be taken as the final word on this topic. Because it is a community-based sample rather than a clinically ascertained sample, the difference between its results and the study of Alexopoulous could be due to sampling differences.

P.V. Rabins, M.D., M.P.H.

References

1. Reifler BV. Mixed cognitive-affective disturbances in the elderly. *J Clin Psychiatry* 47:354–356, 1986.
2. Alexopoulous GS, Myers BS, Young RC, et al: The course of geriatric depression without 'reversible dementia': A controlled study. *Am J Psychiatry* 150:1393–1399, 1993.

Qualitative Magnetic Resonance Imaging Findings in Geriatric Depression: Possible Link Between Later-onset Depression and Alzheimer's Disease?

Greenwald BS, Kramer-Ginsberg E, Bogerts B, et al (Long Island Jewish Med Ctr, Glen Oaks, NY; Albert Einstein College of Medicine, New York)
Psychol Med 27:421–431, 1997 3–10

Background.—Depression in elderly patients may be related to pathologic changes in the brain. Elderly patients were examined with qualititative MRI to evaluate specific brain regions, in a case-control study.

Methods.—Thirty elderly persons with depression (per *Diagnostic and Statistical Manual of Mental Disorders*, ed 3, revised and Hamilton Depression Rating Scale criteria) were matched with 36 elderly control subjects without depression. Clinical data included cerebrovascular risk factors and age at onset of first depressive episode (early onset at age 60 or younger, late onset at older than 60). Magnetic resonance imaging scans were obtained throughout the coronal plane in 3 × 1–mm contiguous slices. An investigator blinded to the image source used a 4-point qualitative scale (normal to severe) to grade brain findings in these instances: lateral ventricle enlargement, third ventricle enlargement, global cortical atrophy, medial temporal atrophy, and caudate atrophy.

Findings.—Elderly depressed patients and their matched controls had no significantly different brain findings in any region examined. However, when the elderly patients with early-onset depression were compared with those with late-onset depression, the latter had more abnormalities; this difference was significant in the left caudate and left medial temporal regions. In the depressed group as a whole, data supported a significant relationship between left medial atrophy and cognitive impairment. The MRI findings did not correlate with cerebrovascular risk factors.

Conclusions.—Structural brain changes were nonspecific for assessing depression in these elderly patients. However, the significant changes in the left medial temporal region in elderly patients with late-onset depression may indicate that such patients have undetected Alzheimer's disease, and further research is warranted. Given the lack of correlation between cerebrovascular risk factors and brain changes, other pathophysiologic contributions are at work.

▶ The struggle to find consistent differences on MRI scans in elderly depressive patients continues. In this study of 30 elderly individuals with major depression and 36 controls, there were no significant differences based on regional analyses. However, late-onset cases had greater left medial temporal and left caudate abnormality than early-onset cases.

The authors review some of the reasons for the many conflicting findings in the literature. These include differences in samples and differences in techniques. The lack of consistency is frustrating, but the evidence that there are structural brain changes in elderly individuals with major depression is clear. One reason for inconsistency that the authors do not cite is that many studies, including this one, do not state hypotheses a priori but do not correct for multiple comparisons.

The interesting findings in this study are the links between medial temporal atrophy, caudate atrophy, and later age of onset as well as the correlation between greater atrophy in these structures and cognitive dysfunction. As the authors note, atrophy in these structures has been reported in other studies of elderly depressive patients. They suggest that atrophy in these structures may identify individuals at risk for dementia on follow-up.

Quantitative measurements are now the norm in neuroimaging studies. It will be important to determine whether these findings can be confirmed in prospective quantitative examinations. Long-term follow-ups to determine the prognostic significance of these findings will be of great interest.

P.V. Rabins, M.D., M.P.H.

Suicidal Ideation Among Older Primary Care Patients

Callahan CM, Hendrie HC, Nienaber NA, et al (Indiana Univ, Indianapolis; Ricard L Roudebush VA Med Ctr, Indianapolis)

J Am Geriatr Soc 44:1205–1209, 1996 3–11

Objective.—Suicide is the ninth leading cause of death in the U.S., and the elderly have the highest rate. Although identifying patients at risk has focused on characteristics of suicidal ideation, such patients are rare. The frequency of ideation, the severity of depressive symptoms and functional impairment, and the 1-year mortality were studied in a group of older patients with significant symptoms of depression.

Methods.—Between January 1991 and July 1993, 301 patients age 60–102 with depression and a random sample of 101 patients without depression were included in a randomized clinical study to identify and refer patients with suicidal ideation on the basis of responses to the HAM-D test. Demographic and clinical characteristics of patients with depressive symptoms and no suicidal ideation, depressive symptoms and suicidal ideation, and patients with no depressive symptoms and no suicidal ideation were statistically compared. Patients were followed for 12 months.

Results.—Fourteen of the 301 patients with CES-D scores of at least 16 were categorized as suicidal at sometime during the study period and reported suicidal ideation. The prevalence of suicidal ideation based on CES-D scores between 12 and 16 was estimated to range from 0.7% to 1.2% for this cohort. All 14 patients had an affective disorder, and all but 1 had a moderate to severe functional impairment. Four of 14 patients were diagnosed with major depression. Suicide plans consisted of handgun for 4 patients, medication overdose for 3, car accident in 2, and handgun or car accident in 1. There were no significant differences between depressed suicidal patients and depressed non-suicidal patients with respect to age, sex, race, education, alcoholism, cognitive impairment, or depressive scores. There were no deaths during the study.

Conclusion.—The prevalence of suicidal ideation in this cohort ranged from 0.7% to 1.2%, but approached 5% in the group with major depressive symptoms. The only way to identify patients with suicidal ideation is to ask them whether they are having such thoughts, particularly if they have symptoms of depression or anxiety.

▶ This study examines the relationship between suicidal ideation and depression in a sample of patients identified in a primary care group practice. Its finding that all patients with suicidal ideation have some symptoms of a depressive disorder is important. Equally important is the finding that only 4 of 14 patients with suicidal ideation met diagnostic criteria for major depression; that is, a majority of patients with suicideal ideation and depressive symptoms did not meet standardized criteria and are at higher likelihood of being undiagnosed if a rigid definition of major depression is required for treatment.

Although this study finds an association between depressive symptoms and suicidal ideation, it can not be used as evidence that all individuals who commit suicide suffer from major depression. Indeed, although research shows that upwards of 90% of individuals who commit suicide do suffer from either a mood disorder or substance abuse disorder, a small percentage, not all individuals do. Nevertheless, this study is very important in showing that among those attending a general practice the association is high. The importance of this reinforces the finding noted by Eli Robins more than 35 years ago: a significant proportion (about 75% in most studies) of individuals who successfully commit suicide have visited their primary care physician in the prior several weeks.[1]

Fortunately, none of the patients identified as having suicidal ideation had committed suicide. Therefore, we can not yet conclude that earlier recognition of depression will lower the high suicide rates in older individuals. However, this suggestion is plausible enough to suggest that major efforts should be made to identify individuals at risk for suicide, to carefully assess them for treatment of depression, and to carefully observe their progress or lack thereof.

P.V. Rabins, M.D., M.P.H.

Reference

1. Robins E, Murphy GE, Wilkinson RH, et al: Some clinical consideration in the prevention of suicide based on a study of 124 successful suicides. *Am J Public Health* 49:888–899, 1959.

Attempted Suicide by Chinese Elderly in Hong Kong

Chiu HFK, Lam LCW, Pang AHT, et al (Chinese Univ, Hong Kong)
Gen Hosp Psychiatry 18:444–447, 1996 3–12

Introduction.—Despite the strong association between age and suicide, nonfatal suicide behavior in the elderly has been a neglected area of research. There is a lack of information about the Chinese elderly, who reportedly have a higher rate of suicide than Indian or Malay elderly. In China, the suicide rate for the general population was 13.3 per 100,000, and for the elderly population, it was 40 per 100,000 in 1994. The elderly suicide rate in China is double that of the United States. The characteristics of a sample of elderly individuals who attempted suicide were examined, along with the rate of subsequent repetition and completed suicide.

Methods.—During a 2½ year period, 55 elderly individuals with suicidal attempts in a psychiatric unit in Hong Kong were studied. They were followed up by telephone and letter to examine the rate of repetition and to determine their current condition. Researchers also obtained information from relatives and examined medical notes and death registries.

Results.—During the follow-up portion, 43 patients or 78.2% were successfully contacted. There were 34 women and 21 men. Thirty-one were married, 16 widowed, 5 divorced or separated, and 8 were single. The mean age was 72.8 ± 6.7 years. Self-injury accounted for 72.7% of the suicidal attempts and drug overdose accounted for 27.3%. Ingestion of corrosive or detergent was the most common means of self-injury (32.5%), followed by jumping from a height (16.3%), wrist-cutting (11.6%), hanging (9.3%), and drowning (7%). Psychotropic drugs (60%) were the most common drugs used with benzodiazepines accounting for 77.8% of attempts. Significant physical illness, mainly cardiovascular, respiratory, or other chronic physical problems, was seen in the majority of patients (76.4%). A mood disorder was evident in nearly half (49.1%) of the patients. Of the 55 patients, 2 attempted further suicide and 3 committed suicide within a year.

Conclusion.—In Hong Kong, attempted suicide among the elderly is a major problem. A decline in the elderly's socioeconomic status has resulted in the past decades from the absence of a pension system, and the changing structure of the family from an extended to a nuclear one, together with the erosion of traditional Chinese norms and expectations of filial piety. Prospective studies of the factors associated with attempted and completed suicide in Chinese elderly are necessary to formulate rational preventive and therapeutic strategies.

► The high rates of suicide among the elderly are of major public health concern. The significant variability in rates across cultures and nations suggests that culture must play an important role in the genesis of suicidal behavior. This study focuses on a case series of individuals hospitalized in Hong Kong. There are more women than men. Approximately half the patients suffered from a mood disorder but 36.4% had no psychiatric illness. This latter figure is higher than that reported in Great Britain and the United States.

One useful piece of data is the follow-up of 78.2% of cases; 5.5% committed suicide and 3.6% had made another attempt. All completed suicides occurred within 1 year of the index attempt. The number of completed suicides was too small to analyze statistically.

Cultural influences on the behavior of suicide are significant but some elements appear to be present in suicide across cultures. For example, there is a strong relationship between suicide and major depression everywhere. On the other hand, there are large differences by sex and method of attempt, and the latter is linked to likelihood of completion. The high prevalence of depression throughout the world suggests that many suicides are potentially and appropriately preventable. Clinicians not only must be alert to the high rates of suicide in elderly individuals with major depression but also must emphasize to the public the rarity of suicide as a rational act.

P.V. Rabins, M.D., M.P.H.

Major Depression and Refusal of Life-sustaining Medical Treatment in the Elderly

Hooper SC, Vaughan KJ, Tennant CC, et al (Hornsby Ku Ring Gai Hosp, Sydney, Australia; Royal North Shore Hosp, Sydney, Australia; Univ of Western Sydney, Australia)

Med J Aust 165:416–419, 1996 3–13

Objective.—Despite the advances in medical treatment that allow very sick patients to remain alive much longer, many refuse such treatment. The effect of depression on decisions to refuse treatment has not been studied. Results of a study on the effect of recovery from major depression on decisions about life-sustaining treatment in a group of patients in an Australian community psychogeriatric service are reported.

Methods.—Between October 1994 and January 1995, 22 patients (4 men), average age 76.9 and referred to the service for DSM-IV major depression, were included in the prospective case survey. The intensity of depression was measured on the Geriatric Depression Scale (GDS). Desire for life-sustaining treatment was assessed before and 6 weeks after treatment for depression. Recovery from depression was evaluated clinically at follow up. Baseline and follow-up score (after an average of 88.5 days) were compared statistically by means of the paired *t* test.

Results.—Four patients had been referred previously. Twelve were treated at home, 8 at an inpatient psychiatric facility, and 2 in a medical ward. Depression was severe in 5 patients, moderate in 16, and mild in 1. The mean GDS score decreased significantly from 24.4 at baseline to 16.7 at follow-up. Eighteen patients had improved GDS scores, and 12 of these were recovered. After treatment for depression there was a significant increase in desire for life-sustaining medical intervention, the number of medical interventions, and for "good prognosis" illness among all patients.

Conclusion.—There is an association between major depression and refusal of life-sustaining medical treatment in the elderly. After treatment for depression, patients are significantly more likely to desire life-sustaining medical intervention.

► Advanced directives have been promoted in the United States as a method of improving patient autonomy by clarifying the types of medical care that individuals would like to receive in the future if they were to develop life-threatening illnesses. Although many individuals have completed advanced directives, a majority have not. Much of the research in this area has focused on why people are not completing such directives. Some research has shown that there is significant variability over time in how individuals would like their advanced directives expressed.

Questions raised about advance directives are of particular interest to geriatric psychiatrists (1) because the patients they are treating often have significant medical and psychiatric co-morbidity, (2) because psychiatrists are experts in assessing whether individuals have capacity to make judgments, and (3) because the most common disorders treated by geriatric psychiatrists—major depression and dementia—can impair individuals' abilities to assess information and make choices. This study from Sydney, Australia, partially confirms and extends previous work done by Linda Ganzini and her colleagues at the VA hospital in Portland, Oregon. Ganzini and coworkers have shown that individuals with severe depression are at high likelihood of changing their preferences for basic treatment once they recover from the depression and that this change is almost always in the direction of desiring more medical care and a higher degree of intervention when they are not depressed.[1] This study by Hooper and coworkers complements that work. It confirms Ganzini's major finding (in a sample from another country) that individuals desire more life-sustaining treatments when they recover from a major depression. It also broadens the applicability of the results because it contains more women than the Ganzini studies. (Because the Ganzini studies have been done at the VA there were few women; in this study 82% of the subjects were women.) However, this study also differs from the Ganzini study in an important way. The finding that individuals with moderate depression are also likely to change their desires differ from Ganzini's findings which were limited to those with severe major depression.

These studies have important implications for clinicians and advocates for the elderly. They strongly suggest that any individual who is depressed should be urged not to complete an advance directive while depressed. Ideally, the document would have been completed earlier but individuals who have had depressions and who desire to complete such a document should do so when they are recovered. Because the prevalence of depression in the medically ill may be as high as 20%, these studies also raise the question of how carefully individuals completing advance directives in a medical setting should be screened for depression. Because screening questionnaires are not widely used or well accepted, this approach is not a solution. Perhaps the best we can do now is to alert clinicians to this issue and urge them to assess whether individuals are depressed when completing advanced directives.

An issue not addressed by either study is the meaningfulness of advance directives. This has received surprisingly little debate since they were proposed by the President's Commission as a solution to the widely perceived inadequacy of discussion between patients and their physicians on such an important issue. Studies such as this one should sensitize policy makers, clinicians, and the public at large to the fact that legislative solutions to difficult ethical and clinical matters are not easily solved by legislation or a piece of paper. Attention from both clinicians and researchers to increase patient autonomy, improve the comfort of clinicians and patients in discussing these difficult issues, and increase the involvement of family members in decisions about life-sustaining treatments in the severely ill should supplement efforts to increase rates of advance directives.

P.V. Rabins, M.D., M.P.H.

Reference

1. Lee M, Ganzini L: The effect of recovery from depression and preferences for life-sustaining therapy in older persons. *J Gerontol* 49:M15–M21, 1994.

High Relapse Rate After Discontinuaton of Adjunctive Medication for Elderly Patients With Recurrent Major Depression

Reynolds CF III, Frank E, Perel JM, et al (Univ of Pittsburgh, Pittsburgh, Pa)
Am J Psychiatry 153:1418–1422, 1996 3–14

Background.—Older patients may benefit as much from treatment with antidepressant medication as younger patients, although the response may be slower and such patients tend to relapse. This phenomenon raises questions about the use of adjunctive or augmented pharmacotherapy to bring about remission in patients who respond slowly or partially to primary pharmacotherapy. Unanswered questions about this issue include the percentage of older patients with depression who may need adjunctive medication, what happens after adjunctive treatment, whether patients given augmentation are more or less likely to relapse than patients not given augmentation, and how long adjunctive medication should be used.

Methods.—Outcome in 158 older patients with late-life recurrent major depression was examined: 39 patients received adjunctive medication during acute-phase pharmacotherapy because of a slow or partial response to nortriptyline, and 119 patients received no such adjunctive treatment. Adjunctive medication consisted of lithium, perphenazine, or paroxetine. Inpatient care was provided for 28 patients during acute-phase treatment.

Results.—The rate of response to acute therapy was lower in patients given adjunctive medication. Also, in these patients the relapse rate was higher during continuation therapy and the rate of sustained remission lower than that in patients who did not receive augmented therapy.

Conclusions.—In older patients with late-life recurrent major depression, augmentation therapy should be discontinued slowly to help prevent early relapse. These patients should also be monitored carefully during this time. It is possible that the combination of medication is more important than the actual dose in maintaining mental health in these patients.

▶ This descriptive study provides useful data regarding the discontinuation of adjunctive or augmentation pharmacotherapy in older individuals with recurrent major depression.

Some of the results seem predictable and almost circular. For example, the group given adjunctive medication had poorer response rates to initial therapy. Because adjunctive therapy usually indicates treatment-resistant cases, this finding seems tautologic. The higher relapse rates and lower rates of full recovery in patients given adjunctive treatment also demonstrate that patients requiring this treatment have a more severe form of mood disorder.

The finding that 52% of individuals relapsed after discontinuation of the augmentation treatment is important new information, and suggests that clinicians should be cautious in discontinuing such treatments. The authors suggest that augmentive treatments be tapered slowly when discontinuation is being considered. They also suggest that these treatments must be continued in many patients. This information adds to other data[1] suggesting that many patients require maintenance antidepressant treatment after an initial response. Future research will help us identify which patients should continue augmentive treatments, which patients should continue on primary antidepressant treatments, and which patients can stop treatment and when this discontinuation can be done with low likelihood of relapse.

P.V. Rabins, M.D., M.P.H.

Reference

1. Kupfer DJ, Frank E, Perel JM, et al: Five year outcome for maintenance therapies in recurrent major depressives. *Arch Gen Psychiatry* 49:769–773, 1992.

Estrogen Replacement and Response to Fluoxetine in a Multicenter Geriatric Depression Trial

Schneider LS, and the Fluoxetine Collaborative Study Group (Univ of Southern Calif, Los Angeles)

Am J Geriatr Psychiatry 5:97–106, 1997 3–15

Introduction.—Estrogen replacement therapy (ERT) may enhance mood-related symptoms and even facilitate effects of antidepressant medication. The effect of ERT on clinical response to fluoxetine was evaluated in 367 women aged 60 years or older who met DSM-III-R criteria for current unipolar major depression.

Methods.—Seventy-two women receiving ERT and 295 not receiving ERT were randomly and "blindly" assigned to either fluoxetine, 20 mg daily, or placebo for 6 weeks. Illness severity was measured weekly using the observer-rated, 21–item Ham-D (Ham-D_{21}) and the self-rated Geriatric Depression Scale.

Results.—Patients receiving ERT had a significantly greater treatment effect than patients receiving placebo. Patients receiving ERT and fluoxetine had greater Ham-D percentage improvement, compared with patients receiving ERT and placebo. Patients not on ERT did not experience significant benefit from fluoxetine, compared with patients not on ERT who received placebo.

Conclusions.—It may be that ERT or its lack may affect antidepressant response in appropriate age groups of women. More trials are needed before a definitive statement can be made regarding the use of ERT as an antidepressant alone or as an augmenter of antidepressant treatment in elderly female patients.

► This is a retrospective analysis that needs to be interpreted cautiously. Nevertheless, the case report literature contains reports that estrogen therapy can improve mood,[1] and a rapidly growing literature suggests that ERT may improve cognition and diminish the risk of developing dementia. This study suggests that greater attention needs to be given to the concomitant use of estrogen in drug trials in the study of antidepressant drugs.

Estrogen has multiple biological actions, and some of these have little or nothing to do with its action on the reproductive function. Estrogen is likely to act in several areas of the brain and upon several neurotransmitter systems.

However, it would be a mistake to use this retrospective analysis to recommend that estrogen replacement be used as an augmentive therapy in major depression. Prospective clinical trials are needed before any such recommendation can be made. The authors note this in their discussion but also note that it will be difficult to carry out such studies. They suggest that similar data might be present in other clinical trial databases, and some confirmation could be sought by reanalyzing such data sets.

P.V. Rabins, M.D., M.P.H.

Reference

1. Sherwin BB: Estrogen and refractory depression, in Amsterdam JA (ed): *Advances in Neuropsychiatry and Psychopharmacology*, vol 2. New York, Raven Press, 1991, pp 209–218.

Dementia

The Pathogenesis of Alzheimer Disease: An Alternative to the Amyloid Hypothesis

Terry RD (Univ of California—San Diego, La Jolla)
J Neuropathol Exp Neurol 55:1023–1025, 1996 3–16

Introduction.—Although various cellular structures are involved in Alzheimer's disease (AD), few reports have applied the principles of cell biology to this condition. Most of the discussion has focused on the effects of amyloid on brain tissue, to the exclusion of other potentially important causative mechanisms. The various chemical and structural changes of the brain that lead to dementia in AD were reviewed.

Pathogenesis of Alzheimer's Disease.—Most authors believe that amyloid deposition is the key pathogenetic mechanism of AD. This author believes that the condition is better explained on the basis of cytoskeletal abnormality. All 4 genes identified as being associated with AD are involved with the cytoskeleton. All cases of AD show destabilization of the cytoskeleton, with deficiency of formed microtubules within neurons and the formation of paired helical elements made of hyperphosphorylated tau. Axoplasmic flow would be disrupted by the loss of the microtubule system. Poor flow and dystrophic neurites would lead to synaptic loss, the consequences of which would include neuronal death. Synaptic loss would lead to topographic disconnections and characteristic dementia. Rather than being a central causative factor, amyloid plays only a peripheral role in this pathogenetic schema (Fig 1).

Discussion.—The author proposes that the cytoskeleton, rather than amyloid, plays the key role in the pathogenesis of AD. Destabilization of the cytoskeleton leads to loss of the microtubule system, decreased axoplasmic flow, synaptic degeneration, disconnection of cerebral functions, neuronal death, and, finally, dementia. This is a more coherent and satisfactory explanation than the widely accepted amyloid hypothesis.

► Much of the effort in discovering the pathobiology of AD has focused on abnormalities related to the amyloid precursor protein. This brief paper presents the view of Robert Terry, one of the pioneers in Alzheimer research, that cytoskeletal abnormalities should be studied as a common pathogenetic mechanism for all causes of AD. Terry reviews the evidence that all the known genetic causes lead to abnormalities in Golgi body processing of proteins, and he suggests that this leads to loss of synapses, death of neurons, and the neuropathology of AD.

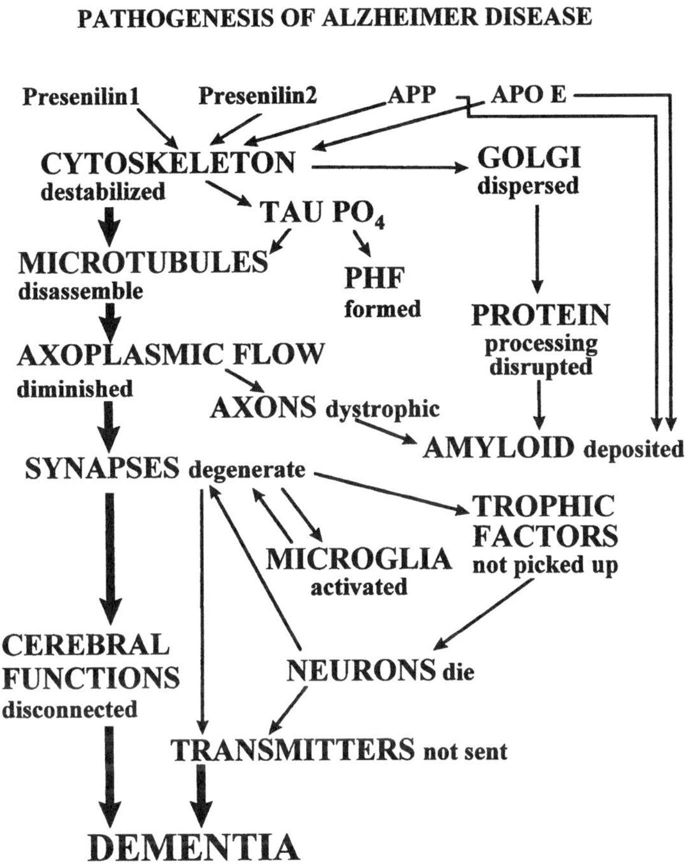

FIGURE 1.—Pathogenesis of Alzheimer's disease. *Abbreviation*: *APP*, amyloid precursor protein; *APO E*, apolipoprotein E. (Courtesy of Terry RD: The pathogenesis of Alzheimer disease: An alternative to the amyloid hypothesis. *J Neuropathol Exp Neurol* 55:1023–1025, 1996. Reproduced by permission from the *Journal of Neuropathology and Experimental Neurology*.)

It now seems clear that AD is best characterized as a syndrome in which multiple causes are operative. How and why these multiple causes lead to the pathology of AD are not known. Terry was the first to describe the neurofibrillary tangle as consisting of paired helical filaments. This article reminds us that the tangle—which is more unique to Alzheimer than is the plaque—deserves continued attention.

P.V. Rabins, M.D., M.P.H.

A Population-based Study on the Incidence of Dementia Disorders Between 85 and 88 Years of Age

Aevarsson O, Skoog I (Univ of Göteborg, Sweden)
J Am Geriatr Soc 44:1455–1460, 1996 3–17

Background.—There are fewer studies on the incidence than on the prevalence of dementia. Data on the incidence of dementia in the very elderly are particularly rare. Most of the available data suggest that the incidence of dementia increases in very old age. There is little information on the incidence of different types of dementia. The incidence of dementia from 85 to 88 years of age was assessed in a 3-year follow-up study.

Methods.—The prospective cohort study comprised a systematic sample of a birth cohort living in one Swedish city, whether in the community or in an institution. The subjects were age 85 at baseline and 88 when studied at follow-up. The evaluations included neuropsychiatric and neuropsychologic tests, interviews with key informants, and laboratory and imaging studies, included head computed tomography. Alzheimer's disease, vascular dementias, and other forms of dementia were diagnosed according to standard criteria.

Results.—The study began with an at-risk population of 347 nondemented subjects—243 women and 104 men. Adequate data were collected in about 92% of this group. Eighteen percent of subjects became demented during follow-up—the incidence of dementia was 61 per 1000 per year for men and 103 per 1000 per year for women. For specific types of dementia, incidence was 36 per 1000 per year for Alzheimer's disease, 39 per 1000 per year for vascular dementia, and 9 per 1000 per year for other types of dementia. By the end of the study, the severity of dementia was moderate to severe in most affected subjects.

Conclusions.—Nearly one tenth of elderly people who are nondemented at baseline will develop dementia between the ages of 85 and 88. The findings confirm the magnitude of dementia in the very old, which is the fastest-growing segment of the population. Each new case of dementia should be carefully evaluated to identify potentially treatable causes.

▶ One of the important remaining questions in the epidemiology of Alzheimer's disease and other dementias is whether incidence rates (the number of new cases per year) continues to increase after age 85 or 90. It is now well established that incidence rates are approximately 0.25% at age 65 and double every 5 years; thus, by age, incidence rates are approximately 4% per year. This study of a representative sample of cognitively normal 85-year-old residents of Gothenberg, Sweden, is a well-designed study and indicates that the incidence rate of dementia between ages 85 and 88 is 9%. Therefore, between age 85 and 90, incidence rates of dementia continue to rise with increasing age. This is an important finding and has relevance to such basic questions as, "What is normal aging?" and "What is the likely effect of the increasing life expectancy and the increasing number of individuals living into their early and mid-ninth decade on the prevalence of dementia?"

One finding that has been consistent from the Scandinavian studies but is not confirmed in U.S. studies is that the number of cases with Alzheimer's dementia and with vascular dementia is similar. In this study, the incidence of each is 6.3% to 6.9% per year. However, these diagnoses were based on clinical data and neuroimaging studies. Even though there is a high degree of reliability (i.e., agreement) among those making diagnoses in the study, there is no neuropathologic information of the validity of their diagnoses. The authors' statement, "Distinguishing between Alzheimer's disease and vascular dementia is often difficult" is certainly true; in fact, no research center has published a study to demonstrate that it can reliably diagnose vascular dementia when neuropathologic studies are used as the standard. Therefore, the rates of vascular dementia reported may not be accurate. On the other hand, the reliability of diagnosing dementia is in the acceptable range and their overall incidence figure (9%) is likely to be an accurate one.

P.V. Rabins, M.D., M.P.H.

Longitudinal Assessment of Symptoms of Depression, Agitation, and Psychosis in 181 Patients With Alzheimer's Disease

Levy ML, Cummings JL, Fairbanks LA, et al (Univ of California, Los Angeles; West Los Angeles VA Med Ctr; Sigma Tau Pharmaceuticals, Gaithersburg, Md)

Am J Psychiatry 153:1438–1443, 1996 3–18

Introduction.—Neuropsychiatric disturbances (such as depression, psychosis, and agitation) in patients with Alzheimer's disease are associated with earlier institutionalization and a greater burden for caregivers. The longitudinal course of these symptoms has not been adequately defined. Patients with probable Alzheimer's disease in the placebo control group of a large clinical trial were observed for episodes of depression, psychosis, and agitation.

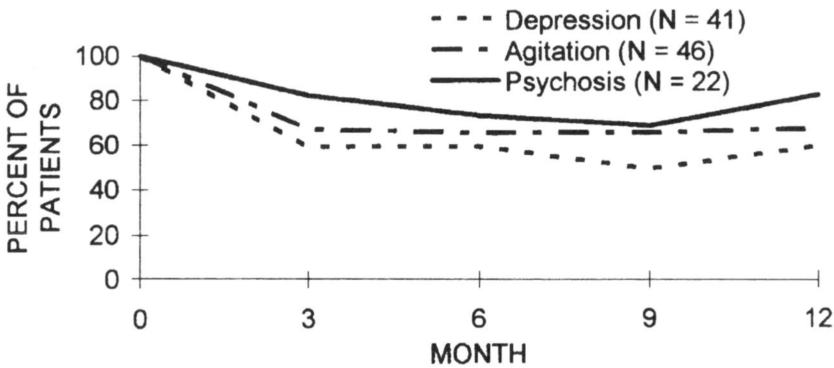

FIGURE 2.—Recurrence of neuropsychiatric symptoms at each assessment period in patients with Alzheimer's disease who had these symptoms at study onset. (Courtesy of Levy ML, Cummings JL, Fairbanks LA, et al: Longitudinal assessment of symptoms of depression, agitation, and psychosis in 181 patients with Alzheimer's disease. *Am J Psychiatry* 153:1438–1443. Copyright 1996, the American Psychiatric Association. Reprinted by permission.)

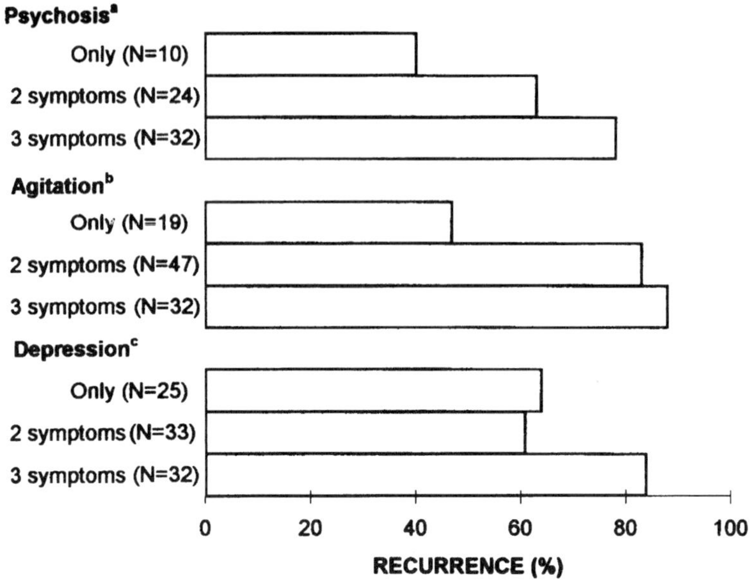

[a]Linear trend: χ^2=5.21, df=1, p<0.05.
[b]Linear trend: χ^2=9.27, df=1, p<0.01.
[c]Linear trend: χ^2=3.14, df=1, p=0.08.

FIGURE 3.—Rate of recurrence of neuropsychiatric symptoms among 181 patients with Alzheimer's disease. *Asterisk* indicates following linear trend: $\chi^2 = 5.21$, $df = 1$, $p < 0.05$. *Dagger* indicates following linear trend: $\chi^2 = 9.27$, $df = 1$, $p < 0.01$. *Double dagger* indicates following linear trend: $\chi^2 = 3.14$, $df = 1$, $p = 0.08$. (Courtesy of Levy ML, Cummings JL, Fairbanks LA, et al: Longitudinal assessment of symptoms of depression, agitation, and psychosis in 181 patients with Alzheimer's disease. *Am J Psychiatry* 153:1438–1443. Copyright 1996, the American Psychiatric Association. Reprinted by permission.)

Methods.—A total of 181 of 215 patients with probable Alzheimer's disease who were in the placebo arm of a drug trial completed all 5 scheduled assessment visits. Patients were evaluated every 3 months during the observation period using the Alzheimer's Disease Assessment Scale, the Mini-Mental State examination, the Activities of Daily Living scale, the Instrumental Activities of Daily Living scale, the Clinical Global Impression scale, and the Clinical Dementia Rating scale. The frequency, incidence, and recurrence of neuropsychiatric symptoms were calculated.

Results.—The recurrence rates of depression, agitation, and psychosis were 85%, 93%, and 95%, respectively (Fig 2). Patients with multiple symptoms had significantly higher rates of recurrence (Fig 3). Female patients had more symptoms than male patients. Patients with lower Mini-Mental State scores had higher rates of depression and significantly higher rates of agitation and psychosis. Older patients ages 76–87 had more psychosis, less depression and agitation, and slower cognitive decline. There was an association between psychosis and more rapid cognitive decline. Agitation was associated with rapid functional deterioration.

Conclusions.—When neuropsychiatric symptoms are present in patients with Alzheimer's disease, they recur frequently. Variability of symptoms was observed with age, sex, and rate of illness progression.

▶ The high prevalence of so-called non-cognitive, behavioral and emotional symptoms in Alzheimer's disease is well established. This article demonstrates that once they occur, such symptoms are frequently persistent or recurrent. This is an important finding and adds urgency to the search for direct treatments of these symptoms. The findings that patients with psychosis had more rapid cognitive decline and that agitation is associated with more rapid functional decline underscores the urgency of treatment.

There has been no consistent relationship between the prevalence of specific symptoms and the severity of cognitive disorder in other studies. This study found high rates of depression, agitation and psychosis among the patients with Mini Mental scores of 12–17. This is the most severe level of cognitive impairment in this study but moderately severe in comparison with other studies.

Figures 2 and 3 illustrate 2 important findings: (1) recurrence or persistence occurs in a majority of patients, and (2) these symptoms rarely occur in isolation. The authors also found that women are more likely than men to be agitated and to have multiple symptoms. This is somewhat surprising because agitation/aggression is usually said to be more of a problem for men.

The authors identify the major limitations of this study. As with most similar studies, this is a selected sample of individuals seen at primary assessment centers for possible participation in a drug study. Even if prevalence is lower in the community, persistence and recurrence are likely to be prevalent there as well.

P.V. Rabins, M.D., M.P.H.

Delusions and Hallucinations in Alzheimer's Disease: Results From a Two-Year Longitudinal Study

Haupt M, Romero B, Kurz A (Universität Düsseldorf, Germany; Universität München, Germany)

Int J Geriatr Psychiatry 11:965–972, 1996 3–19

Introduction.—Delusions and hallucinations are important features of Alzheimer's disease. However, the prevalence of psychotic symptoms in dementia and their association with the progression of cognitive and functional impairment are open to debate. A longitudinal study of psychotic symptoms in Alzheimer's disease is reported.

Methods.—The study included 78 out-patients with clinically diagnosed Alzheimer's disease, according to the ICD-10 draft research criteria. The frequency of psychotic symptoms was evaluated annually. These assessments were done with a specific scale for measurement of delusions and hallucinations in Alzheimer's disease, the BEHAVE-AD. The patients were followed up for 2 years. Associations were sought between the frequency of psychotic symptoms and the severity and progression of cognitive and functional impairment.

Results.—Half of the patients with mild Alzheimer's disease had delusions, the most common being the delusion that people had stolen things. The frequency of delusions decreased as the disease progressed. Delusional symptoms were significantly associated with the rate of progression in cognitive and functional decline. Hallucinations were less frequent than delusional symptoms, but became more frequent as Alzheimer's disease progressed. Visual hallucinations were more common than auditory hallucinations. There was no link between the presence of hallucinations and the rate of disease progression.

Methods.—Many patients with Alzheimer's disease have psychotic symptoms. Patients who have psychotic symptoms early in the course of disease may be at greater risk of rapid disease progression, including a greater likelihood of institutionalization. These patients should receive psychopharmacologic treatment, and the family should receive counseling about how to manage the psychotic symptoms.

▶ Although the reported prevalence of hallucinations and delusions in Alzheimer's disease varies widely, the "lifetime prevalence," that is, the likelihood that an individual will experience such a symptom during the course of his or her disease, approximates 66%.[1] This prospective study used well-accepted, standardized instruments, the BEHAVE-AD, CAMCOG, and MMSE, and the Dementia Behavior Scale, a measure of functional impairment, and reexamined subjects 3 times. Multiple regression analyses revealed that the presence of delusions predicted a more rapid decline in both cognition and function. This is an important finding because it is well known that these symptoms correlate with higher levels of family distress. The results should spur researchers to find better treatments for these symptoms as well as try to better understand the genesis.

The authors note that some studies find that delusions become increasingly prevalent with worsening severity of dementia, whereas others do not. They correctly point out that the source of patients can influence prevalence of delusions and severity of dementia (with higher prevalence found in referral and psychiatric centers) and that the range of severity of dementia can affect whether severity correlates with other phenomena. Intriguingly, they found correlations with severity only at 1 of 3 observations over a 2-year period. This finding suggests that prevalence and correlates of hallucinations and delusions are likely to depend on how frequently they are asked about and the setting in which the study is being done.

Although neuroleptic drugs are widely used to treat hallucinations and delusions in dementia, evidence for their effectiveness is weak. It is not surprising, therefore, that there is no evidence that treating these symptoms slows progression. The intriguing reports by Cummings et al.[2] that cholinesterase inhibitors may improve these symptoms is exciting because they suggest that drugs that improve cognitive performance may also diminish noncognitive symptoms; perhaps these drugs will also be shown to slow progression, thereby having multiple benefits.

P.V. Rabins, M.D., M.P.H.

References

1. Chen JY, Stern Y, Sano M, et al: Cumulative risks of developing extrapyramidal signs, psychosis or myoclonus in the course of Alzheimer's disease. *Arch Neurol* 48:1141–1143, 1991.
2. Cummings JL, Gorman DG, Shapira J: Physostigmine ameliorates the delusions of Alzheimer's disease. *Biol Psychiatry* 33:536–541, 1993.

Psychiatric Features in Diffuse Lewy Body Disease: A Clinicopathologic Study Using Alzheimer's Disease and Parkinson's Disease Comparison Groups

Klatka LA, Louis ED, Schiffer RB (Univ of Rochester, NY; Walter Reed Army Med Ctr, Washington, DC; Columbia Univ, NY)

Neurology 47:1148–1152, 1996 3–20

Introduction.—Diffuse Lewy body disease (DLBD) is a form of dementia accompanied by cortical Lewy bodies. Its cognitive and some of its extrapyramidal characteristics have been well described; however, relatively few reports have addressed its psychiatric manifestations. The psychiatric features of DLBD were compared with those of Alzheimer's disease (AD) and Parkinson's disease (PD).

Methods.—The study included 28 patients with DLBD, 58 with AD, and 26 with PD. All diagnoses were confirmed at autopsy. The psychiatric features at any time during the illness were assessed in each group. The main outcome measures were the percentages of patients with depression, hallucinations, and delusions, with the latter 2 categories being further classified by type.

Results.—Depression was found in 50% of patients with DLBD and 58% of patients with PD compared with 14% of patients with AD. The percentage of patients with hallucinations was 61% for DLBD, 54% with PD, and 34.5% with AD. Delusions were noted in 57% of patients with DLBD and 53% of those with AD compared with 15% of those with PD. Paranoid delusions were the most common type in patients with DLBD, but other types were present as well. Overall, at least one psychiatric feature was found in 96% of DLBD patients, 77% of PD patients, and 65.5% of AD patients. The DLBD and PD groups had more men than women; the AD group had more women than men (Table).

Conclusions.—Psychiatric features, including depression, hallucinations, and delusions, are very common in patients with DLBD. The presence of these features should be a key diagnostic criterion for DLBD. This is the largest group of DLBD patients studied to date.

TABLE.—Demographic characteristics of subjects

	DLBD	AD	PD
Number of subjects	28	58	26
Men	18	13	17
Women	10	45	9
Mean age at time of death (y), ± SD	78.1 ± 9.6	80.8 ± 8.5	74.9 ± 8.2
Mean duration of illness (y), ± SD	9.5 ± 4.9	9.2 ± 4.7	14.5 ± 6.6
Depression (%)	14 (50.0)	8 (13.8)	15 (57.7)
Hallucinations (%)	17 (60.7)	20 (34.5)	14 (53.8)
Delusions (%)	16 (57.1)	31 (53.4)	4 (15.4)

(Courtesy of Klatka LA, Louis ED, Schiffer RB: Psychiatric features in diffuse Lewy body disease: A clinicopathologic study using Alzheimer's disease and Parkinson's disease comparison groups. *Neurology* 47:1148–1152, 1996. Copyright American Academy of Neurology. Used with permission of Lippincott-Raven.)

▶ Although the neuropathologic features of what is now called Lewy body dementia (LBD) were described in 1961 by Okazaki et al.,[1] the clinical relevance of this disorder has been noted for only 10 years, and operational criteria have been available for only 5 years. This large series of neuropathologically diagnosed cases of LBD, AD, and PD confirms that hallucinations are more prominent in LBD than in patients with AD and that they are equally prevalent in PD. Conversely, the study found high but similar prevalences of delusions in both LBD (57.1%) and AD (53.4%). One finding of this study that has not been widely reported is that depressive symptoms were also common in LBD (50%), the same rate as found in PD cases (57.7%) but significantly greater than the percentage found in AD cases.

The authors importantly note that the major limitation of this study is that the psychopathology was determined retrospectively. It is also possible that the cases were not matched for severity of disease.

One important note for recognizing LBD is the extreme caution that should be exercised when prescribing neuroleptic antipsychotic drugs for such patients, even though there is a high prevalence of hallucinations and delusions in LBD; a descriptive literature suggests that they might be more likely to develop PD. This is an issue that bears further study. It may also be important to make the distinction between LBD and AD for treatment studies. Although one study has suggested that cholinesterase inhibitors might benefit patients with LBD,[2] it seems plausible that LBD and AD will have different etiologies and therefore different treatments. Not properly distinguishing between the two diagnostic groups might dilute a treatment effect in experimental trials.

P.V. Rabins, M.D., M.P.H.

References

1. Okazaki H, Lipkin LE, Aronson SM: Diffuse intracytoplasmic ganglionic inclusions (Lewy type) associated with progressive dementia and quadriparesis in flexion. *J Neuropathol Exp Neurol* 20:237–244, 1961.
2. Levy R, Eagger S, Griffiths M, et al: Lewy bodies and response to tacrine in Alzheimer's disease. *Lancet* 343:176, 1994.

Alzheimer's Disease and Apolipoprotein E ϵ4 Allele in Older Drivers Who Died in Automobile Accidents

Johansson K, Bogdanovic N, Kalimo H, et al (Karolinska Inst, Huddinge, Sweden; Turku Univ Hosp, Finland)

Lancet 349:1143–1144, 1997 3–21

Background.—The risk for fatal automobile accidents is greater for elderly drivers age 65 and older. Most fatal accidents occur at intersections, which demand the driver's focused attention. Are elderly patients who die in automobile accidents more likely to have cognitive impairment? The apolipoprotein E ϵ4 phenotype and the brain regions associated with Alzheimer's disease were examined in elderly drivers killed in automobile accidents.

Methods.—Neuropathologic sections were examined from 98 elderly drivers who had been killed in traffic accidents during a 2.5-year period in Sweden and Finland. Stained sections were examined for pathologic changes in the middle frontal cortex and the angular parietal gyri. For 70 of the 98 patients, the apolipoprotein E ϵ4 phenotype was determined by microsequencing. Age- and sex-matched patients were selected from previous studies for use as controls.

Findings.—One third of the elderly patients who died in automobile accidents had histologic confirmation of Alzheimer's disease. In another one fifth of such patients, the histologic findings were suggestive of Alzheimer's disease. In another 17% of patients, the parietal or frontal cortices contained at least one neurofibrillary tangle. The apolipoprotein E ϵ4 phenotype was found significantly more often in the patients who were killed than in their matched controls. The older the patient, the greater the number of neuritic plaques.

Conclusions.—Incipient Alzheimer's disease could have been present in as many as 53% of these elderly drivers. Previous research has shown that drivers with dementia have more accidents. Thus, cognitive performance should be constantly monitored in elderly patients who continue to drive so as to avoid the risk of automobile accidents.

► Making recommendations about continued driving is one of the most difficult clinical issues faced by the physician caring for a person with Alzheimer's disease (AD). Although many studies document that individuals with AD have higher rates of accidents than age-matched normal individuals, and others demonstrate the correlations between impaired cognitive impairment and poor performance on simulated driving, the question of whether patients with early AD should drive remains a vexing and controversial one. This case-controlled study examined the neuropathologic abnormalities in Swedish and Finnish drivers aged 65 years and older and found that more than half of those killed in motor vehicle accidents met neuropathologic criteria for likely or definite AD. The apolipoprotein E ϵ4 genotype was more prevalent in killed drivers than in controls.

The study cannot identify the percentage of killed drivers who had clinically obvious AD. Nevertheless, the finding that almost half the drivers had significant neuropathologic evidence of AD is much higher than the expected rate of 10% to 20% prevalence in a cohort with a mean age of 75. It is certainly possible that many of these individuals had clinically obvious AD and would have fallen into the group that a clinician would advise that they not drive, but it is also possible that many of those dying had undetected AD. This study would be more useful if the authors had contacted families and determined whether they were aware of symptoms of AD, whether any clinician had advised against driving, and whether these subjects had had prior accidents or other evidence that they might be at risk. Nevertheless, the study supports the contention that individuals with early or mild AD who are still driving are at increased risk of having automobile accidents. The article does not note injuries or deaths sustained by others, but it is likely that this risk involves not only the individual but also other drivers and pedestrians.

P.V. Rabins, M.D., M.P.H.

The Predictive Value of Dementia Screening Instruments in Clinical Populations

Flicker L, Logiudice D, Carlin JB, et al (Univ of Melbourne, Australia; Natl Ageing Research Inst, Parkville, Australia; Royal Children's Hosp, Melbourne, Australia; et al)

Int J Geriatr Psychiatry 12:203–209, 1997 3–22

Background.—Some screening instruments for cognitive impairment have been developed for use in research settings or specific clinical situations. These include the Folstein Mini-Mental State Examination (MMSE) and the Abbreviated Mental Test Score (AMT). Other instruments have been developed that rely on simple cognitive instruments and other questions to obtain diagnostic information. There are other instruments that use informants to document the presence of cognitive decline. One such instrument is the Informant Questionnaire for Cognitive Decline in the Elderly (IQCODE). The positive and negative predictive value of screening tests have the most impact on clinicians. To determine the positive and negative predictive values, it is necessary to know the prevalence of dementia in the target population and the sensitivity and specificity of the test.

Methods.—There were 2 groups of subjects: 299 subjects referred to a memory clinic (memory clinic subjects), 216 of whom had dementia; and 78 randomly selected subjects who had been referred to an aged care assessment team (ACAT subjects), 32 of whom had dementia. The sensitivity, specificity, and positive predictive value of the MMSE, AMT, and IQCODE were determined, as well as the correlation between tests.

Results.—The correlation between the MMSE and AMT was 0.86 for memory clinic subjects and 0.87 for ACAT subjects. The correlation between the MMSE and IQCODE was −0.56 for memory clinic subjects and −0.65 for ACAT subjects. The correlation between the AMT and IQCODE was −0.54 for memory clinic subjects and −0.62 for ACAT subjects. The sensitivity and specificity of the AMT and MMSE was lower in memory clinic subjects than in ACAT subjects. A sensitivity of 78% and a specificity of 88% were used to determine the positive predictive value. The positive predictive value in clinical situations ranged from 70% in individuals older than 75 admitted to acute teaching hospitals, to 84% in individuals referred to ACATs, inpatient geriatric liaison patients, and individuals in acute geriatric units. The positive predictive value was 45% in the general population older than 80–84.

Discussion.—These instruments are useful in clinical situations or screening programs that meet strict criteria. The use of these tools in the general population is not supported because it is likely that the tests will produce more false positives than true cases of dementia.

▶ The development of treatments for Alzheimer's disease and other common dementias has brought increased urgency to the development of techniques for earlier recognition. To date, no study has demonstrated that any biological marker or any clinical test has adequate sensitivity, specificity, and positive predictive value to be used for early recognition. Unfortunately, this study replicates these findings. They demonstrate that neither the MMSE, AMT, nor the IQCODE has sufficient psychometric properties when used in individuals referred to memory clinics or geriatric assessment teams. These findings suggest that neither a clinically based questionnaire nor a brief cognitive assessment (MMSE or AMT) will be adequate alone.Their failure is best illustrated by the author's statement that these tests are more likely to produce a false positive than a true case of dementia. This is an unacceptable characteristic of any screening test.

On the other hand, the findings do suggest that these instruments are useful in the acute medical hospital and for the screening of patients who are seeking admission to long-term care facilities. It may well be that different instruments or different combinations of approaches (e.g., neuroimaging, biochemical markers, and cognitive testing) will be necessary in different settings. Future work should begin to examine combining markers and methods. A AHCPR panel has recently suggested 6 "symptoms that may indicate dementia." Although they have face validity, it is ironic that they are the most visible contribution of a panel that was supposed to make recommendations based on existing studies. This highlights the need for further research into an important topic.

P.V. Rabins, M.D., M.P.H.

Questionable Dementia: Clinical Course and Predictors of Outcome

Devanand DP, Folz M, Gorlyn M, et al (New York State Psychiatric Inst, New York; Columbia Univ, New York)

J Am Geriatr Soc 45:321–328, 1997 3–23

Background.—The number of cognitively impaired, nondemented persons seeking medical care is increasing. The clinical course and outcome predictors in outpatients with cognitive impairment who do not meet the criteria for dementia at the initial assessment were explored.

Methods.—One hundred twenty-seven cognitively impaired patients in a memory disorders clinic were classified as having "questionable dementia" (QD). Seventy-five were followed for at least 1 year. Baseline neuropsychologic assessment was performed in 62.

Findings.—At the final assessment, 41.3% of the patients met the diagnostic criteria for dementia. Twenty-seven of these 31 patients had possible or probable Alzheimer's disease (AD). Of the remaining patients, 44% were classified as not demented, and 14.7% continued to have "uncertain" dementia. The final diagnosis of dementia was associated with increased age but not duration or follow-up, Clinical Dementia Rating, or modified Mini-Mental State Examination (mMMS) scores. The final diagnosis of dementia was predicted by low scores on the mMMS delayed recall subtest; consistent long-term retrieval on the Selective Reminding Test; category naming for animals; and the WAIS-R digit symbol, picture arrangement, and block design subtests. The sensitivity and specificity for mMMS delayed recall were 66.7% and 71.4%, respectively; for the other 5 neuropsychological subtests together, 66.7% and 66.7%, respectively; and for the 6 tests together, 81% and 76.9%, respectively. The predictive accuracy for the final diagnosis of AD was similar.

Conclusion.—In patients with QD, a low score on the mMMS delayed recall item may be a useful predictor of the diagnosis of dementia on follow-up. Good predictive accuracy may be achieved by combining a screening instrument such as the mMMS with specific neuropsychological testing.

► This is a descriptive study that presents useful information on a clinically challenging presentation: the patient who presents with mild cognitive impairment. As reviewed in the introduction to the article, some studies have suggested that most individuals with this presentation go on to a progressive dementia, whereas others find a more variable outcome. In this study, a definite dementia developed in 42.3% of individuals followed for a minimum of 1 year.

What is clinically useful and somewhat new is the identification of tests that correlate with the development of dementia. The delayed recall items on the mMMS showed approximately the same sensitivity and specificity as several other in-depth neuropsychological tests, including the WAIS-R digit symbol, picture arrangement, and block design tests. The combination of the neuropsychological tests and the mMMS together was slightly more sensitive and specific. As the authors note, this suggests that a strategy in which the mMMS is used as a screen with individuals who are impaired on delayed memory items then referred for neuropsychological testing will be helpful in identifying those individuals with mild impairment who are likely to progress to AD and other dementia.

The greatest drawback to this study is that 40% of the subjects were lost to follow-up. Although these subjects were not significantly different from those who remained in the study, this is a large dropout rate, and it raises the possibility that the percentage of individuals progressing to dementia might be significantly different from the 41.3% reported. Nevertheless, the study emphasizes the need for better means of identifying which of these individuals has early dementia. The development of treatments such as vitamin E, selegeline, and cholinesterase inhibitors demands that AD be recognized earlier. Although there are not yet data suggesting that earlier intervention would delay progression, this is a plausible hypothesis that should be tested in very mildly impaired patients.

P.V. Rabins, M.D., M.P.H.

Sharing the Diagnosis: A Survey of Memory Disorders Clinics, Their Policies on Informing People With Dementia and Their Families, and the Support They Offer

Gillard J, Gwilliam C (Univ of Bristol, England)

Int J Geriatr Psychiatry 11:1001–1003, 1996 3–24

Introduction.—The issue of sharing the diagnosis of dementia with the patient remains under debate. A questionnaire was sent to 20 memory disorders clinics in England, Scotland, and Eire to determine how much information is shared with patients in whom dementia is diagnosed. Sixteen clinics completed and returned the questionnaire.

Methods.—The questionnaire focused on 3 areas: developing guidelines, information given and language used when talking to patients and their caregivers, and availability of back-up services.

Results.—Six of 16 clinics (37.5%) had guidelines regarding how much information is shared with patients who have dementia diagnosed. Of these 6, only 1 had written guidelines. Patients were informed of their specific diagnosis in 9 clinics (56%), likely progression of disease in 12 clinics (75%), speed of progression of disease in 7 clinics (43%), and content of dementia and its manifestation in 5 clinics (31%). In 4 clinics (25%), staff members would not routinely discuss any of the above-mentioned information with the patient, but would respond honestly if the patient asked directly. Clinic staff members were divided regarding with whom, how, when, and where to share information about the diagnosis of dementia. Clinics did not always have information available regarding available services and benefits. Wright and Lindesay found that only 1 of 20 clinics had an in-house social worker.

Conclusions.—The debate about truth telling in dementia is becoming more open. Many clinics refer their clients to organizations like the Alzheimer's Disease Society, but there seems to be a big gap between information about a service and use of that service by patients and caregivers. There is a national lack of information and counseling support for persons with dementia. Adequate information and backup is needed for patients with whom the diagnosis of dementia has been shared.

▶ I am frequently asked whether I discuss the diagnosis of Alzheimer's disease or dementia with the patient. This brief submission reviews the practice of 16 memory disorder clinics in England, Scotland, and Ireland. The most striking feature is the variability among clinics. While 56% do tell patients the diagnosis, another 25% would not unless the patient asked. A third or less of clinics have either formal or informal guidelines about informing patients.

This is a clinically important issue. Drickamer and Lachs[1] discussed the ethical dimensions of this question 5 years ago but the question remains a vexing one to many clinicians. The variability and practice on this issue emphasized the relative uniqueness of dementia, because almost all clinicians (except those in France and Japan) would discuss a diagnosis of any other disease with the affected adult. This is an example of an issue in which there is no single right or wrong answer. Explicit public debate about care issues such as this should serve to improve the care of individuals with dementia. A central challenge of the care of the patient with Alzeheimer's disease is the support of personhood in spite of the disease's destruction of the person. This requires constant vigilance. However, it must be balanced with the potential harm of informing the patient. In the opinion of this reviewer, the ethical decision requires an evaluation of each individual patient's capacities, impairments, and social situation.

P.V. Rabins, M.D., M.P.H.

Reference

1. Drickamer M, Lachs M: Should patients with Alzheimer's disease be told their diagnosis? *N Engl J Med* 326:947–951, 1992.

Ethics of 'Informed Consent' in Dementia Research: The Debate Continues

Agarwal MR, Ferran J, Ost K, et al (Univ of Liverpool, England)
Int J Geriatr Psychiatry 11:801–806, 1996 3–25

Introduction.—In the treatment of Alzheimer's disease, there has been a dramatic increase in phase-3 drug trials as a result of recent developments in research. The patient and caregiver or next of kin usually gives informed consent; however, for patients who are incapable of giving their consent, agreement from only their caregiver or next of kin is sought. In a group of patients with Alzheimer's disease participating in a phase-3, double-blind, placebo-controlled treatment trial, the issue of informed consent was examined.

Methods.—A legal test of capacity to consent to treatment was proposed by the Law Commission in the United Kingdom. There were 15 patients with Alzheimer's disease who were asked to fill out questionnaires to determine whether they fulfilled the criteria for capacity to give informed consent. A similar questionnaire was given to their caregivers to assess their understanding of the patients' capacity to consent and to determine whether consent was a true choice.

Results.—None of the subjects were able to fulfill all the criteria for the congnitive or function test. Four caregivers indicated that the subjects could not make the decision to participate in the study, and the caregivers had to make that decision independently. As side effects from the treatment were negligible, the caregivers opted to have treatment provided to the subjects.

Conclusion.—Unless a caregiver has been appointed by a judicial forum to act as a proxy for a subject, there is no legal provision for a caregiver to give consent on a subject's behalf. More consideration needs to be given to caregivers in the decision-making process. On the issue of consent remaining valid throughout the course of a long-term trial, clarification is needed because of the problem of deteriorating congnitive functions, particularly short-term memory.

▶ This article examines the level of agreement between subjects with dementia participating in a randomized controlled trial (presumably of an anti-dementia drug) and compares a clinical determination of the decisional capacity of the person with dementias to the caregiver's predictions of decisional capacity. Although this is a very small sample, the article is indicative of the kinds of studies that can be done to improve our understanding of the decision-making process in the cognitively impaired. The authors operationalize the capacity to consent to research into 8 questions. Their findings demonstrate that none of the patients in the study fulfilled all criteria for decisional capacity and that more than half of the patients did not fulfill 50% of the criteria. They also administered a modified version of this questionnaire to caregivers and asked them to rate the capacity of the research subject. As in other studies, the surrogates overestimated capacity in each area, although only on average did so in 2 of 15 individuals. The fact that surrogates overestimate capacity is a consistent finding, and likely to be generalized to all studies of the cognitively incapacitated, at least in North America and Great Britain.

The authors' conclusions seem reasonable. First, it is very unlikely that a "single test" can be developed to assess capacity to consent to research participation. Second, further thought and attention needs to be given to the role of proxy consent, particularly that given by caregivers. Another issue the authors highlighted is that many of the research subjects were unaware that they were involved in an ongoing drug study. This raises the need for re-assessment of consent to participate in research over time in longitudinal studies. This article and the article by Karlawish and Sachs[1] suggest that similar ethical issues are being raised in the United States and in England. It is likely that there will be wide variability of opinion on this topic in different cultures and countries. Continued debate and attention will be important.

P.V. Rabins, M.D., M.P.H.

Reference

1. Karlawish JHT, Sachs GA: Research on the cognitively impaired: Lessons and warnings from the Emergency Research Debate. *J Am Geriatr Soc* 45:474–481, 1997.

An Observational Study of Sexual Behavior in Demented Male Patients

Zeiss AM, Davies HD, Tinklenberg JR (VA Palo Alto Health Care System, Calif; Stanford Univ, Calif)

J Gerontol 51A:M325–M329, 1996 3–26

Introduction.—Concerns about inappropriate sexual behavior in patients with Alzheimer's disease frequently appear in lay and professional literature, but the actual incidence is not known. The incidence of sexually appropriate, ambiguous, and inappropriate behaviors was determined in male patients with Senile Dementia of the Alzheimer's Type.

Methods.—Research subjects were 40 men, age 60–98, with a dementia diagnosis who were living in an institutional setting. Research subjects were observed for 1-minute intervals at 9 different times of the day, and sexually appropriate, inappropriate, and ambiguous behaviors were coded.

Results.—Behaviors were recorded with high reliability. Across the 9 observational time points, research subjects averaged 0.43, 1.48, and 0.83 sexually appropriate, ambiguous, and inappropriate behaviors, respectively. The scores were not evenly distributed across patients because only 18% of research subjects ever displayed sexually inappropriate behavior. Most instances of inappropriate behavior were brief and minor. Sexually inappropriate behavior was seen in only 1.6% of observed 1-minute time segments.

Conclusions.—Inappropriate sexual behavior was infrequently observed in men with dementia who were institutionalized. It may be that some of the lore regarding sexually disinhibited behavior in patients with dementia may have less to do with inappropriate behavior and more to do with self-care deficits, like appearing in public incompletely dressed.

▶ As the authors note, previous cross-sectional and retrospective studies have found that sexual problems are rare in patients with Alzheimer's disease. This is a prospective study that examined the prevalence of inappropriate sexual behavior in 40 residents of a long-term VA facility. The greatest strength of this paper is that data are based on direct observation. However, the low frequency of these behaviors and the fact that even trained observers had some difficulty distinguishing between "appropriate," "inappropriate," and "ambiguous" behaviors underlies the challenge of this particular topic. It is certainly possible and perhaps even likely that sexual behaviors occurred but were not observed. This is a problem with the method of direct observation of an infrequent occurrence. Nevertheless, the low prevalence is certainly accurate.

There are little data on effective therapies of these behaviors and little understanding of whether therapy is needed. Suggested "treatments" range from ignoring the behavior, moving the patient to a more private location, or using pharmacotherapy. The techniques reported in this article would be ideal for determining the effectiveness of therapies. Because inappropriate sexual behavior does put others at risk, the identification of effective therapies could benefit a significant number of patients and caregivers.

P.V. Rabins, M.D., M.P.H.

Impaired Incentive Learning in Treated Parkinson's Disease

Charbonneau D, Riopelle RJ, Beninger RJ (Queen's Univ, Kingston, Ont)

Can J Neurol Sci 23:271–278, 1996 3–27

Objective.—Animal studies suggest that dopamine dysfunction not only affects locomotor control but also incentive motivational learning, that is, the shaping of behavior through rewards. This form of learning has been linked to the dopaminergic mesolimbic pathway and more recently to the nigrostriatal pathway. There is an increasing emphasis on the cognitive deficits of patients with Parkinson's disease (PD). The performance of patients with PD on incentive learning and stimulus-stimulus associative learning tasks was evaluated.

Methods.—The study included 32 patients with idiopathic PD, 25 healthy controls, and 32 patients with arthritis. All groups were matched for age and education, and the PD and arthritis groups were similar in terms of self-reported physical disability. Patients in the PD group were taking dopaminergic replacement therapy. Two tests were performed: a word-paired associate task, on which the subjects received no performance feedback; and an operant avoidance task, which measured incentive learning to avoid the aversive stimulus of losing money. Both tasks were performed on a computer.

Results.—The 2 control groups performed equally well on the operant avoidance task, whereas the PD group had impaired performance on this task. The 3 groups were similar in their performance on the paired-associate learning test.

Conclusions.—Patients with PD show an impairment in incentive learning. These patients may have nigrostriatal dopamine dysfunction affecting incentive learning but not paired-associate learning. The findings suggest that dopamine may be involved in some forms of learning and memory, and may reflect differences between tonic and modulated function in the nigrostriatal system.

▶ Impaired initiative is common in many psychiatric and neurologic disorders. Understanding its pathophysiology might lead to better treatments of this difficult to manage symptom. This study found a distinction between "incentive learning" and paired-associate learning in patients with PD but not in controls with arthritis. The authors conclude that this links this symptom to dopamine deficiencies in the nigrostriatal system.

Clinically, patients with PD have difficulty initiating activity. Because PD is a disease of the basal ganglia, the authors' hypothesis is plausible. Maximal dopamine replacement therapy does not correct the impaired performance, and the other memory task, which is presumably dependent on an intact hippocampus, is performed normally. These facts also support the hypothesis that the deficit is linked to a specific neuropathologic process. Therefore, this study adds to the large database suggesting that damage to the basal ganglia can impair initiative and mental flexibility and that such deficits may be found not only in PD, but in other diseases with potential dopaminergic involvement such as the mood disorders and schizophrenia.

Studies such as this have major limitations, however, and it is important that they be noted. It is possible that the task on which the 2 groups differ is more difficult or more sensitive. If this were the case, then the lack of a finding on the paired-associate learning task would reflect characteristics of that test rather than differential impairment on neuropsychological functions or a different neurophysiology of the 2 tasks. Also, there is a timed element to the avoidance task, and it is possible that it is slowness or some other aspect of the testing process rather than the neuropsychological paradigm of incentive learning that is impaired. Another limitation that the authors discuss is that the attempt to localize neuropsychological tests is fraught with danger. For example, they note that impairments in "frontal lobe functioning" have been reported in patients with PD. Because there are nigrofrontal pathways, and many other neural systems are connected to these structures, it is premature to conclude that specific structures or neurotransmitters are involved in the cognitive task being studied. Nevertheless, this study does add to a growing body of knowledge associating the basal ganglia and frontal lobe to disorders of initiative. It would be intriguing to determine whether these findings can be confirmed on functional neuroimaging.

P.V. Rabins, M.D., M.P.H.

Miscellaneous

A Family Intervention to Delay Nursing Home Placement of Patients With Alzheimer Disease

Mittelman MS, Ferris SH, Shulman E, et al (New York Univ; Columbia Univ, New York; New York State Psychiatric Inst)

JAMA 276:1725–1731, 1996 3–28

Objective.—Although deterioration occurs in every patient with Alzheimer's disease (AD), the rate of progression varies. Most families prefer to keep the patient out of the nursing home if possible, but this requires considerable assistance for the caregiver. Previous studies have suggested that psychosocial interventions may be able to prevent or delay nursing home placement of patients with AD. A comprehensive support and counseling program for the families of patients with AD was studied for long-term effectiveness in postponing or preventing nursing home placement.

Methods.—The randomized, controlled trial included 206 spouse-caregivers of patients with AD. All patients were living at home at the start of the study. The families came from a broad range of socioeconomic backgrounds. The caregivers were randomly assigned to treatment and control groups. The treatment group received 6 counseling sessions, 2 individual and 4 family. Counseling was task oriented, with a focus on promoting communication, teaching problem-solving techniques, and improving support for the caregiver. All patients in the treatment group were required to join a regular support group. Also, counselors were continuously available to help in crises and as the patient's symptoms changed. The control group received the normal services offered to the families of AD patients. The 2 groups were compared until the family member with AD was admitted to a nursing home.

Results.—On Kaplan-Meier survival analysis, the median adjusted time to nursing home placement was 1,203 days for the treatment group vs. 874 days for the control group. By intention-to-treat analysis in a Cox proportional hazard model, the adjusted relative risk of nursing home placement was 0.65 for the treatment group. Thus, caregivers in the treatment group were two thirds as likely to place their family member in a nursing home as those in the control group, after adjustment for caregiver sex, patient age, and patient income. The treatment program had the largest effect on placement rate for patients with mild to moderate dementia (relative risk 0.18 to 0.38, respectively).

Conclusions.—With comprehensive support and counseling, caregivers may be able to keep family members with AD out of the nursing home longer. Such programs are most likely to be effective for patients in the mild to moderate stages of dementia, when nursing home admission is least appropriate. The cost effectiveness of the study intervention is being analyzed. Convincing the family members to take advantage of available counseling, education, and support will be a challenge for the future.

▶ This paper extends the findings of a study previously reported by this group. It is a much more detailed and refined analysis of their study that determined the effectiveness of counseling to caregivers of patients with AD. The findings that placement was delayed by almost 1 year and that the likelihood of placement of one third lower in the group randomly assigned to active treatment make a strong case for the provision of educational and counseling services to the caregivers of persons with dementia.

Although one might question whether delay in nursing home placement is always better, most families and most patients state that they would like to avoid nursing home care if possible. Clinicians often see placement as beneficial to both patient and caregiver. Certainly from both the "consumer" and cost points of view this demonstration of a delay in placement should be seen as quite positive.

The limitations of the study are important to note. It was done in a university center and the study was unblinded. Blinding is not possible in such a study, and the fact that the caregivers were randomly assigned and that there was a comparison group blunt this criticism somewhat. The authors state that the counselors frequently encouraged caregivers to place patients when it seemed in the caregiver's or patient's best interest, suggesting a behavior that parallels that of most clinicians. The counseling was provided by clinicians with advanced degrees; such individuals, particularly with the expertise of this team, are not likely to be available in many communities. It will be interesting to determine whether the intervention provided in this study can be effectively provided in other settings.

The program includes scheduled counseling sessions with a focus on management of specific noncognitive problems at the beginning of treatment, counseling by telephone on an "as-needed basis" thereafter and attendance at support groups.

Dementia remains one of the major public health problems of this era. Advances are being made on the basic research front while pharmacologic agents for cognitive impairment are just coming to market. This important study powerfully demonstrates that clinicians have much to offer both patients with dementia and their caregivers.

P.V. Rabins, M.D., M.P.H.

Truly Late Onset of Eating Disorders: A Study of 11 Cases Averaging 60 Years of Age at Presentation

Beck D, Casper R, Andersen A (Duke Univ, Durham, NC; Stanford Univ, Calif; Univ of Iowa, Iowa City)

Int J Eat Disord 20:389–395, 1996 3–29

Introduction.—Traditionally, adolescents and young adults comprise the population with eating disorders. To assert control over non–weight-related aspects of life, to relieve dysphoria, or to avoid conflicts about sexual issues, some use dietary restrictions. The diagnostic criteria for anorexia nervosa are self-induced starvation, morbid fear of fatness, and denial of the seriousness of the low body weight. Bulimia is diagnosed when there is a history of uncontrolled binge behavior associated with a fear of weight gain. Eleven patients who began to have an eating disorder either during or after their mid-life were evaluated.

Methods.—Patients were chosen for this study from 3 university hospital programs if their eating disorder began after the age of 40 and if they met the criteria for an eating disorder.

Results.—The patients ranged in age from 46 to 80, and the onset of their eating disorder had a range from 42 years to 77 years. One 60-year-old woman weighed 62 pounds and her ideal weight was 131–135 pounds. She was married and had a major depression. An 80-year-old woman had low weight and binge behavior. Her husband forbade her to have a breast reduction for her size 46 DD breasts, for which she suffered physical and social discomfort. After her husband died, when she was 73, she dieted strenuously and lost about 60 pounds. She had a fear of fatness and scored high on the Drive for Thinness subscale of the Eating Disorders Inventory. She did not want treatment.

Conclusion.—Whenever self-starvation or binge-purge behaviors become entrenched as sustaining behaviors for alleviating psychodyamic conflicts, mood disorders, or interpersonal distress, age itself should not be considered a barrier. In later life, weight loss is frequently associated with depression. A pattern was found among the patients who were ridiculed about their weight in childhood and who remained sensitive about their weight in later life. Co-morbid affect disorders, such as perfectionism, frequently accompany the eating disorders. Three patients had a history of sexual abuse.

► This article reports a case series of individuals with anorexia nervosa or bulimia nervosa that developed in middle and late life. The cases are intriguing because these disorders almost always start in adolescence and seem linked to developmental issues, both psychological and biological, that emerge at that time. The authors make a convincing argument that these cases are typical except for age of onset. The core psychological features—fear of fatness, self-induced starvation, and lack of recognition of the seriousness of the condition—are present in these late onset cases just as they are in cases with early onset. Another similarity is the high rates of co morbid mood disorder and obsessionality in the early and late onset cases.

It is fascinating that some of the precipitants of anorexia nervosa and bulimia nervosa reported in young individuals are present in these cases, although they sometimes may have occurred even decades before. For example, criticism directed toward being overweight is shared in both early and late onset cases. Change in environment (entering college in the young and moving in the old) and loss of relationship are also common precipitants regardless of age of onset. Treatment is challenging in these cases as it is in young individuals.

Although it is possible that the late onset patients were symptomatic in early life but denied or had forgotten this, this explanation seems unlikely. The senior authors are well known experts and explored this issue as much as possible. These cases thus alert clinicians to include anorexia nervosa in the differential diagnosis of weight loss in the elderly. Perhaps they can also provide leads in the search for etiologic factors.

P.V. Rabins, M.D., M.P.H.

Epidemiology of Psychiatric Disorders in Elderly Compared With Younger Adults With Learning Disabilities

Cooper S-A (Univ of London)

Br J Psychiatry 170:375–380, 1997 3–30

Introduction.—There is limited information on psychiatric disorders among elderly people with learning disabilities, and it is not known how the prevalence of psychiatric disorders changes with age. For clinicians and service planners, this issue is important in view of the increasing life span of people with learning disabilities. The epidemiology of psychiatric disorders among elderly individuals compared with younger adults with learning disabilities was examined.

Methods.—There were 134 individuals who were 65 or older with learning disabilities living in a defined geographic area who had a comprehensive psychiatric examination using a semi-structured rating scale. They were compared to a randomly selected control group of 73 adults age 20–65 with learning disabilities who were also from the same geographic area.

Results.—A greater prevalence of psychiatric morbidity was found among elderly individuals with learning disabilities (68.7%) compared to the younger controls (47.9%). There were higher rates for depression and anxiety disorders. The rate for depression among the elderly was 6% compared to 4.1% for controls and the elderly had a 9% rate of anxiety disorder compared to 5.5% for the controls. Dementia was common. Among the elderly, the rate was 21.6% compared to 2.7% in the controls. In the 2 groups, there were equal rates of schizophrenia or delusional disorders, behavior disorders, and autism. The elderly group exhibited agoraphobia more commonly than the controls.

Conclusion.—The need for psychiatric services increases for people with learning disabilities as they age. Both groups may have common etiologic factors, such as underlying brain damage, epilepsy, genetic syndromes, psychiatric disorders, and family history of psychiatric illness. Support from learning disabilities psychiatric services must be more available to the elderly population with learning disabilities.

▶ Elderly individuals with mental retardation have received little attention, in part because they have higher early life mortality and are thus less likely to live to older age. As the elderly population expands and as the treatments of medical psychiatric morbidities improve, the absolute number of individuals could increase quite rapidly. The prevalence of psychiatric morbidity among older individuals with mental retardation was examined in a geographically defined area in Great Britain.

This study used the case register method. In this approach, the sample consists of all individuals in a geographic area who have come to the attention of any agency. Thus, the weakness of this approach is that individuals who have come to the attention of agencies are different than individuals who do not and that it is not a random sample of affected individuals. The fact that only 0.25% of the residents in Leicestershire County have been identified in this manner suggests that there are many uncounted individuals. In spite of this major limitation, the study is notable because it is one of the very few using any kind of epidemiologic approach that examines the important issue of concomitant psychiatric morbidity in the mentally retarded.

The principal finding of the study is that psychiatric morbidity is more common in older individuals with mental retardation than in younger individuals. These higher rates are accounted for by dementia (not very surprising), depression, and anxiety. The overall rate of psychiatric disorder among the elderly (68.7%) is quite high, and the over-representation of generalized anxiety and depression suggests that there is a significant prevalence of treatable psychiatric morbidity in this population which is not being treated.

The mentally retarded elderly are understudied. As more individuals with mental retardation live into their 70s and 80s, it is likely that many of the social and family supports that they have maintained throughout their life will be lost. Meeting the needs of these individuals will be a challenge in the coming decades.

P.V. Rabins, M.D., M.P.H.

Risk Factors for Late-Life Insomnia in a Representative General Practice Sample

Morgan K, Clarke D (Univ of Sheffield, England; Leicester General Hosp, England)

Br J Gen Pract 47:166–169, 1997 3–31

Introduction.—Insomnia is widely reported and widely treated, but few reports have focused on its natural history. The risk of insomnia onset associated with selected health and lifestyle factors was determined using data from an 8-year longitudinal trial.

Methods.—Data were collected from the 25 general practitioners serving noninstitutionalized individuals age 65 and older living within survey areas of the Nottingham Longitudinal Study of Activity and Aging. Data were collected from interview questionnaires of 1,042, 690, and 410 elderly individuals in 1985, 1989, and 1993, respectively, regarding health, lifestyle, demographic, psychological well-being, and quality of sleep. The risks of insomnia onset were evaluated in relation to selected factors.

TABLE 1.—Logistic Regression Estimation of Risks for Insomnia

Factor	Odds ratio	95% Confidence interval	P value
Age	0.99	0.94–1.06	0.98
Female gender	1.18	0.59–1.85	0.63
Morale (per unit change)	0.98	0.92–1.05	0.59
Bereavement	0.44	0.03–1.07	0.07
Anxiety (higher)	1.01	0.13–1.91	0.99
Depression	4.41	3.32–5.43	0.01
Living alone	0.51	0.09–1.14	0.11
Body weight (high)	0.84	0.19–1.47	0.79
Physical activity			
Intermediate	2.89	1.91–3.62	0.02
Low	2.94	2.14–3.64	0.01
Physical health scale			
(Per unit change)	1.19	1.06–1.31	0.02
(Lower scale scores)	4.3	2.90–5.80	0.01

(Courtesy of Morgan K, Clarke D: Risk factors for late-life insomnia in a representative general practice sample. *Br J Gen Pract* 47:166–169, 1997.)

Results.—At baseline, 802 individuals (78.8%) did not meet criteria for insomnia and were considered to be at risk. At first follow-up in 1989, insomnia was observed in 84 individuals who were insomnia-free in 1985, giving an overall incidence rate per person-year of 3.1%. Three factors in 1985 were significantly and independently related to incident insomnia detected in 1989: psychometric ratings consistent with depressed mood, health index scores indicating lower health status, and moderate and low levels of physical activity (Table 1). Physical, not mental ill health was the most significant risk factor. The best outcomes occurred in individuals in whom insomnia was not preceded by poor physical health.

Conclusions.—Depressed mood was clearly a major risk for insomnia, but only in a minority of research subjects. Poor physical health was shared by more individuals with incident insomnia, suggesting that late-life insomnias may be more likely to originate in somatic rather than psychiatric ill health. Assessment of risk factors of insomnia could easily be incorporated into the yearly physical examination.

▶ Insomnia is a challenging clinical problem and a common complaint. In this study of individuals attending a general practice, both depression and physical morbidity increase the risk of developing incident (new onset) insomnia. This demonstrates that older individuals with new-onset sleep complaints should undergo a thorough psychiatric and medical assessment.

The authors also looked at the outcome associated with the psychiatric and physical disorders in each of the incident cases. Physical illness appears to have predated many more incident cases than depressed mood, but this analysis does not address the question of causality. We would not expect individuals who have new cases of insomnia caused by depression to be depressed before the onset of insomnia. That is, insomnia is often an early sign of depression. What is clear from this analysis is that in individuals in whom physical ill health precedes insomnia, mortality rates are high (52.2%

in this study), whereas fatality rates appear lower (the numbers are too small to do statistical analysis) in individuals whose depressed mood preceded onset of insomnia or in individuals who had neither depression nor physical illness before the onset of insomnia.

It remains to be seen whether improved recognition of depression and more aggressive treatment of underlying physical disorders would diminish morbidity. Importantly, this article demonstrates that patients with new-onset insomnia should be carefully assessed for both medical and psychiatric illness and that these comorbidities need to be aggressively treated when recognized.

P.V. Rabins, M.D., M.P.H.

Older and More Moral: Age-related Changes in Performance on Piagetian Moral Reasoning Tasks

McDonald L, Stuart-Hamilton I (Worcester College of Higher Education, England)

Age Ageing 25:402–404, 1996 3–32

Introduction.—Much of the research on moral reasoning has arisen from Piaget's work. Most of the current knowledge about moral development in older adults is based upon extrapolation. It seems to be assumed that because older children and adolescents perform correctly on Piaget's moral tasks, adults will do the same. Three different age groups participated in Piaget's moral reasoning tasks to determine how older individuals perform compared with younger cohorts.

Methods.—Of 110 research subjects, 44 were teenagers, 37 were middle-aged, and 29 were older adults. All participants completed a written version of Piaget's moral reasoning tasks that assessed lying, carelessness, collective responsibility, stealing, punishment, immanent justice, equality and authority, and justice between children. The higher the score, the higher the level of moral reasoning.

Results.—Significant overall differences were noted between age groups. The pattern of responses was not uniform in 1 direction. Teenagers consistently scored lower, but the nature of the age group difference was mixed. Teenagers and middle-aged groups differed significantly on "total carelessness" and "stealing" scales. There were significant differences between teenagers and middle-aged individuals and teenagers and older individuals on the "justice between" scale.

Conclusions.—Teenagers had a lower level of moral reasoning on some tasks, compared with older adults. All groups gave lower numbers of "high" responses than even Piaget would have predicted. It is possible that Piaget was wrong when he predicted that the developmental process achieved a certain level and did not change.

▶ This article uses an unusual approach to assess 3 important questions about the study of the aging process: Do all cognitive functions decline with age? If there are differences between young and old individuals, are these because of age or cohort difference? And third, do older individuals have more wisdom than younger individuals?

This study is based on the Piagetian concept of moral judgment. While the concept of moral judgment has come under fire in recent years because of its inherent cultural biases, nevertheless, within this relatively homogeneous group, the analysis offers some information about the 3 questions posed above. Unfortunately the study has several limitations that need to be noted before too much is made of the results: the subjects were volunteers, with individuals being recruited from school and older individuals from senior citizen center activity groups or newspaper advertisement. Nevertheless, the findings that older individuals are "more moral" supports the hypothesis that the elderly have greater "wisdom" than younger individuals. The authors are right in noting that this could be either an age difference or cohort difference. What is ironic is that this explanation is usually used to explain studies in which younger individuals perform better than older individuals, whereas in this study the converse is true. The concept of "wisdom" has been difficult to operationalize. This study suggests that it is a topic worth exploring.

P.V. Rabins, M.D., M.P.H.

Development, Testing, and Validation of Two Scales Measuring Nursing Home Management of Subjects With Mental Disorder

Ooi WL, Sherwood S, Murphy K, et al (Hebrew Rehabilitation Ctr for Aged, Research and Training Inst, Boston)
J Clin Epidemiol 49:1381–1388, 1996 3–33

Introduction.—More than 65% of residents of nursing homes have 1 or more of the following: dementia, psychosis, depression and anxiety disorder, alcohol/drug abuse, or other mental disorders. A cross-sectional investigation of 1,017 residents from a proportionate random sample of nursing facilities in Delaware was conducted to determine the prevalence of mental disorders and to define distinguishing characteristics. How the nursing process is used to care for elderly residents with cognitive, mood, behavioral problems, or other markers of mental disorder was also evaluated.

Methods.—An exploratory factor analysis was conducted on 11 frequently encountered nursing management strategies used with 808 residents with some degree of mental disorder.

Results.—Two factors emerged and 2 scales were subsequently created to measure the basic approaches used by health professionals to manage resident behavior: *Encouragement* (derived from 6 variables) and *Control* (derived from 5 variables). Internal consistency of these scales was determined using alpha reliability levels. Multiple regression was used to identify cognitive, behavioral, and mood correlates for each scale. Similar findings were observed at another long-term care facility that was used to attain replication and validation.

Conclusions.—The *Encouragement* and *Control* scales may be used to measure prevalent and potentially useful nursing strategies in caring for the complex needs of older adults who are debilitated and have cognitive, mood, or behavior problems.

▶ There are 1.7 million individuals in nursing homes in the United States, and approximately 1 million of those individuals have dementia. Yet, we know surprisingly little about good nursing home care. This is an important study that focused on strategies used by staff to manage cognitive mood and behavior problems in the long-term care setting. The authors used 2 large cohorts to first develop and then confirm that 2 major factors, encouragement and control, are used by staff to manage difficult behaviors. Validation of this categorization is provided by the finding of correlations between one of these nursing strategies and specific behavior problems.

One of the difficulties in improving care in nursing homes has been a lack of understanding of the process of care in these institutions. The schema and instruments reported in this study should help those interested in studying this large and needy group. The next steps include a determination of the effectiveness of these strategies, how they are used in both non-pharmacologic as well as pharmacologic interventions, how their appropriate use can be fostered, and how they can be taught. It will be important to recognize that there is wide variability in the needs of individual patients and in the capacities of individual care providers. Flexibility and other personality characteristics of the caregiver may also be predictors of successful use of these interventions.[1]

P.V. Rabins, M.D., M.P.H.

Reference

1. Rabins PV, Fitting MD, Eastham J, et al: Emotional adaptation over time in caregivers for the chronically ill elderly. *Age Ageing* 19:185–190, 1990.

Assessing Attentiveness in Older Hospital Patients: Global Assessment Versus Tests of Attention

O'Keeffe ST, Gosney MA (Royal Liverpool Univ Hosp, England)

J Am Geriatr Soc 45:470–473, 1997 3–34

Introduction.—Delirium occurs commonly in older individuals with acute illness. Impaired attentiveness is a cardinal symptom of delirium. Attentiveness may be evaluated by using tests of attention or clinical judgement to make a global assessment. The relationship between global assessment of attentiveness and tests of attention was evaluated in 110 patients admitted to an acute geriatric unit.

Methods.—Two experienced geriatricians made assessments of attention within 90 minutes of each other upon patient admission. One physician rated global attentiveness on a 10-cm visual analogue scale after a 2-minute general conversation with the patient. The other physician administered 4 tests of attentiveness (Digit Span Forwards [DSF], Digit Span Backwards [DSB], Vigilance 'A' test [VAT], and a timed Digit Cancellation Test [DCT]) and determined whether patients met DSM-3 criteria for delirium or dementia.

Results.—Twenty-three patients were unable to participate in all tests of attention. Of the remaining 87 patients, 18 had delirium and 17 were demented. There were no differences between patients who were demented and those with delirium in VAT, DSF, or the Folstein Mini-Mental State Examination (MMSE). All other comparisons between patients with delirium or dementia and between delirious patients and those with neither delirium or dementia were significant. With the exception of DSF, all tests of attention were significantly correlated with the global rating.

Conclusions.—Global assessment may be considered a valuable tool for determining attentiveness in patients with dementia or delirium.

▶ Delirium is a perplexing condition for many clinicians. Many find it difficult to understand the criteria, and there is wide skepticism about the reliability and validity of diagnosis. This brief article addresses a very important aspect of the issue. One clinician rated "attentiveness" based on a 2-minute general conversation with the patient. Agreement between this brief assessment and a clinician who used traditional criteria for determining the presence of delirium was relatively high.

The primary implication of this study is that the criterion "altered level of consciousness and inattention" can be reliably identified. It remains to be demonstrated that this reliability can be accomplished in groups of practicing physicians. Methods for teaching clinicians how to assess level of consciousness and attention are needed as well.

P.V. Rabins, M.D., M.P.H.

Research on the Cognitively Impaired: Lessons and Warnings From the Emergency Research Debate

Karlawish JHT, Sachs GA (Univ of Chicago)

J Am Geriatr Soc 45:474–481, 1997 3–35

Introduction.—A debate is raging in emergency research regarding whether existing federal research regulations permit research involving individuals who cannot provide informed consent. This debate could affect research in the psychiatric, neurology, and geriatric fields. Pertinent journal articles, books, regulations, and court cases that deal with this controversy were reviewed, and similarities between emergency research and research on the cognitively impaired were examined.

The Problem.—Two agencies within the federal Department of Health and Human Services (HHS) regulate the conduct of human research: the Office for Protection from Research Risks and the Food and Drug Administration (FDA). Most populations are well represented by regulations written 2 decades ago, but new interests in research and changing times have stimulated attention to populations once considered off limits. The FDA guidelines do not provide for waiver of informed consent. Emergency research and research involving patients who are cognitively impaired have been historically controversial because of conflicting interpretations of research regulations.

Proposed Solution.—New proposed FDA guidelines for emergency research do not address the issues of minimal risk or deferred consent. They do address advance informed consent; a broad role for family in approving a research subject's participation; replacement of a threshold of permissible risks—called minimal risks—with a more sensible balancing of risks and benefits; and a role for the community in research approval.

Conclusions.—Many of the same problems exist for research of patients who are cognitively impaired that existed for emergency research. Research involving patients who are cognitively impaired may cease if steps similar to those taken for emergency research are not used.

▶ Recent cases in New York State and California have brought public scrutiny to the question of informed consent to participate in research of the cognitively impaired. Those 2 cases involve patients with major medical illnesses, but many of the issues are also relevant to individuals with cognitive disorders. This article reviews the recent changes in regulations that allow decisionally-impaired individuals seen in emergency departments to be included in research, and compares this issue with research in emergency setting and research in non-emergent settings. The article highlights ethical concerns, the major potential solutions, consent before the development of decisional incapacity, the use of families to give consent, and the need for attention to potential benefits and risks. One of the solutions suggested by this article is greater involvement of the general public. The authors of this article (and others) suggest that this would bring greater scrutiny to the process, better protection to cognitively impaired individuals and, at the same time, encourage needed research.

Because dementia causes so much devastation to both patients and families, it is easy to overlook the protections needed to minimize the risks of research. A broadened public debate can only improve the current situation. This article is a useful start in that process.

P.V. Rabins, M.D., M.P.H.

Predictors of Antipsychotic Withdrawal or Dose Reduction in a Randomized Controlled Trial of Provider Education

Meador KG, Taylor JA, Thapa PB, et al (Vanderbilt Univ, Nashville, Tenn)

J Am Geriatr Soc 45:207–210, 1997 3–36

Background.—The Nursing Home Reform Amendments of 1987 (OBRA-87) sought to narrowly restrict the use of antipsychotic medications for long-term care residents, resulting in renewed attention to the

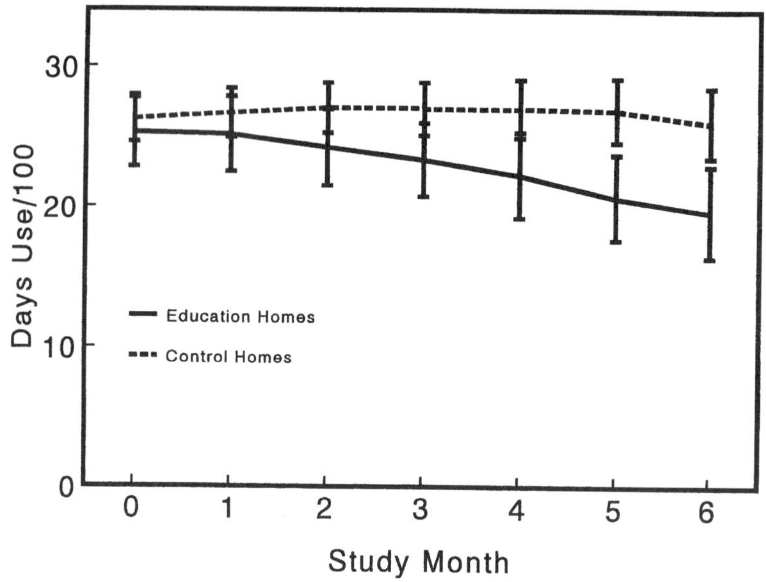

FIGURE 1.—Antipsychotic use (mean days of use per 100 days of residence in the home in 6 educational intervention (*solid line*) and 6 control (*broken line*) homes. Means are calculated for the 30-day period preceding the start of the study (month 0) and the 6 subsequent 30-day periods (months 1 to 6). *Bars* represent standard errors of the mean, calculated with the home as the unit of analysis. (Courtesy of Meador KG, Taylor JA, Thapa PB, et al: Predictors of antipsychotic withdrawal or dose reduction in a randomized controlled trial of provider education. *J Am Geriatr Soc* 45[2]:207–210, 1997.)

management of behavioral manifestations of dementia in nursing homes. A randomized, controlled trial investigated a provider education program after implementation of OBRA-87 in nursing homes that continued to have high rates of antipsychotic use.

Methods.—Twelve Tennessee nursing homes participated in the study. Six received the educational intervention, and 6 served as controls. A total of 1,152 patients were assessed at study enrollment and at 6 months. A cohort analysis of 133 baseline antipsychotic users in 5 intervention nursing homes able to implement the recommendations of the educational program was performed.

Findings.—After the educational intervention, antipsychotic use declined from 25.3 days per 100 at baseline to 19.7 days per 100 by the sixth month, a 23% decrease compared with the control homes. Medications were withdrawn from 33% of 133 baseline antipsychotic users. Baseline factors that predicted successful withdrawal were low antipsychotic dose, no use of benzodiazepines or antidepressants, and behavioral symptoms score less than the median. However, although another 22 patients had dose decreases of 50% or more, none of the withdrawal predictors were associated with dose reductions (Fig 1).

Conclusion.—Focused provider educational programs may facilitate the reduction of antipsychotic use in nursing homes beyond that attributable to regulatory changes. Substantial dose reduction may be possible in patients who are poor candidates for total antipsychotic withdrawal, which should reduce the risk of adverse antipsychotic effects.

► Because neuroleptic drugs have high rates of side effects, are associated with adverse outcomes such as falls and hip fractures, and can lead to tardive dyskinesia, many efforts have been aimed at decreasing their use in the elderly and in nursing homes. This study demonstrates the benefits of an educational intervention directed toward professionals practicing in nursing homes: physicians, nurses, and nursing assistants. The elements of the program are similar to those that would be provided by psychiatric consultants in this setting: an assessment to determine whether there is a medical cause of the behavior disorder, suggestions for the nonpharmacologic management of behavior problems, and trials of withdrawal in patients who were neither violent nor psychotic. Strengths of the study include its design and the large number of patients involved. It uses a classic randomized clinical trial design and included more than 1,000 patients.

The principal findings were that this focused intervention reduced, but did not eliminate, the use of neuroleptic drugs in the nursing home and that the reduction persisted for 6 months. It would be useful to determine whether benefits persisted for longer periods and whether such a program needs to be repeated. The high turnover in nursing assistants suggests that repeated presentations might be necessary.

The 23% decrease in the use of neuroleptic drugs in the intervention homes demonstrates that a significant number of individuals required the continuation of these drugs. However, one quarter of the patients who continued to receive neuroleptics were able to undergo a 50% or greater dosage reduction. Thus, it is likely that neuroleptic drugs are necessary and beneficial in the nursing home setting but that careful attention to underlying cause and ongoing education can lessen their use.

P.V. Rabins, M.D., M.P.H.

New Evidence on Benzodiazepine Use and Falls: The Time Factor

Neutel CI, Hirdes JP, Maxwell CJ, et al (Risk Management & Regulatory Affairs, Ottawa, Ont; Univ of Waterloo, Kitchener, Ont; SCOHS-Elisabeth Bruyère Pavilion, Ottawa, Ont, et al)

Age Ageing 25:273–278, 1996 3–37

Objective.—It has been suggested that use of benzodiazepine (BZD) drugs may be an important risk factor for falls in the elderly. Although several studies have looked at the associations between individual BZDs and the risk of falls or fractures, most have been retrospective and recall based. A prospective cohort study was performed to evaluate the risk of fall-related injury associated with BZD use, including the impact of duration of BZD use.

Methods.—A study population of 321,422 was identified from a group of linked health care databases, including information on 468 hospitalizations for injuries caused by falls. Patients with a filled prescription for a BZD sedative or tranquilizer were considered exposed and were matched to nonexposed controls. Incidence rates for fall-related hospitalization were calculated, comparing the effects of risk factors among exposed and nonexposed patients. The effects of time since BZD prescription were assessed as well.

Results.—The incidence of fall-related hospitalization within 28 days after prescription was 26/10,000 for subjects using BZD sedatives, 12/10,000 for those using BZD tranquilizers, and 9/10,000 for nonexposed controls. Such hospitalizations were more frequent in older people and for women. On multivariate analysis, the risk of falls was still elevated for BZD users; however, the odds ratio was higher for men than for women. The risk of falls was greatly increased by a history of treatment for alcohol abuse—by nearly 11-fold for men and fourfold for women. Falls were most likely to occur within 15 days after the prescription fill date—odds ratios were 3.6 for BZD sedatives and 2.6 for BZD tranquilizers. Thereafter, the risk decreased with time. Odds ratios for falls were highest with flurazepam and triazolam, 3.4 and 2.7, respectively. Odds ratios were 2.2 for oxazepam, 2.0 for lorazepam, and 1.8 for diazepam.

Conclusions.—BZD drugs are an important risk factor for fall-related hospitalization. The risk is greatest in the first few weeks after BZDs are prescribed. The mechanisms responsible for BZD-related falls in the elderly should be investigated further. Alternatives to BZD use must be studied as well.

► BZDs are well-known risk factors for falls in the elderly. This study demonstrates that the risk of falls is highest within 2 weeks of a BZD being started. The authors' demonstration that drugs with longer half-lives (e.g., flurazepam and triazolam) were associated with the highest risk of falling supports the widely held clinical belief that BZDs with shorter half-lives (e.g., oxazepam and lorazepam) might be safer.

There is still controversy about the appropriate use of BZDs in the elderly. They are not recommended for the primary treatment for anxiety disorder nor is their efficacy in treating behavior or sleep disorders in the dementias established. Nevertheless, many physicians find them to be efficacious, and it is likely that they will continue to be prescribed in these situations. This study suggests that increased scrutiny for falls should take place when BZDs are started and that vigilance is particularly important at the initiation of therapy.

P.V. Rabins, M.D., M.P.H.

4 Geriatric Neurology

Introduction

As in years past, this section of the YEAR BOOK focuses on common neurological disorders in the elderly—namely, dementia, vascular disease, Parkinson's disease (PD), and a variety of miscellaneous conditions. Although these disease categories are treated separately, it is often difficult to organize them into these discrete categories. For example, much attention is now being paid to the relationship between vascular pathology and Alzheimer's disease (AD). Moreover, we have known for years that PD and AD overlap. Patients with PD become demented and patients with AD may develop parkinsonian symptoms. Nevertheless, we approach these disorders in a traditional way and begin our discussion with dementia, perhaps the most threatening neurological condition of the aging.

From a basic scientific perspective, probably the most exciting work continues to be in the area of genetics. This year more attention was paid to the basic biology of apolipotrotein E (ApoE) and the epidemiology of ApoE ε4 status in relation to AD. At the same time that this work was being done, commercial testing for ApoE ε4 and the presenilin 1 mutations was being advanced. New studies have demonstrated that in patients who come to autopsy, the specificity of ApoE ε4 status is rather high, although the sensitivity is not as great. However, it is still a problem to figure out how to use ApoE testing in clinical practice, if at all.

First, the average patient in a geriatrician's office does not come to autopsy, which suggests that we need to be careful about making generalizations from the risk information obtained in selective samples of patients who come to autopsy at academic centers. This is particularly important because age and ethnic background appear to affect the degree to which ApoE status modifies the risk of getting AD. Moreover, it seems that ApoE ε4 status may make one more vulnerable to neurological sequellae in other diseases, such as Lewy body dementia, as well as vascular conditions. Whereas this increases the importance of the basic science discovery, it may detract from the diagnostic utility of ApoE testing.

Perhaps the greatest problem with the clinical use of this genetic test is that it is difficult for physicians and patients to understand and use the information. Without adequate physician education and patient and family counseling, the probability information may be difficult to interpret and may lead to unnecessary anguish. ApoE testing of one member of a family has implications for others, hence the need for family counseling.

Another aspect of dementia that received attention this year is the topic of noncognitive symptoms. We are still trying to understand the biology of these conditions, partly by looking at noradrenergic mechanisms. A variety of studies are underway that will help us better understand how to use new antidepressants and neuroleptics in treating these important symptoms in different kinds of dementias.

The whole area of vascular dementia is being reexamined. There is great dissatisfaction with the current diagnostic criteria and great interest in improving them, in part because of the likelihood that medications to treat vascular dementia will be developed in the near future. Mixed dementia is receiving the greatest scrutiny, because it seems to be clear that pure vascular dementia is relatively rare, whereas mixed dementia is quite common. Part of the process will be to understand the different mechanisms by which damage to blood vessels can cause stroke and to understand the role of vascular pathology in producing AD.

Donepezil (Aricept) has been approved in the United States and other countries and is quickly replacing tacrine as the first line of therapy for AD. Unfortunately, not much has been published on donepezil making it difficult for the average physician to be aware of the scientific foundation for this change in practice. Potential efficacy differences between tacrine and donepezil are probably small. However, donepezil is given once a day, requires little titration, causes few gastrointestinal side effects, and does not require bimonthly blood tests.

A variety of other cholinesterase inhibitors are working their way toward approval. For example, Excelon was submitted in March 31, 1997. Trials of muscarinic agonists are proving to be somewhat less successful than expected. The hope was that compared with cholinesterase inhibitors, selective M1 agonists would produce better cognitive improvement with fewer side effects. However, it remains to be seen whether any of these medications can achieve this goal.

With regard to stroke, the revolution continues in trying to reinvent the disease in the minds of the general population and healthcare providers, now that death and disability can be prevented by early thrombolitic therapy. The notion of "brain attack" has been developed to help individuals realize that the acute onset of neurological symptoms needs as urgent a response as heart attack. However, stroke will continue to be a common cause of disability in the elderly, requiring us to focus on the whole process of care, not just the care provided after acute presentation in the emergency room. This year we offer a series of articles on the process of stroke care, including prevention and rehabilitation. Changes in systems of care can be as important as changes in medications to improve outcomes.

With regard to PD, there was some concern this year about the possibility that selegeline (deprenyl) might actually *increase* mortality. Deprenyl is not proven to slow progression of disease, as originally claimed, but it can be used as an adjunctive drug. Moreover, additional monoaminoxidase inhibitors such as lazabemide are being developed, which may be added to the therapeutic armamentarium.

In summary, we continue to make slow progress in geriatric neurology, helping patients and primary care physicians deal with disorders that threaten quality of life. Attempts to improve the biological treatment of these conditions are meeting with some success. However, changes in the way we care for patients will provide as much (or more) enhancement of quality of life than the medications we can foresee in the near future.

Peter J. Whitehouse, M.D., Ph.D.

Dementia

GENETICS AND EPIDEMIOLOGY

Apolipoprotein E and Cognitive Change in an Elderly Population
Hyman BT, Gomez-Isla T, Briggs M, et al (Harvard Med School, Boston; Univ of Iowa, Iowa City)
Ann Neurol 40:55–66, 1996 4–1

Introduction.—The ϵ4 genotype of the apolipoprotein E (apoE) gene is overrepresented in subjects with late-onset familial Alzheimer's disease (AD), suggesting that it may be a risk factor for AD. Conversely, the ϵ2 genotype is underrepresented, suggesting that it may be a protective factor. However, the AD risk associated with apoE genotype is unknown. The risk of cognitive impairment associated with the apoE ϵ4 and ϵ2 genotypes was evaluated in a general population study.

Methods.—The analysis included 1,899 subjects aged 65 years and older who were participants in the Iowa 65+ Rural Health Study, one of the Established Populations for Epidemiologic Study of the Elderly. Cognitive function and other aspects of health were prospectively evaluated at baseline and at 4 to 7 years of follow-up. Apolipoprotein E genotype was determined by polymerase chain reaction. The effects of apoE genotype on cognitive function, as indicated by a delayed recall task, were evaluated by multiple regression and logistic regression analyses.

Results.—The apoE ϵ4 and apoE ϵ2 genotypes were both significant predictors of performance on the delayed recall task at follow-up. The effects were fairly modest, with odds ratios for cognitive impairment of 1.37 for apoE ϵ4 and 0.53 for apoE ϵ2. Genotype had more of an effect on cognitive change in women than in men. Eighty-five percent of subjects with the apoE ϵ4/4 genotype showed no impairment on a screening test of mental status.

Conclusions.—Cognitive decline is more likely for elderly people with the apoE ϵ4 genotype and less likely for those with the apoE ϵ2 genotype. However, even subjects with 2 apoE ϵ4 alleles are likely to be unimpaired when they reach old age. Thus apoE genotyping is not likely to be a useful tool in diagnosing or assessing the prognosis of cognitive decline in individual subjects. The biologic interactions leading to apoE ϵ4-associated risk remain to be clarified.

► The controversy continues surrounding the use of apoE in diagnostic testing. There is no question that individuals with the ϵ4 allele are overrepresented in patient populations with AD, and similarly there is evidence that ϵ2 is underrepresented. However, Athena Neuroscience and Dr. Allen Roses have claimed that the diagnosis of AD is now a diagnosis of inclusion, that apoE ϵ4 testing should be used as part of a diagnostic battery.

The problem is that the evidence for the value of apoE is usually produced from rather unusual populations of individuals who come through autopsy at university medical centers. This population-based study concludes that the risks are much smaller than originally reported. Thus, the sensitivity, specificity, and positive predictive values of apoE tests in clinical practice may be less than in academic studies. For example, 85% of elderly subjects who were ϵ4/ϵ4 scored in the unimpaired range. One needs to be careful about using apoE testing as a prognostic indicator (i.e., in individuals who are older but not showing any symptoms) as opposed to a diagnostic indicator (i.e., in individuals who are suffering from AD).

Another problem with apoE testing is that physicians, patients, and families may not be able to correctly interpret the results. Individuals may consider a positive result to be definitive evidence that they have AD or that the disease will develop. Moreover, there are major unresolved issues about who will pay for the test and about confidentiality when an insurance company knows an individual's apoE status. Thus, I continue to recommend a conservative approach, namely, that the test should not be used except perhaps in a few unusual circumstances. For example, if one were considering a brain biopsy or a shunt for NPH, it might be reasonable to include in one's risk benefit equation whether the patient is ϵ4/ϵ4 or ϵ2/ϵ2.

P.J. Whitehouse, M.D., Ph.D.

Apolipoprotein E in Alzheimer's Disease Risk and Case Detection: A Case-Control Study

Kukull WA, Schellenberg GD, Bowen JD, et al (Univ of Washington, Seattle; Seattle Veteran Affairs Med Ctr)

J Clin Epidemiol 49:1143–1148, 1996 4–2

Background.—Studies of the genetic factors underlying Alzheimer's disease (AD) are based primarily on large, early-onset families with many affected persons. Genetic factors associated with late-onset AD have been more difficult to identify. The association between the ϵ4 allele of the apolipoprotein E gene (apoE ϵ4) and AD was investigated in this study, and the feasibility of using apoE ϵ4 genotyping as a test for AD was determined.

Methods.—The subjects for this case-control study were drawn from 23,000 elderly enrollees in one large health maintenance organization. Two hundred thirty-four patients with probable AD identified between 1987 and 1993 and 304 cognitively intact control subjects matched for age, sex, and race were studied. All were age 60 or older. Blood samples were analyzed for apoE genotypes. Data were also obtained from patient interviews, diagnostic examinations, or medical record review.

Findings.—Compared with persons with no ϵ4, heterozygotes for ϵ4 had a crude odds ratio of 3.1 for AD. Homozygous ϵ4 persons had an odds ratio of 34.4 for AD. Having one ϵ4 allele was 0.52 sensitive and 0.74 specific as an AD indicator. Homozygous ϵ4 genotype had a sensitivity and specificity of 0.23 and 0.99, respectively. Although the presence of cardiovascular disease differed in case and control subjects, this did not confound or modify the association between apoE ϵ4 and AD.

Conclusions.—The apoE ϵ4 allele appears to be a significant risk factor for AD. However, homozygous or heterozygous ϵ4 genotype cannot be used as a screen or diagnostic marker for AD because many true cases would be missed and many normal persons misclassified as having AD.

► A test for apoE ϵ4, along with assays for cerebrospinal fluid levels of $A\beta_{40}$ and τ, is being marketed as an adjunct for diagnosing AD. One of the problems in the initial launch of this test was that the data on sensitivity and specificity were obtained only in populations of patients who were research subjects, often at academic centers who had an autopsy. This study reflects the experience of a managed care organization and calculates sensitivity and specificity figures that are much lower than those in the smaller samples from academic centers. As found before, the sensitivity is lower than the specificity and at a level that is not likely to make one consider the test diagnostic. Please note that, all subjects in this study were white; the odds ratios may be different in other ethnic groups.

P.J. Whitehouse, M.D., Ph.D.

A Prospective Study of Cognitive Health in the Elderly (Oregon Brain Aging Study): Effects of Family History and Apolipoprotein E Genotype

Payami H, Grimslid H, Oken B, et al (Oregon Health Sciences Univ, Portland; Veteran's Affairs Med Ctr, Portland, Ore)

Am J Hum Genet 60:948–956, 1997 4–3

Objective.—The "oldest old" are the most rapidly expanding age group in the population. They also have the highest prevalence of dementia—20% to 40% among individuals older than 85. There are few data on the genetic factors affecting cognitive function in the very elderly. Advancing age, apolipoprotein E (*apoE*) genotype, and a family history of dementia are the main risk factors for late-onset Alzheimer's disease. The effects of the 2 genetic risk factors on cognitive function among the very elderly were studied.

Methods.—The prospective study included 114 white research subjects who, at age 75, were in good physical health and had intact cognitive function. The mean age was 86. During an average follow-up of 4 years, they were monitored by neurologic, psychometric, and neuroimaging studies in the course of their participation in the Oregon Brain Aging Study, a prospective study of aging's effects on the nervous system. The findings were analyzed to determine the effects of *apoE* genotype and family history of dementia on the incidence and onset age of cognitive decline.

Results.—During follow-up, 25% of research subjects met the criteria for cognitive impairment. The baseline level of physical health was not a protective factor against cognitive decline. As the research subjects aged, the rate of cognitive decline increased markedly. Patients with the *apoE* ϵ4 genotype or a family history of dementia had an earlier age of onset of dementia. The effect of family history was independent of that of *apoE* ϵ4. With adjustment for age, the risk of dementia for research subjects with either *apoE* ϵ4 or a family history of dementia was 9 times higher than for those with neither risk factor.

Conclusions.—In the oldest old, the genetic risk factors for Alzheimer's disease—*apoE* genotype and family history of dementia—continue to affect the risk of dementia. This is in contrast to previous studies suggesting that the effect of these factors decreases after age 75. The incidence of cognitive decline increases with age among research subjects who are cognitively intact at age 75.

▶ The utility of *apoE* testing in clinical practice has been challenged on a number of grounds. One issue is whether the increase in susceptibility associated with the ϵ4 allele differs with age. This study suggests, however, that the predictive value of *apoE* ϵ4 continues into later ages. Nevertheless, other studies have shown age, sex, and ethnic effects, which weaken the easy application of this test in clinical practice.

P.J. Whitehouse, M.D., Ph.D.

Genetic Factors for the Development of Alzheimer Disease in the Cherokee Indian

Rosenberg RN, Richter RW, Risser RC, et al (Univ of Texas, Dallas; Univ of Oklahoma, Tulsa; Health Services Division of the Cherokee Nation, Tahlequah, Okla)

Arch Neurol 53:997–1000, 1996 4–4

Background.—The apolipoprotein E *ϵ4 *(apoE*ϵ4)* allele is well established as a risk factor for the development of Alzheimer disease (AD). Among white European populations, the heterozygous form of this allele is present in 40% to 50% of patients with a diagnosis of late-onset AD. African-Americans, however, appear to have a reduced risk of AD with the presence of the *ϵ4 allele. A study of members of the Cherokee Nation of northeastern Oklahoma compared the genetic degree of Cherokee ancestry, the *apoE* allele type, and development of AD.

Methods.—Study participants were 26 patients with AD and 26 controls with no history of cognitive decline. All were age 65 or older.

Patients and controls were grouped according to the genetic degree of Cherokee ancestry and the presence or absence of an *apoE*ϵ4* allele. Multivariate logistic regression analysis was used to determine the risk associated with the genetic degree of Cherokee ancestry. Investigators also examined whether AD results from the same or different genetic factors and risks as those found in other American genetic groups.

Results.—Compared with controls, the group of patients with AD contained more women (88% vs 58%) and tended to be older. Patients and controls differed significantly in average genetic degree of Cherokee ancestry. Eleven controls, but only 2 patients with AD, were 100% Cherokee. Patients fell more often into the categories with a low degree of Cherokee ancestry (less than 25% and 25% to 49%), whereas controls were found more frequently in the categories with a higher genetic degree of Cherokee ancestry (50% to 74% and at least 75%). An *apoE*ϵ4* allele was found in 46% of patients versus 23% of controls. The inverse relationship between genetic degree of Cherokee ancestry and AD was independent of the **ϵ4* allele status and diminished with increasing age.

Discussion.—The Cherokee Indian is genetically different from both European and African-American populations. Findings of this study indicate that as the genetic degree of Cherokee increased, the risk for development of AD was reduced. This protective effect declines with increasing age. A further implication of these findings is that complex protective and disease-causal genetic factors for AD may exist in other racial groups.

▶ This article illustrates the complexities of using genetic testing in a diverse country such as the United States. The authors found that a greater degree of Cherokee ancestry reduced the risk of Alzheimer's disease. This effect appeared to be independent of apolipoprotein E subtype, and it diminished with age. Similar approaches might be adopted in genetically diverse communities, such as so-called African Americans, who overlap considerably in genetic makeup with other pools, including so-called Caucasian Americans. It becomes difficult to estimate the protective factors and risk factors for any individual in one's office whose genetic makeup may come from many different populations.

P.J. Whitehouse, M.D., Ph.D.

APOE Genotyping and Response to Drug Treatment in Alzheimer's Disease

Richard F, Helbecque N, Neuman E, et al (IRIS, Courbevoie, France; Inst of Psychiatry, London; Institut Pasteur de Lille, France)

Lancet 349:539, 1997 4–5

Background.—The consensus on apolipoprotein E (*apoE*) genotyping in Alzheimer's disease (AD) suggests that this test may be of some value in predicting response to AD drug treatments. The relationship of *apoE* genotyping and treatment responses was studied in a multicenter, double-blind, placebo-controlled trial of the drug S12024 in the treatment of AD.

Methods and Findings.—Four hundred four patients with probable AD in 6 countries were assigned to placebo or 100 or 300 mg daily of S12024 for 12 weeks. The patients were stratified according to the presence or absence of the *apoE ϵ4* allele. In patients with the *ϵ4* allele, S12024 significantly decreased the reduction in the Mini Mental State Examination score, compared with placebo. However, in patients without the *ϵ4* allele, S12024 did not have any detectable effect.

Conclusion.—A different predisposition to drug response occurred based on *apoE* genotype in this preliminary study of the effect of S12024. Additional research is needed to confirm the slower cognitive deterioration with S12024 in patients with the *ϵ4* allele.

▶ In recent months, investigators have been making attempts to relate *apoE* status to therapeutic responsiveness to various medications. With tacrine, reports have been made on both sides of the equation, i.e., that individuals with the *ϵ4* allele are either more or less responsive to tacrine. This brief article concerns a drug that is under development for treatment of AD, S12024. It is another illustration of this post hoc attempt to try to determine therapeutic responsiveness to an agent. Such studies are important because many families tend to think that genetic susceptibility testing, or other testing, may be useful only if it predicts therapeutic responsiveness or leads to a new therapy. However, at what point would we not offer medication to someone just because that person had a decreased risk for responsiveness to the drug, based on genetic tests? Better prospective studies are needed before such information can be incorporated into clinical practice.

P.J. Whitehouse, M.D., Ph.D.

Atherosclerosis, Apolipoprotein E, and Prevalence of Dementia and Alzheimer's Disease in the Rotterdam Study

Hofman A, Ott A, Breteler MMB, et al (Erasmus Univ, Rotterdam, The Netherlands; Univ of Antwerp, Belgium)

Lancet 349:151–154, 1997 4–6

Introduction.—The 2 major subtypes of dementia are Alzheimer's disease (AD) and vascular dementia. There appears to be an association between the apolipoprotein E (apoE) ϵ4 allele and AD, and evidence exists for a role of atherosclerosis in patients with vascular dementia. It is uncertain, however, if atherosclerosis is involved in the cause of AD. This question was examined in a population-based cross-sectional study of 284 patients with dementia and 1,698 individuals age 55 and older who had negative screening results for dementia.

Methods.—The study was conducted in a suburb of Rotterdam between March 1990 and July 1993. Dementia was assessed by a 3-phase approach: screening with a brief cognitive test, cognitive and neurologic testing of those who had positive screening results, and a detailed examination of those whose results suggested dementia. Analysis was restricted to the 284 of 474 cases of dementia with an onset of less than 3 years. Dementia was diagnosed according to *DSM-III-R*. Atherosclerosis was indicated by US assessment of vessel wall thickness and plaques of the carotid arteries. A measure of generalized atherosclerosis was the ratio of ankle/brachial systolic blood pressure. Apolipoprotein E polymorphisms were evaluated in 246 patients and 928 controls.

Results.—In the group with dementia, 207 (73%) had a diagnosis of AD and 50 (18%) had vascular dementia; other dementias were present in 27 (10%). All indicators of atherosclerosis were significantly associated with all dementia, with AD, and with vascular dementia. The odds ratios were similar for all dementia and for AD (range 1.3 to 1.9) and greater for vascular dementia (range 1.9 to 3.2). Associations were also observed between the apoE ϵ4 allele and all dementias, AD, and vascular dementia. Increases in the degree of atherosclerosis were accompanied by increases in the odds ratios of all dementia, AD, and vascular dementia. Study participants with both the apoE ϵ4 genotype and high atherosclerosis scores had odds ratios of 4.5 for dementia, 3.9 for AD, and 19.8 for vascular dementia.

Conclusion.—Dementia and its 2 major subtypes, AD and vascular dementia, were found to be associated with atherosclerosis. The association between atherosclerosis and dementia is particularly strong in those with the apoE ϵ4 genotype.

▶ The relationships between vascular dementia and Alzheimer's disease are complex. First, many individuals may have both disease processes causing their cognitive impairment. Second, even in pure AD, abnormalities of blood vessels have been reported, including amyloid angiopathy and changes in the innervation of blood vessels and some of the associated transporter proteins. We know that apoE subtypes can affect one's risk for vascular disease in general as well as AD. This population-based study explored, for the first time, the relationships among AD, vascular dementia, and apoE. All indicators of atherosclerosis increased the likelihood of dementia, and apoE ϵ4 status had an additive effect.

P.J. Whitehouse, M.D., Ph.D.

Apolipoprotein E ϵ4 and the Risk of Dementia With Stroke: A Population-based Investigation

Slooter AJC, Tang M-X, van Duijn CM, et al (Columbia Univ, New York; Erasmus Univ, Rotterdam, The Netherlands; Univ of Antwerp, Belgium)

JAMA 277:818–821, 1997 4–7

Introduction.—People with the ϵ4 allele of the apolipoprotein E gene (*apoE*) are at elevated risk for Alzheimer's disease (AD). However, the role of *apoE* in patients with dementia who have also had strokes—defined as either vascular dementia (VaD) or AD with cerebrovascular disease (AD with CVD)—is unclear. The *apoE* genotype was investigated in patients with dementia who have also had strokes.

Methods.—The study included data from 2 population-based studies, 1 Dutch and 1 American. Comparisons were performed between 187 patients with dementia who had had strokes and 507 controls of similar age and ethnicity. The frequencies of various *apoE* alleles were compared between groups, and adjustments were made for age, sex, residency, and education. The extent to which the risk of dementia with the risk of having a stroke could be attributed to the *apoE* ϵ4 allele was estimated.

Results.—The *apoE* ϵ4 allele was more frequent in patients with dementia and strokes than in controls. The risk of dementia with a stroke was 7 times higher in research subjects homozygous for *apoE* ϵ4 than in those homozygous for *apoE* ϵ3 (odds ratio [OR], 6.9). For those with *apoE* ϵ4 heterozygosity, the risk was doubled (OR, 1.8). The increased risk associated with *apoE* ϵ4 held regardless of dementia with stroke subtype, age, or sex. For African-American and Hispanic patients, the risk was greatest with *apoE* ϵ4 homozygosity. An estimated 41% of the risk of dementia plus the risk of having a stroke was attributed to the *apoE* ϵ4 allele: 33% for patients with VaD and 44% for those with AD with CVD.

Conclusions.—Individuals with the *apoE* ϵ4 allele are at increased risk for dementia with strokes and their subtypes, VaD and AD with CVD. The findings suggest some shared susceptibility between patients who have dementia with strokes and those who have AD. Another explanation is that patients with AD may be included among those classified as having dementia with strokes—including those meeting the current definition of VaD.

► Is the ϵ4 allele of *apoE* useful as a specific diagnostic test for AD? Clearly, in studies of patients from academic centers, there is an association between *apoE* ϵ4 and AD as diagnosed at autopsy. However, relatively fewer studies have been done on other types of dementia. This article demonstrates that, in a population-based study, *apoE* ϵ4 increased the risk for VaD as well. The authors rightfully include the caveat that, without autopsy, we do not know whether the patients with "VaD" in fact had AD.

P.J. Whitehouse, M.D., Ph.D.

► The number of recent publications on the relationship between *apoE* and the *apoE* ϵ4 genotype, dementia, and outcomes is staggering. This well-designed, important study demonstrates that patients with clinically diagnosed VaD or clinically diagnosed "mixed" dementia (here called AD with CVD) are more likely to have ϵ4 genotype. In addition, their finding tht ϵ4 homozygotes had an odds ratio of 6.9% while heterozygotes had an odds ratio of 1.8% suggests that there might be a "dose-response" relationship; that is, the greater the dose of the ϵ4 genotypes the greater the risk of developing dementia. The most parsimonious conclusion is that *apoE* genotype influences risks of developing dementia not only from AD but from vascular disease as well. The findings that *apoE* genotype also influences recovery after traumatic brain injury[1] and is a risk factor for the dementia pugilistica[2] suggest that the ϵ4 allele increases the risk of dementia from multiple causes. Perhaps it influences brain plasticity in response to a variety of trauma.[1, 2] The implications of this hypothesis, were it confirmed, is that modification of this genetic risk factor might protect against brain injury due to a variety of causes and may have implications for recovery from many central nervous system injuries.

P.V. Rabins, M.D., M.P.H.

References

1. Roberts GW, Gentleman SM, Lynch A, et al: Amyloid protein deposition in the brain after severe head injury. *J Neurol Neurosurg Psychiatry* 57:419–425, 1994.
2. Jordan BD, Relkin MR, Ravdin LD, et al: Apolipoprotein E ϵ4 associated with chronic traumatic brain injury in boxing. *JAMA* 278:136–410, 1997.

Evidence That the 42- and 40-Amino Acid Forms of Amyloid β Protein Are Generated From the β-Amyloid Precursor Protein by Different Protease Activities

Citron M, Diehl TS, Gordon G, et al (Harvard Med School, Boston; Athena Neurosciences Inc, San Francisco)

Proc Natl Acad Sci USA 93:13170–13175, 1996 4–8

Background.—Early in the course of Alzheimer's disease (AD), cerebral deposition of the amyloid β($A\beta_{40}$) protein occurs. Normally, 90% of all Aβ released from cells is of the 40-amino acid form. However, in AD this form appears to be involved only in the later stages. The major constituent of amyloid plaques in AD is the longer, more amyloidogenic 42-residue form of Aβ($A\beta_{42}$), which accounts for only 10% of normally secreted Aβ. Thus inhibition of $A\beta_{42}$ is an important therapeutic goal in AD. It is assumed that γ-secretase is the protease responsible for generating the C termini of both $A\beta_{40}$ and $A\beta_{42}$. The effects of γ-secretase inhibition on β-amyloid precursor protein processing were studied.

Methods and Results.—The in vitro study used the calpain inhibitor MDL 28170, which is thought to be a direct inhibitor of γ-secretase. Conditioned medium of various cell lines was immunoprecipitated with antibodies specific to $A\beta_{40}$ and $A\beta_{42}$. The results showed that MDL 28170 mainly reduced $A\beta_{40}$ and $p3_{40}$, with little effect on A_{42} and $p3_{42}$.

Conclusions.—Surprisingly, the $A\beta_{40}$ and $A\beta_{42}$ C termini appear to be generated by different proteases. This finding raises the possibility of finding compounds that specifically block the $A\beta_{42}$ peptide, which is pathogenic in AD, without blocking general β-amyloid precursor protein metabolism. This could offer a more promising approach to reducing plaque amyloid burden in AD.

▶ The Holy Grail of the baptists (individuals who are religiously committed to β-amyloid protein) is to prevent the damage caused by amyloid in the nervous system. This religious sect tends to ignore the variable evidence that amyloid is toxic and that neurofibrillary tangles (the religious icon of the tauists) are more closely associated with cell death in autopsy material. However, $A\beta_{40}$ now appears to be involved in pathogenesis, although found in lower concentrations than the $A\beta_{40}$ form. This article demonstrates that a particular compound, MDL 28170, may act selectively on the metabolism of the $A\beta_{40}$ and $A\beta_{42}$ forms. This work offers some evidence that selective therapeutic agents could actually be produced.

P.J. Whitehouse, M.D., Ph.D.

Correlative Memory Deficits, Aβ Elevation, and Amyloid Plaques in Transgenic Mice

Hsiao K, Chapman P, Nilsen S, et al (Univ of Minnesota, Minneapolis; Univ of Wales, Cardiff; Mayo Clinic, Jacksonville, Fla)

Science 274:99–102, 1996 4–9

Objective.—Although the presence of amyloid plaques in brain tissue is commonly used in diagnosing Alzheimer's disease (AD), other changes are also present and may be better related to dementia. The amyloid in senile plaques is derived from the larger amyloid precursor protein (APP), of which the APP_{695} isoform is the most abundant. Several mutations in APP have been identified in families with early-onset AD. A transgenic mouse model of AD with overexpression of the APP_{695} is reported.

Methods and Findings.—The transgenic mice were produced with human APP_{695} containing a double mutation, Lys^{670} →Asn, Met^{671} →Leu, isolated from a family with early-onset AD. The resulting mice had nearly 6 times the level of brain APP expression as did nontransgenic controls. In the transgenic mice, learning and memory in spatial reference and alternation tasks was normal at 3 months of age but significantly impaired at 9 to 10 months. As the behavioral changes appeared, so did a fivefold increase in Aβ(1-40) and a 14-fold increase in Aβ(1-42/43). The cortex and limbus of mice with elevated Aβ showed numerous Aβ plaques that stained with Congo red dye.

Conclusions.—The development of transgenic mice with behavioral, biochemical, and pathologic abnormalities similar to those seen in AD is reported. Deficits in learning and memory develop as the mice age, along with markedly increased amounts of Aβ and number amyloid plaques and Aβ deposits. This model may be useful for studying the physiology and neurobiology of AD.

► Do we have an animal model for AD? We certainly have models of certain aspects of the pathogenesis of AD (e.g., animals with cholinergic deficiencies have been helpful in developing cholinesterase inhibitors). However, to develop more fundamental interventions, we need animal models that include pathologic hallmarks, namely senile plaques and neurofibrillary tangles. Moreover, we presumably need these models of disease pathogenesis to be associated with behavioral abnormalities.

In this study, a transgenic mouse overexpressing the 695 amino acid isoform of human Aβ developed learning and memory problems after normal performance at 3 months of age. This does appear to model a dementia, and the amount of dementia was correlated with the appearance of plaques. I should point out that this animal does not appear to have neurofibrillary tangles. Moreover, it is not clear that the mechanism of cell dysfunction in this animal is quite the same as would be found in human beings. Nevertheless, this research does represent a step forward in the development of animal models that might help us develop medications with more fundamental effects on pathogenesis.

P.J. Whitehouse, M.D., Ph.D.

RAGE and Amyloid-β Peptide Neurotoxicity in Alzheimer's Disease

Yan SD, Chen X, Fu J, et al (Columbia Univ, NY; Sun Health Research Inst, Sun City, Ariz; Berlex Biosciences, Richmond, Calif; et al)

Nature 382:685–691, 1996 4–10

Introduction.—Neurotoxic amyloid-β peptide plays a key role in the pathology of Alzheimer's disease. It acts directly by inducing oxidant stress and indirectly by activating microglia. Previous reports have suggested a specific cell-surface acceptor site that would focus the effects of amyloid-β peptide on target cells; however, no such receptor has been identified. The "receptor for advanced glycation end products" (RAGE) is identified as the receptor mediating the effects of amyloid-β peptide in Alzheimer's disease.

Findings.—Experimental studies identified a polypeptide of molecular mass ~50K that bound synthetic amyloid-β. This peptide proved identical to RAGE, which previous reports identified as a central cellular receptor for advanced glycation end products. Further experiments demonstrated that RAGE mediated interaction between amyloid-β protein and endothelial cells and neurons, producing cellular oxidant stress. Interaction with microglia led to cellular activation, with cytokine production, chemotaxis, and haptotaxis. Enhanced RAGE expression was noted in Alzheimer's disease, in affected neurons, in microglia, and in the vasculature.

Conclusions.—The RAGE receptor may play an important pathophysiologic role in Alzheimer's disease. Engagement of RAGE may have diverse effects, depending on the nature of the ligand, cell maturation, and the microenvironment. This receptor promotes neurite growth and normal development during the fetal and perinatal periods and may be involved in the disposal of physiologic levels of amyloid-β peptide in later life. However, sustained cellular oxidant stress may result from engagement of RAGE by cortical neurons in the presence of higher levels of amyloid-β peptide. This interaction could have harmful effects on cellular function and organic homeostasis.

▶ Mixing metaphors somewhat, one might say that the search for the holy grail in AD is to find a unified theory. In the physics and metaphysics domain, perhaps one could say that the search for the Nobel Prize will depend on finding the element that soothes the religious arguments between the taoists (those who think that tao is critical to pathogenesis), the baptists (those who think that amyloid protein is the key element), and other religious adherents. It may be that RAGE is part of this process. Many groups have been trying to define the normal function of the amyloid precursor protein, and part of this quest has been to identify the receptor with which it binds. So far the only receptors that have been claimed to play any role are substance P and the serpin-enzyme complex (SEC receptors). However, many other proteins, including apolipoprotein E and extracelluar matrix proteins, also bind to amyloid-β.

The appeal of this article is its ties to yet another popular hypothesis about cell death and AD, that is to say, the accumulation of oxidant stress. The RAGE receptor is the receptor for advanced glycation end products, which might be involved in pathogenesis and cell death in AD, as a number of groups have suggested. Thus, this paper links amyloid-β to oxidant stress, microglia activation, and other components of the pathogenesis of AD, and it suggests some potential common links between them.

P.J. Whitehouse, M.D., Ph.D.

Effect of Oestrogen During Menopause on Risk and Age at Onset of Alzheimer's Disease

Tang M-X, Jacobs D, Stern Y, et al (Gertrude H Sergievsky Ctr, New York; Taub Ctr for Alzheimer's Disease Research, New York; Columbia Univ, New York; et al)

Lancet 348:429–432, 1996 4–11

Introduction.—Reports are conflicting regarding the beneficial use of estrogen as a treatment for Alzheimer's disease in elderly women. It has been shown that estrogen promotes the growth of cholinergic neurons, stimulates the secretase metabolism of the amyloid precursor protein, and may interact with apolipoprotein E. All 3 factors may affect risk of Alzheimer's disease. The effect of estrogen use on the development of Alzheimer's disease was evaluated in 1,124 nondemented elderly women participating in a community-based investigation on aging.

Methods.—Participants underwent an interview that included history of estrogen use, clinical assessment, and a battery of neuropsychological tests. Medical records were reviewed for pertinent information.

Results.—Women who had Alzheimer's disease were significantly older and had significantly fewer years of education. Age at menopause did not differ regarding development of Alzheimer's disease. Of 1,124 women, 156 reported using estrogen an average of 6.8 years after the onset of menopause. Estrogen users were significantly younger, had significantly higher education levels, and were significantly more likely to have had a hysterectomy or early onset of menopause, compared with nonusers. Significantly fewer black women had used estrogen, compared with white and Hispanic women. Women who had used estrogen were significantly less likely to have Alzheimer's disease, compared with nonusers. The age at onset of Alzheimer's disease was significantly higher in estrogen users, compared with nonusers. Women who used estrogen for 1 year or less had a lower risk of Alzheimer's disease, and women who took estrogen for longer than 1 year had a significantly lower risk, compared with nonusers. There was a significant linear trend observed between duration of estrogen use and disease risk. Of 23 women still taking estrogen at the time of enrollment, none had Alzheimer's disease. Women with the ϵ4 allele of apolipoprotein E (*apoE*ϵ*4*) genotypes had a significantly higher risk for Alzheimer's disease, compared with women with other genotypes. The relative risk of developing Alzheimer's disease was lower in women with heterozygous genotype *apoE*ϵ*4* who used estrogen, compared with women with heterozygous genotype *apoE*ϵ*4* who did not use estrogen. The estimated annual incidence rates of Alzheimer's disease were 2.7% and 8.4%, respectively, for estrogen users and nonusers.

Conclusions.—Estrogen use may delay the onset and decrease the risk of Alzheimer's disease. Women with a history of long-term estrogen use had the lowest risk for Alzheimer's disease. The next step is a prospective investigation of estrogen use in perimenopausal women and its effect on Alzheimer's disease, once more data are available on the safety, dosage, and duration of estrogen treatment required.

► One of the strengths of this study is that it was longitudinal and community based. Even following adjustment for differences in education, ethnic origin, and *apoE* genotype, a so-called protective effect of estrogen was determined.

This is the type of report that makes clinicians wonder whether they should be prescribing estrogen to their patients with dementia or perhaps to women at risk for dementia. Some small clinical trials have suggested that estrogen has a beneficial effect in patients with Alzheimer's disease, and some have shown cognitive-enhancing properties of estrogen in normal aging women. Several prospective studies are under way, supported by the Women's Health Initiative and the National Institute on Aging Cooperative Study Group. A purist would wait until these studies were available, knowing well the potential foolishness of following purely epidemiologic trials. However, in my own view, for a woman who is receiving or might receive estrogen for other reasons (i.e., osteoporosis or cardiovascular disease), a possible positive effect on the brain ought not to be forgotten by the clinician.

P.J. Whitehouse, M.D., Ph.D.

Polyunsaturated Fatty Acids, Antioxidants, and Cognitive Function in Very Old Men

Kalmijn S, Feskens EJM, Launer LJ, et al (Natl Inst of Public Health and the Environment, Bilthoven, The Netherlands; Erasmus Univ, Rotterdam, The Netherlands; Netherlands Inst for Health Sciences, Rotterdam, The Netherlands)

Am J Epidemiol 145:33–41, 1997 4–12

Objective.—Cognitive impairment can develop in patients with atherosclerosis and thrombosis as a result of cerebral infarcts or white matter hyperintensities. Oxidative stress is believed to play a major role in the process of atherogenesis. Dietary factors can increase oxidative stress, such as a high intake of polyunsaturated fatty acids or a low intake of antioxidants. Thrombosis may be reduced by a high intake of n-3 polyunsaturated fatty acids, the main source of which is fish. However, it is unknown how these dietary factors affect cognitive function. The link between polyunsaturated fatty acid and antioxidant intake and cognitive function was investigated in a community-based, longitudinal study of older men.

Methods.—The men, age 69–89, were participants in a Dutch longitudinal study of risk factors for chronic diseases. Cognitive impairment was assessed by the 30-point Mini-Mental State Examination (MMSE) in 1990 and again in 1993. The 1990 sample included 476 men. The cross-check dietary history method was used to estimate food intake in 1985 and 1990. Associations between dietary factors and cognitive function were analyzed by logistic regression, and potential confounders were taken into account.

Results.—In 1990, 32% of men had cognitive impairment on the MMSE, as indicated by a score of 25 or less. Fifteen percent of men had cognitive decline from 1990 to 1993, as indicated by a drop of more than 2 points. After adjustment for confounders—including age, education, smoking, alcohol consumption, and energy intake—a high intake of linoleic acid was significantly associated with cognitive impairment (odds ratio [OR], 1.76 for highest vs. lowest tertile of intake). Cognitive impairment was unrelated to n-3 polyunsaturated fatty acid intake. However, a high level of fish consumption was linked to a reduced risk of cognitive impairment (OR, 0.63) and cognitive decline (OR, 0.45). The level of cognitive function was unrelated to beta-carotene, vitamin C, vitamin E, or flavonoid intake.

Conclusions.—Elderly men with a high intake of linoleic acid may be at elevated risk for cognitive impairment, whereas those with a high level of fish consumption may be protected against cognitive impairment. No protective effect of antioxidant drugs is apparent, however. The findings should be interpreted with caution and should be confirmed in larger, prospective studies.

► In a variety of diseases, including Alzheimer's disease and atherosclerosis, oxidative stress is believed to be a major contributor to the disease process. Studies of antioxidants suggest potential therapeutic benefits, and basic science studies imply a role for free radicals in causing the cellular damage. The interesting question is whether dietary exposure to polyunsaturated fatty acids and antioxidants may alter the risk of these diseases.

In this study, the authors looked at the relationship between dietary consumption of these substances and cognitive performance. They suggest that atherosclerosis may lead to cognitive impairments via infarcts or white matter hyperintensities, although the relationship between white matter hyperintensities and cognition is unclear. Nevertheless, they do find that intake of linoleic acid, a polyunsaturated fatty acid, was associated with cognitive impairment, and that a high intake of fish, which includes certain polyunsaturated fatty acids, may lower risk. Although it is difficult to obtain this kind of retrospective dietary information and the authors are appropriately conservative about interpreting their findings, the study does illustrate the importance of examining lifelong dietary habits and their relationship to age-related diseases.

P.J. Whitehouse, M.D., Ph.D.

Effects of Alzheimer's Disease Severity on Cerebrospinal Fluid Norepinephrine Concentration

Elrod R, Peskind ER, DiGiacomo L, et al (Univ of Washington, Seattle)
Am J Psychiatry 154:25–30, 1997 4–13

Background.—Autopsies of subjects with Alzheimer's disease (AD) show loss of noradrenergic neurons in the locus ceruleus. In contrast, previous reports have suggested that measures of central noradrenergic activity increase with the severity of AD in living patients. Cerebrospinal fluid norepinephrine is a useful indicator of CNS noradrenergic activity. The effects of AD severity and of normal aging on CSF norepinephrine were determined.

Methods.—Four groups of subjects underwent lumbar puncture: 49 patients with mild to moderate AD, 25 patients with advanced AD, 42 normal elderly subjects, and 54 normal young adults. The patients with advanced AD were identified by a Mini-Mental State score of less than 12. Levels of norepinephrine in CSF and plasma were measured by a sensitive single-isotope radioenzymatic assay.

Results.—Mean CSF norepinephrine level was 279 pg/mL in the patients with advanced AD, 198 pg/mL in those with mild to moderate AD, 219 pg/mL in normal elderly subjects, and 154 pg/mL in normal young subjects. In the patients with AD, the Mini-Mental State score was significantly negatively correlated with CSF norepinephrine concentration. The difference in CSF norepinephrine concentration was not significantly different between normal elderly subjects and patients with mild to moderate AD. The 3 groups of elderly subjects had higher levels of norepinephrine in both CSF and plasma and higher mean arterial blood pressure than the young subjects did.

Conclusions.—Patients with mild to moderate AD continue to show the high concentrations of CSF norepinephrine associated with normal aging, even though they are losing locus ceruleus neurons. As their disease progresses, the CSF norepinephrine level continues to increase. High levels of brain noradrenergic activity may play a role in the agitation or cognitive deficits observed in patients with advanced AD.

▶ Despite the recent focus on the molecular biology of Alzheimer's disease and proteins such as amyloid and tau, neurotransmitters are still the means by which neurons communicate and they are important in AD. The loss of locus ceruleus neurons has been clearly documented, although cell loss can be variable. Moreover, cell loss can occur in this structure as a function of normal aging. Yet in this study, norepinephrine concentrations were higher in patients with advanced AD. As the authors surmise, this may represent some alteration in the turnover metabolism of noradrenaline in AD. This activity may contribute to clinical symptoms such as agitated behavior or cognitive deficit.

P.J. Whitehouse, M.D., Ph.D.

Linkage of Frontotemporal Dementia to Chromosome 17: Clinical and Neuropathological Characterization of Phenotype

Yamaoka LH, Welsh-Bohmer KA, Hulette CM, et al (Duke Univ, Durham, NC; VA Med Ctr, Durham, NC)

Am J Hum Genet 59:1306–1312, 1996 4–14

Background.—Frontotemporal dementia (FLDEM) is a degenerative dementia characterized by behavioral and neuropsychological symptoms that reflect frontal lobe dysfunction. Neuropathologic investigations have demonstrated nonspecific degeneration of the neocortex and subcortical nuclei. Frontotemporal dementia appears to be inherited as an autosomal dominant disease with age-dependent penetrance. Recent single-family studies have discovered 2 distinct chromosomal regions, 17q21 and a chromosome 3 locus, linked to non-Alzheimer's disease FLDEM. A novel large, multigenerational family (DUK1684) with clinical and neurologic characteristics of FLDEM is described. Linkage analysis was performed to determine whether the dementia occurring in members of this kindred was allelic with any of the other FLDEM syndromes that have been previously described.

Methods.—This family was referred to Duke University Medical Center. Affected members of this kindred were assessed through medical history, neurologic examination, and neuropsychological testing. Simple-tandem-repeat polymorphisms were typed for individual family members using polymerase chain reaction. Linkage analysis was performed assuming autosomal dominant inheritance with age-dependent penetrance using the VITESSE program package.

Results.—The proband, DUK1684/39, had symptom onset at age 52, beginning with depression, personality changes, and physical complaints. These initial symptoms progressed to apathy and amotivation, interspersed with irritable explosions. Neuropsychological examination demonstrated naming, visuoperception, and executive function impairments. Brain MRI was normal. These findings were not consistent with a diagnosis of Alzheimer's disease. The patient's condition continued to deteriorate. Among other affected individuals in this kindred for whom information is available, initial symptoms were cognitive in 5, behavioral in 5, and extrapyramidal in 1. The average age of onset was 55, with a duration of 9 years. The most common symptoms were impaired judgment, problem solving, perseveration, insight, and social awareness. Microscopically, neuronal loss and gliosis were most prominent in the temporal lobe, third nerve nucleus, and substantia nigra. Senile plaques, tangles, and Pick bodies were not detected. Gross examination of the brain of 1 patient revealed some atrophy of the frontal, parietal, occipital, and temporal lobes and severe ventricular dilatation. There was severe neuronal loss as well as moderate pigment incontinence in the substantia nigra. Linkage analysis demonstrated that the most likely location for the mutated gene in this family was the 17q21 chromosomal region.

Conclusions.—This report describes a novel kindred (DUK1684), inheriting a progressive, neurodegenerative FLDEM-like disease, linked to locus 17q21. Comparison of the clinical, pathologic, and linkage characteristics of this family with those of other chromosome 17-linked families with FLDEM suggests that these families are allelic. The understanding of the pathophysiology and phenotype variation within this disease awaits the identification and characterization of this mutated gene and its product.

▶ Frontal lobe dementia is a degenerative dementia that causes cognitive impairment in the elderly. Clinically, it is characterized by cognitive impairment that affects executive abilities, such as goal setting and self-monitoring. Moreover, changes in personality and perseverative behaviors are common. Exciting recent genetic research into this disorder has characterized loci on chromosomes 17 and 3. This article characterizes 1 such family with localization to chromosome 17. I expect that in the future, more specific chromosome abnormalities will be identified, which, it is hoped, will contribute to our understanding of the range of molecular biological lesions that can cause cognitive impairment in the elderly.

P.J. Whitehouse, M.D., Ph.D.

Preparing for Presymptomatic DNA Testing for Early Onset Alzheimer's Disease/Cerebral Haemorrhage and Hereditary Pick Disease

Tibben A, Stevens M, de Wert GMWR, et al (Erasmus Univ, Rotterdam, The Netherlands; Univ Hosp Dijkzigt, Rotterdam, The Netherlands; Inst of Bioethics, Maastricht, The Netherlands)

J Med Genet 34:63–72, 1997 4–15

Purpose.—Hereditary Pick's disease (HPD) and familial Alzheimer's dementia and cerebral hemorrhage (FAD-CH) are primary degenerative brain diseases, with an average onset in the fourth to sixth decades of life, for which there is no specific treatment. Through genetic mutational or linkage analysis, both of these diagnoses can now be confirmed. Presymptomatic testing, as offered for patients with Huntington's disease, is also a possibility. The impact of presymptomatic testing for these hereditary presenile dementias was assessed in families at risk.

Methods.—The study sample comprised 21 people at risk for the APP-692 mutation that causes FAD-CH and 43 at risk for HPD. Each research subject was at 50% risk. Each participant completed a general medical examination, neurologic examination, neuropsychological tests, brain MRI, a clinical psychological assessment, and an attitudinal survey. The goal was to determine the patients' ability to cope with being at risk for these diseases, how the disease influenced various aspects of their lives, and their attitudes toward presymptomatic testing.

Findings.—Although 64% of the research subjects said they would request presymptomatic testing if it were available, two thirds did not believe that they were ready to be tested yet. Major reasons cited for doing the test in both groups were to make a contribution to basic research, to inform their children, to plan for the future, and to relieve uncertainty. If the results were to be unfavorable, the participants expressed concern about the problems the disease would create for spouses and children. Most of the research subjects believed that an unfavorable result would not have a negative impact on their personal mood and relationships.

One third of the participants felt that prenatal testing should be performed when 1 parent was at risk for the disease. Thirty-five percent said they would encourage their children to have the test before starting a relationship, and 44% would encourage their children to do so before starting a family. Thirty-seven percent said they would recommend that their children choose prenatal diagnosis. Worry over potential symptoms was greater for research subjects at risk of HPD than for those at risk of FAD-CH. This was related to the disruptive impact of loss of inhibition in patients affected by HPD.

Conclusions.—The findings lay the groundwork for presymptomatic testing programs for families at risk for 2 kinds of hereditary presenile dementia. An integral part of such testing programs will be adequate counseling and the availability of resources to help the families deal with the test results. The results have implications in many different areas, including participation in pedigree linkage studies, acceptability of presymptomatic testing programs, prenatal testing, genetic discrimination, and genetic research in health care.

► Genetic testing for dementia will increase in visibility and complexity during the next several years. Commercialization continues, starting with the marketing of the Athena Neuroscience Presenilin I test. In addition, other susceptible loci are being characterized, although the premature commercialization of these tests may affect our trust in the data being presented.

This article focuses on a specific population of individuals who are at risk for 2 rather rare degenerative dementias. However, the lessons can be generalized to other populations. In this Dutch population, it was good to see that the reason almost 50% of individuals took the test was to further basic research. However, that mode is very different from clinical counseling because, in many basic research programs, there is no communication of the information to the individuals concerning their own status. Also, many individuals may indicate interest in a commercial test, but when it becomes available, they may be less likely to have the test once the risks and benefits are explained. This reversal of position is common in patients with other diseases, such as Alzheimer's disease and Huntington's disease.

I agree wholeheartedly with the conclusion of the article, which is that there is a need for further counseling and resources to deal with the impact of test results. There is also a need for more general public discussion about the ethics and public policy implications of genetic testing in neurodegenerative conditions.

P.J. Whitehouse, M.D., Ph.D.

Diagnosis and Assessment

Do Cognitive Complaints Either Predict Future Cognitive Decline or Reflect Past Cognitive Decline?: A Longitudinal Study of an Elderly Community Sample

Jorm AF, Christensen H, Korten AE, et al (Australian Natl Univ, Canberra)
Psychol Med 27:91–98, 1997 4–16

Background.—Whether cognitive complaints are related to longitudinal measures of cognitive performance is unknown. Data from a 2-wave longitudinal study of one group of elderly community dwellers were analyzed to determine whether cognitive complaints predict subsequent cognitive decline or reflect past cognitive decline.

Methods.—The first wave of interviews was done in 1990–1991, and the second wave in 1994. Data were available for 945 subjects during the first wave and for 507 for the second wave. Cognitive complaints and cognitive function were evaluated at these times.

Findings.—Cognitive complaints reported during the first wave of interviews did not predict future cognitive changes on the Mini-Mental State Examination, an episodic memory test, or a test of mental speed. Cognitive complaints reported at the second interview were also unassociated with past cognitive changes on these tests, after adjustment for anxiety and depression. Cognitive complaints did not predict mortality after adjustment for anxiety and depression or future dementia.

Conclusions.—Cognitive complaints apparently do not predict cognitive change in the next 3.5 years or relate to cognitive change in the preceding 3.5 years, after adjustment for anxiety and depression. These findings do not support the inclusion of cognitive complaints in the diagnostic criteria for proposed disorders such as age-associated memory impairment, mild cognitive disorder, and cognitive decline associated with aging.

► The base rate of memory complaints among aging geriatricians and their patients is quite high. The question is how much attention we should pay to these complaints, along with objective assessment of changes in memory or cognition. This article provides some additional evidence that memory complaints really are not valid to predict cognitive loss. Certainly we should not ignore these complaints—in fact, they may signal psychological problems more than dementia. However, we should recognize that many factors aside from objective performance play into whether memory complaints indicate a serious neurologic disease.

P.J. Whitehouse, M.D., Ph.D.

A 5-Year Longitudinal Study of the Mini-Mental State Examination in Normal Aging

Jacqmin-Gadda H, Fabrigoule C, Commenges D, et al (Institut Natl de la Santé et de la Recherche Médicale, Bordeaux, France)

Am J Epidemiol 145:498–506, 1997 4–17

Background.—The Mini-Mental State Examination (MMSE) is widely used as a screening test for dementia. Cross-sectional studies have linked the MMSE score to educational level, lifetime occupation, and age. Most longitudinal studies to date have evaluated the progression of cognitive impairment in small samples of patients with dementia. This 5-year longitudinal study used the MMSE to monitor cognitive functioning in community-dwelling elderly individuals without dementia.

Methods.—The study sample comprised 2,537 French individuals aged 65 years or older and living at home at baseline. They were participants in a larger prospective study of normal and pathologic cerebral aging. The MMSE was administered at baseline and again at 1, 3, and 5 years later. The course of the MMSE score over time was analyzed by a random effects linear regression model. Whether the sociodemographic factors linked to low MMSE scores in cross-sectional studies were also associated with the rate of cognitive decline was also determined.

Results.—The linear model demonstrated an increase in MMSE score between baseline and year 1: by 0.60 points for research subjects age 65 at baseline and 0.83 points for those age 85. This was followed by a slight decline from year 1 to year 5: 0.02 points for research subjects age 65 and

0.57 points for those age 85. The first-year rise was attributed to the stress of testing at baseline or to a learning effect at year 1; less-educated research subjects had a larger increase. From year 1 to year 5, older and less well-educated research subjects had a greater decline in MMSE scores. The cross-sectional effect of age was greater than the longitudinal effect of time, probably because of a cohort effect or a practice effect.

Conclusions.—Elderly research subjects without dementia show a very slight decline in MMSE scores during follow-up. The results suggest that the aging process does not affect the various cognitive processes measured by the MMSE. Although more research is needed to clarify the implications for screening, a declining MMSE score may be a useful indicator of risk of dementia over the subsequent few years.

▶ There is renewed attention to the notion of screening populations of older individuals for early signs of dementia. This is a complicated topic that this article helps us to understand better. First, we can see that improvements in MMSE scores occurred during the first time period, perhaps because of practice effects or reduced anxiety from having participated in the experimental situation previously. Scores then declined very slowly but in a way that was more pronounced for older and less well-educated research subjects. In the United States, a variety of organizations and pharmaceutical companies are making the MMSE available to primary care physicians. These physicians must be aware of the kind of data presented in this article, which will allow them to judge the performance of their patients and avoid raising unnecessary concern or, on the other hand, missing early dementia.

P.J. Whitehouse, M.D., Ph.D.

Response of the Pupil to Tropicamide Is Not a Reliable Test for Alzheimer Disease

FitzSimon JS, Waring SC, Kokmen E, et al (Mayo Clinic and Found, Rochester, Minn)

Arch Neurol 54:155–159, 1997 4–18

Background.—In living patients, there is no clear biological marker of Alzheimer's disease. One recent study found that patients with Alzheimer's disease have an exaggerated pupil response to topical instillation of a diluted cholinergic antagonist, apparently because of hypersensitivity to antagonists of acetylcholine neurotransmission. However, pupil sensitivity can be affected by many different factors besides receptor sensitivity. This study sought to confirm the finding of pupil hypersensitivity in patients with Alzheimer's disease.

Methods.—The study included 20 patients with Alzheimer's dementia and 20 cognitively normal controls. Each patient underwent instillation of a weak mydriatic (0.01% tropicamide) or placebo, followed by automated binocular infrared pupillography. Two percent sodium fluorescein was used to trace penetration of the eyedrops into the aqueous humor. The percent change in pupil diameter was compared for patients with and without Alzheimer's disease.

Results.—There was no significant difference in pupil dilation between research subject groups. Neither was there any difference in the rate of ocular penetration by fluorescein.

Conclusions.—This study does not confirm the previously reported finding of pupil hypersensitivity to tropicamide in patients with Alzheimer's disease. Thus, pupil sensitivity would not be a reliable early diagnostic test for Alzheimer's disease.

▶ If I had a nickel for every claim of a new diagnostic test for Alzheimer's disease, I would be wealthy. The pupil test is perhaps the most interesting one to come on the scene recently. It seemed far-fetched from the beginning but received publicity beyond the merit of the original report. This article and others have shown that pupillary hypersensitivity to anticholinergic drugs is not consistently found. Clearly, the pupil test is an example of how we develop diagnostic delirium. Yes, we need better diagnostic tests; however, we do not need to raise the public's expectations until we are firmly assured that the test is not only based on a valid scientific observation but also that the findings can be translated into clinical practice.

P.J. Whitehouse, M.D., Ph.D.

Consistency of Physician Judgments of Capacity to Consent in Mild Alzheimer's Disease

Marson DC, McInturff B, Hawkins L, et al (Univ of Alabama at Birmingham)
J Am Geriatr Soc 45:453–457, 1997 4–19

Introduction.—Patients with Alzheimer's disease (AD) and other progressive dementias eventually lose decision-making capacity and legal competency. Many physicians must make competency judgments concerning patients on a daily basis, particularly in terms of competency to provide informed consent. However, physicians may be inconsistent in their judgment of their patients' capacity to make consent decisions. The reliability of physicians' judgments of capacity to consent was studied.

Methods.—The study included 5 physicians experienced in assessing competency in patients with dementia. They were drawn from the specialties of geriatric psychiatry, geriatric medicine, and neurology. The physicians viewed videotapes of 45 patients responding to a standard consent capacity interview, consisting of a series of clinical history questions, the Mini-Mental State Examination, and a brief clinical vignette with follow-up questions. Twenty-nine of the patients had mild AD, and 16 were normal older adults. Unaware of the patients' diagnoses, the physicians were to judge each patient as competent or incompetent to provide consent. Agreement in judgments between physicians was analyzed.

Results.—The physicians agreed well (98%) in their competency judgments of normal controls. However, judgment agreement for the patients with mild AD was only 56%. Group kappa statistics were 1.00 for controls vs. 0.14 for patients with AD. On logistic regression analysis, judgments varied significantly for those in the AD group but not for those in the control group (χ^2 values were 63.8 for the AD group and 4.1 for the control group). On pairwise analysis of judgments for those in the AD group, the physicians disagreed in 7 of 10 pairs.

Conclusions.—Physicians experienced in making competency determinations vary significantly in their judgments of consent capacity in patients with mild AD. There is little disagreement in judgments of normal older adult controls. Physician judgment should not be considered a "gold standard" for making consent capacity determinations in patients with dementia. Competency judgments might be made more accurate and agreement improved by standardizing the assessment instruments used in making judgments and by offering clinical training on this topic.

Cognitive Models That Predict Physician Judgments of Capacity to Consent in Mild Alzheimer's Disease

Marson DC, Hawkins L, McInturff B, et al (Univ of Alabama at Birmingham)

J Am Geriatr Soc 45:458–464, 1997 4–20

Purpose.—There has been surprisingly little research in the area of competency loss in dementia, including the natural history of loss of competency, factors affecting physicians' decisions regarding competency, and interventions to assist decision-making capacity in patients. Physician judgments are widely accepted as the standard for determining capacity to consent in patients with dementia, yet there have been no studies of how specific cognitive changes in Alzheimer's disease (AD) are related to loss of competency judgments by physicians. Cognitive factors predicting consent capacity, as judged by experienced physicians, were researched.

Methods.—Five experienced physicians made competency decisions regarding 45 patients: 29 with mild AD, as reflected by a Mini-Mental State Examination score of 20 or greater, and 16 normal older controls. These judgments were based on videotaped interviews of the research subjects responding to a standardized consent capacity interview (SCCI). The same patients were also assessed on various neuropsychological measures linked or potentially linked to competency. The physicians' judgments of competency or noncompetency to consent to treatment were made without knowledge of the research subjects' diagnoses or neuropsychological test results. Data on the overall sample were used in stepwise discriminant function analyses (DFAs) to identify neuropsychological variables affecting each physician's competency judgments. These models were then tested for accuracy in classifying competency outcomes by classification DFAs.

Results.—The individual physicians varied in their cognitive models, and the variation was unrelated to the stringency of judgments for patients with AD. Judgments were predicted by delayed verbal recall in 1 physician, by short-term verbal recall in another, by phonemic word fluency in another, and by visuomotor tracking–sequencing in another. The percentages of patients with AD judged incompetent by these physicians were 90%, 52%, 24%, and 14%, respectively. The rates of correct classification by these single-predictor solutions were 93%, 87%, 87%, and 96%, respectively. (The fifth physician judged all research subjects with AD to be competent; therefore, he had no predictor model for incompetence). When 2 predictor solutions were used, rates of successful classification improved to 98% to 100%.

Conclusions.—Physicians' judgments of consent capacity can be described by 2 cognitive models: verbal recall and simple executive function. Under the verbal recall model, physicians are likely to judge patients with mild AD to be incompetent. Under the executive function model, the judgment is more likely to be for competency. Physicians evaluating capacity to consent to treatment in patients with dementia may find it useful to assess the patients' verbal recall and simple executive functions.

▶ These articles continue the helpful work of a group at the University of Alabama that is investigating how to assess the competency of patients with dementia. The first paper (Abstract 4–19) demonstrates that we have a significant problem to deal with, namely, that the reliability of judgments made by different physicians, even those with special competency in assessing patients with dementia, is not good. As the authors recognize, part of the reason is that many physicians are not specifically trained to assess competency, even if they are trained in geriatrics, neurology, or psychiatry. The authors themselves consider the study to be exploratory. A better assessment of physicians' attitudes toward dementia, their perceptions of quality of life, and their personal reactions to cognitive impairment may help to explain the differences among different individuals. In the small group of 5 physicians reported, 2 were more likely to think that individuals were incompetent, whereas 3 may have had a bias toward finding individuals to be competent. This may reflect fundamental issues i.e., whether the physicians are more concerned about safety or are more protective of autonomy.

The second paper (Abstract 4–20) describes work done by a group of psychologists to develop more objective measures of competency, such as neuropsychological measures of cognitive abilities. The authors find that verbal recall and simple executive functions are important to physicians' judgments about competency. This makes sense because we judge an individual by the words and sentences they choose to characterize the problem-solving situation, as well as by their ability to express goals and outline plans.

P.J. Whitehouse, M.D., Ph.D.

Therapies

A Controlled Trial of Selegiline, Alpha-Tocopherol, or Both as Treatment for Alzheimer's Disease

Sano M, for the Alzheimer's Disease Cooperative Study (Columbia Univ, NY; et al)

N Engl J Med 336:1216–1222, 1997 4–21

Introduction.—The monoamine oxidase inhibitor, selegiline, and alpha-tocopherol (vitamin E) may have beneficial effects in patients with Alzheimer's disease. These medications may increase the levels of brain catecholamines and protect against oxidative damage by decreasing neuronal damage, thus slowing the deteriorating progression of Alzheimer's disease. Treatment with selegiline, alpha-tocopherol, or both was evaluated to determine whether these agents could delay time to occurrence of clinical outcomes reflecting functional deterioration in 341 patients with Alzheimer's disease.

Methods.—A double-blind, placebo-controlled, randomized trial was conducted in 23 centers. Patients with Alzheimer's disease were randomly assigned to receive either selegiline 10 mg/day, alpha-tocopherol 2,000 IU/day, both, or placebo for 2 years. Primary outcomes were death, institutionalization, loss of the ability to perform basic activities of daily living, and severe dementia. Measures of cognition, function, behavior, and the presence or absence of extrapyramidal signs were taken on follow-up visits.

Results.—There was a trend toward significant differences among groups in scores on the Mini-Mental State examination. The placebo group scored highest and the alpha-tocopherol group scored lowest. The Mini-Mental State Examination score was highly predictive of primary patient outcome. Median time to primary outcome was 655, 670, 585, and 440 days, respectively, for patients receiving selegiline, alpha-tocopherol, combined therapy, and placebo. There was a significant delay in time to institutionalization in patients taking alpha-tocopherol.

Conclusion.—Treatment with selegiline or alpha-tocopherol or both was helpful in delaying the median time to primary outcome in patients with moderately severe impairment from Alzheimer's disease.

▶ Scientific evidence is increasing that vitamin E plays a role in the prevention of a variety of chronic age-related diseases. This study, conducted by the National Institutes of Aging Cooperative Study, was a randomized control study of both selegiline and vitamin E in moderately severe Alzheimer's disease (AD). Interestingly, both selegiline and alpha-tocopherol appear to delay the development of certain milestones, including death, institutionalization, loss of ability to perform basic activities of daily living, and severe dementia. This study has generated considerable interest and has likely increased the number of individuals with AD who take the medication.

There are several important limitations to the study. First, even though it had a randomized design, there was some mismatching between the groups at entry. If these differences were not statistically corrected, the positive effects of drugs would disappear. Second, there were no apparent effects on cognition, despite changes in global severity and performance of basic activities of daily living. It is possible that the effect may have been on behavior, such as anxiety or depression, but it is puzzling that there were no detectable changes in cognition, given the magnitude of the effect.

In my own clinical practice, I am ambivalent. I inform patients of the study and many decide to take vitamin E. However, from a population perspective, I am concerned. If this study creates an environment in which a majority of patients with AD take vitamin E, we may lose opportunities to study its effect further and establish an appropriate dose. We may need to modify the design of other trials to include vitamin E use as a baseline condition. Moreover, although the economic cost of vitamin E for an individual patient is small, the social costs of widespread use of vitamin E may be greater.

P.J. Whitehouse, M.D., Ph.D.

▶ This is a controversial study that illustrates some of the pitfalls and challenges that face the designers and the implements of randomized control trials. The theoretical underpinning of this study is the hypothesis that oxidative stress and the accumulation of free radicals are involved in the development of cell death in AD. The 2 agents studied, vitamin E and selegiline, have a variety of actions, one of which is antioxidation. The study was designed with functional decline and nursing home placement as the primary outcomes and slower cognitive decline as a secondary outcome.

The groups receiving the active compounds, vitamin E and selegiline, had better outcomes than the placebo group. Surprisingly, and counterintuitively, the combination of vitamin E and selegiline was less effective than either drug alone. If the drugs worked by antioxidant mechanisms, one would predict that the combination would be more effective than either single agent alone unless 1 or both drugs were used at doses that had the maximal benefit as antioxidants or interact in some unknown way to diminish their effectiveness.

Also difficult to understand is the fact that there was no benefit in the cognitive realm. Since cognitive performance and functional performance correlate with each other, it seems likely that improvement in one would lead to improvement in the other if the basic pathophysiology of the dementia were being attacked. Since there was improvement in function and delay in placement but not in cognition, it seems quite possible that the drugs were acting in a fashion that did not affect the primary neuropathology, for example, by affecting a secondary aspect of the disease. One possibility is that they diminish certain behaviors linked to nursing home placement or that they affect neurotransmitters whose impairment is linked with nursing home placement but not cognitive decline.

The analytic techniques used also suggest that caution in interpreting these results is appropriate. Since the placbo group initially had a better cognitive performance, the final outcomes were statistically controlled for by initial Mini-Mental. This is an appropriate strategy since cognitive score is a predictor of the primary outcomes. However, without this statistical correction, there were no significant differences among the treatment groups.

What should the clinician do in the face of a single, relatively well-designed study such as this when the results are not absolutely clear cut? Opinions vary widely. Certainly selegiline has a less desirable side effect profile and is more expensive than vitamin E. Also, nursing home placement is a financially and emotionally undesirable outcome for most people and delaying it by three quarters of a year is clinically meaningful. Some clinicians are recommending that patients with AD take vitamin E in addition to other treatments, whereas others are awaiting further studies before adding the cost of vitamin E and the burden of taking several more pills per day to their patients' responsibilities.

The final conundrum facing the clinician who wants to recommend vitamin E is the dosage. In this study 2,000 mg, a dose more than 10-fold greater than the daily requirement, was used. Two thousand milligrams is unlikely to be harmful, but taking large pills or multiple pills does present a challenge. Therefore, many clinicians are recommending dosages used to prevent cardiovascular disease: 800–1,200 mg daily.

Unfortunately, it is unlikely that other large studies will be funded to replicate this. It is also unclear whether any benefits that might accrue from either vitamin E, selegiline, or both would be additive to the cholinesterase inhibitors that are currently available or those that have been submitted to the FDA for approval. It is exciting that for the first time in history treatments are being developed that appear to impact the progression and adverse outcomes of AD. Hopefully, future studies will be less equivocal, and therapeutic optimism will become the norm.

P.V. Rabins, M.D., M.P.H.

Relationships of Dehydroepiandrosterone Sulfate in the Elderly With Functional, Psychological, and Mental Status, and Short-term Mortality: A French Community-based Study

Berr C, Lafont S, Debuire B, et al (Hôpital de la Salpêtrière, Paris; Université Bordeaux II, France; Hôpital Paul Brousse, Villejuif, France)
Proc Natl Acad Sci USA 93:13410–13415, 1996 4–22

Background.—Dehydroepiandrosterone sulfate (DHEAS) is a steroid secreted by the adrenal cortex. Levels of DHEAS decrease in both men and women with age after reaching maximum levels during the third decade of life. This age-related decline has led some to theorize that serum levels of DHEAS are related to the "normal" changes that occur with aging, as well as diseases such as cancer, atherosclerosis, and dementia. Were this proven, the administration of the free steroid DHEA might have beneficial effects. In a 4-year study of 622 individuals older than 65, data were collected on DHEAS baseline values, changes in levels over time, and the relationship between DHEAS serum concentrations and functional, psychological, and mental status and short-term mortality.

Methods.—The study participants all lived at home. Physical functioning was measured on the Activities of Daily Living scale; those needing help for at least 1 of 6 activities were considered dependent. A global measure of cognitive functioning was obtained with the Mini Mental State Examination. Other standard tests were also administered. Participants were evaluated again at 1, 3, and 5 years after baseline.

Results.—The mean plasma level of DHEAS in the study population was 662 ng/mL (range 49 to 3660 ng/mL). Overall, levels decreased from 742 ng/mL (the mean for those younger than 75) to 589 ng/mL (the mean for those older than 90). Mean levels were significantly higher for the 266 men (835 ng/mL) than for the 356 women (532 ng/mL), although the age-related decrease was greater in men than in women. Women with functional limitation, confinement, dyspnea, depressive symptoms, poor subjective perceptions of health and life satisfaction, and greater number of medications had significantly lower baseline DHEAS levels. Men showed a trend for similar correlations. Cases of incident dementia during follow-up did not differ in DHEAS levels. In men only, lower DHEAS was significantly associated with increased short-term mortality at 2 and 4 years.

Discussion.—Findings confirm the age-related decrease in serum levels of DHEAS, the difference in levels between men and women, and the greater decreases in men after age 65. Associations between DHEAS and measures of physical and mental health were strongest in women, although no relationship was found between DHEAS levels and dementia. Data suggest that studies of DHEAS and aging should continue.

▶ The blood level of dehydroepiandrosterone sulfate (DHEA) decreases with age, and this reduction has been associated with a variety of illnesses. DHEA has become a popular oral supplement that is sold in many health food stores. In this study, the authors found that women with lower DHEA levels had more functional limitation and that men had increased short-term mortality. Although many variables may have accounted for these differences, the authors try to correct for them statistically and conclude, perhaps rightfully, that a randomized, controlled trial of replacement doses of DHEA may be indicated.

P.J. Whitehouse, M.D., Ph.D.

Quality of Life

Quality of Life in Patients With Alzheimer's Disease as Reported by Patient Proxies

Albert SM, Castillo-Castaneda CD, Sano M, et al (Columbia Univ, New York; Johns Hopkins Univ, Baltimore, Md; Harvard Med School, Boston)

J Am Geriatr Soc 44:1342–1347, 1996 4–23

Background.—Although demented patients do not experience the world as healthy persons do, many demented patients do have some kind of "experiential world," about which little is known. The subjective worlds of demented persons are not directly accessible. However, readily observed behaviors may provide insights into these worlds and a basis for assessing quality of life (QOL).

Methods.—One hundred thirty patients with Alzheimer's disease (AD) were included in the multicenter, cross-sectional study. Proxy ratings of the frequency of, opportunity for, and enjoyment of 15 non–activities of daily living (ADL) activities potentially within the ability of a patient were recorded. The frequency of a series of positive and negative affects, as expressed in clearly demarcated facial and bodily expressions, were also rated.

Findings.—Quality of life ratings could be reliably elicited. Family and institutional caregiver ratings differed only in the category of opportunity for patient activity. As the severity of dementia increased, the frequency of activities declined. The frequency of negative affects increased and that of positive affects decreased as dementia severity worsened, but the correlations were not strong. One fourth of the patients were considered to have a high QOL, defined by frequent activity and positive affect. In a multivariate analysis, functional and cognitive status independently predicted QOL among community residents. In nursing home residents, only absence of antipsychotic medication was associated with QOL. Some activity patterns were predicted independently by patient education, a marker of premorbid state.

Conclusion.—Readily observable behaviors offer a basis for determining QOL in demented patients. The data suggest that many assumptions about the experience of dementia should be reassessed. The variability in QOL among the patients studied was determined not only by disease severity but also by caregiver efforts, the different demands of activities, premorbid activity levels, and the presence of behavioral syndromes related to AD.

► The study of QOL in patients with dementia has been neglected. Standard approaches to assessing caregiver burden and caregiver QOL can be applied to caregivers of patients with AD, because their quality of life is clearly affected by the disease. However, standard QOL measures must be used with care in the patients themselves, because their memory, communication, and executive function deficits may make it difficult for them to report on their subjective world. Therefore, several new approaches are being adopted.

In this article, observer measures were used to assess affect. The authors include a useful discussion of assessment problems, especially proxy response. I would urge that researchers continue to develop both observational measures of QOL and assessments of subjective status.

P.J. Whitehouse, M.D., Ph.D.

Stroke

Asymptomatic Carotid Endarterectomy: Patient and Surgeon Selection

Marcinczyk MJ, Nicholas GG, Reed JF III, et al (Lehigh Valley Hosp, Allentown, Pa)

Stroke 28:291–296, 1997 4–24

Introduction.—Carotid endarterectomy (CEA) is a frequently performed vascular surgical procedure that has been recommended for use in patients with asymptomatic disease. However, some reports have questioned whether the Asymptomatic Carotid Atherosclerosis Study (ACAS) and other prospective CEA protocols are applicable to the general population. The authors compare the results in their asymptomatic patients undergoing CEA with those of the ACAS.

Methods.—The study included 277 patients undergoing CEA at the authors' community hospital from 1987 to 1993, the same time at which patients were being enrolled in the ACAS. The authors' results were compared with those achieved in ACAS in terms of mortality, myocardial infarction, and stroke rates. The patients were considered to be in 5 subgroups: 54 patients enrolled in ACAS undergoing surgery, 75 patients eligible for ACAS but not enrolled and operated on by ACAS surgeons, 29 patients eligible for ACAS but not enrolled and operated on by non-ACAS surgeons, 72 patients not eligible for ACAS but operated on by ACAS surgeons, and 47 patients not eligible for ACAS and operated on by non-ACAS surgeons.

Results.—Compared with patients ineligible for ACAS, eligible patients were younger, had more severe carotid stenosis, and had lower incidences of pulmonary and renal diseases. The patient selection criteria used for ACAS eligibility were associated with significantly lower mortality and myocardial infarction rates. The length of stay was shorter for ACAS-eligible patients as well. Surgeons participating in ACAS worked on patients with more severe stenoses and a lower incidence of coronary artery disease than the non-ACAS surgeons did. The ACAS and non-ACAS surgeons achieved similar patient outcomes.

Conclusions.—Patient selection, as performed to determine eligibility for ACAS, has a significant impact on the outcomes of CEA. Hospitals using similar patient selection criteria can expect to achieve outcomes similar to those reported by ACAS for patients undergoing CEA for asymptomatic disease. Morbidity and mortality rates are higher for patients who do not meet the ACAS criteria, and recommendations based on ACAS cannot be extended to these patients.

▶ The ACAS was largely responsible for expanding the use of CEA in asymptomatic patients. This article stresses the importance of 2 factors: patient selection and surgeon selection. Although there were not major differences in mortality for patients operated on by the different surgeons in this particular study, the authors rightfully recognize that surgeons need to meet certain criteria, discussed in the article, before a physician should refer. Patient selection is critical in terms of the degree of stenosis and the presence of coronary artery disease.

P.J. Whitehouse, M.D., Ph.D.

"Just in Time" Decision Making for ICU Care After Carotid Endarterectomy

McConnell DB, Yeager RA, Moneta GL, et al (Portland Veterans Affairs Med Ctr, Ore)

Am J Surg 171:502–504, 1996 4–25

Background.—Active intensive care in the ICU is not needed for many patients undergoing carotid endarterectomy (CE). Whether the need for postoperative care of patients undergoing CE can be established by preoperative assessment and the recovery room course was determined.

Methods.—The preoperative risk factors, recovery room course, and total hospital stay were analyzed in 126 patients receiving postoperative intensive care after CE during a 2-year period when such care was routine. Preoperative evaluation included the presence of cardiac disease, hypertension, severe respiratory disease, diabetes, arrhythmia, renal failure, and Goldman cardiac risk score. The need for acute intensive care was defined as the need for vasoactive, bronchodilator, or antiarrhythmic medication infusion for longer than the recovery room period. Indications for acute intensive care also included treatment for coronary ischemia, myocardial infarction, or perioperative neurologic event, or need for mechanical ventilation or active diuresis.

Findings.—The 126 patients had a total of 132 CEs. Thirty-seven percent needed active ICU care (AIC). When patients requiring AIC were compared with those not requiring AIC, the number of risk factors per patient was the only significant difference. The risk for cardiac morbidity was lower in patients in Goldman cardiac risk class I than in patients in class II and III.

Conclusion.—Preoperative risk evaluation is not helpful in predicting the need for AIC after CE in individual patients. Selecting patients for ICU admission after this procedure can be determined accurately by a short period of recovery room observation.

▶ This retrospective analysis of patients undergoing CE provides useful information concerning selection of patients for ICU admission after such a procedure. The authors emphasize the fact that careful assessment in the recovery room is the best way of deciding about ICU placement (therefore the "just in time" designation). They provide no cost figures in this brief article, but they predict that such a triage system would be a considerable cost saver and, hopefully, would not adversely affect outcomes.

P.J. Whitehouse, M.D., Ph.D.

Transient Cerebral Ischemia: Association of Apoptosis Induction With Hypoperfusion

Vexler ZS, Roberts TPL, Bollen AW, et al (Univ of California, San Francisco)

J Clin Invest 99:1453–1459, 1997 4–26

Background.—Apoptosis is believed to have a major role in the pathogenesis of cerebral ischemia. The exact mechanism of apoptosis is unknown, but studies have suggested that it is triggered by mild or moderate disturbances in microcirculation. The number of cells undergoing apoptosis in areas of the brain with different degrees of cerebral microcirculatory disturbances was analyzed to determine how induction of apoptosis resulting from a transient cerebral occlusion relates to the degree of cerebral microcirculatory compromise.

Methods.—Six young adult cats were used. After 2.5 hours of unilateral middle cerebral artery occlusion and 10 hours of reperfusion, the induction of apoptosis and the influence of the degree of cerebral microcirculatory disturbance were examined. Two noninvasive MRI techniques were used to monitor the disturbances of cerebral microcirculation and to evaluate cytotoxic edema associated with perfusion deficits. The 2 techniques were high-speed echo planar imaging with a bolus of magnetic susceptibility contrast agent and diffusion-weighted imaging. The number of apoptosis-positive cells was counted in anatomical areas with different severities of ischemic injury.

Results.—Anatomical areas with severe perfusion deficits during occlusion and histologic changes 10 hours after reperfusion had significantly more apoptosis-positive cells. Significantly fewer apoptosis-positive cells and no histologic changes were detected in areas with reduced perfusion and perfusion maintained during occlusion. Regions with transient or prolonged subtotal perfusion deficits had a similar number of apoptotic cells.

Discussion.—These findings indicate that apoptosis is induced in the ischemic core and has a major role in the degeneration of neurons associated with transient ischemia. The significance of these results for the pathophysiology of strokes is unknown.

► Apoptosis is a genetic mechanism for causing cell death, which appears to play an important role in both normal development and a variety of disease states. When an insult occurs, it is better that the cell decides to "kill itself" rather than become necrotic, at which stage it expels toxic intracellular contents into the extracellular space. These investigators, using an animal model undergoing a stroke, found more apoptosis in areas in which hypoperfusion had been documented by MRI. The results offer promise for studying the effects of medications that may prevent apoptotic damage and preserve more tissue after a stroke occurs. The authors used the TUNEL (terminal deoxynucleotidyl transferase-mediated deoxyuridine triphosphate-biotin nick end labeling) method, which is commercially available. Whether it is adequate to define apoptosis solely on the basis of this single assay is controversial. However, this study does provide an intriguing model for pursuing therapeutic interventions.

P.J. Whitehouse, M.D., Ph.D.

US National Survey of Physician Practices for the Secondary and Tertiary Prevention of Ischemic Stroke: Medical Therapy in Patients With Carotid Artery Stenosis

Goldstein LB, Bonito AJ, Matchar DB, et al (Duke Univ, Durham, NC; Research Triangle Inst, Research Triangle Park, NC; Univ of Kansas, Kansas City)

Stroke 27:1473–1478, 1996 4–27

Objective.—Although platelet antiaggregants and anticoagulants have long been used for stroke prevention, their value in treating patients at risk for stroke has not been well studied. Results of a study identifying physician practices for stroke prevention in patients with extracranial carotid artery stenosis are presented.

Methods.—A random sample of 2,000 physicians listed in the 1993 American Medical Association's Physician Masterfile under the appropriate primary specialties was surveyed about physician and practice characteristics and availability of procedures and tests. Physicians were also asked how frequently they prescribed anticoagulants and antiaggregates for symptomatic and asymptomatic patients with 50% to 70% and more than 70% stenosis of the carotid artery.

Results.—There were 1,006 responses. The use of aspirin did not depend on the patient's symptomatic or asymptomatic status. Neurologists prescribed aspirin significantly more frequently than did other specialists. More than 85% of physicians prescribed antiaggregants for patients with stenosis. Surgeons reported little or no use of antiaggregants for patients with no surgical contraindications. The use of anticoagulants varied with the patients' symptoms, degree of stenosis, and presence of surgical contraindications. Physicians were 3 times more likely to prescribe anticoagulants for symptomatic patients than nonsymptomatic patients. Physicians were 33% more likely to prescribe anticoagulants for patients with surgical contraindications than for patients without such indications, regardless of symptoms or degree of stenosis. A non–internal medicine primary care physician was 5 times more likely to prescribe anticoagulants than were surgeons. Internists and neurologists were 3.5 and 2 times more likely to prescribe anticoagulants than were surgeons.

Conclusion.—Whereas most physicians would use antiaggregants in patients with stenosis regardless of degree, symptom status, or presence of surgical contraindications, anticoagulant prescribing varied with all 3 variables and with physician specialty. Almost all physicians prescribe antiaggregants for secondary and tertiary stroke prevention, 85% use them for patients with stenosis, but neurologists and internists are 1.5 times more likely than surgeons to use antiaggregants for stroke prevention. Some of these practices are at variance with results of clinical trial data.

▶ Practice variation continues to be a fascinating clue as to how to improve the care of patients with a variety of diseases, including prevention of ischemic stroke. This comparison of internists, neurologists, and surgeons is most interesting for the considerable variation it shows in physicians' use of anticoagulants.

P.J. Whitehouse, M.D., Ph.D.

What Role Do Neurologists Play in Determining the Costs and Outcomes of Stroke Patients?

Mitchell JB, Ballard DJ, Whisnant JP, et al (Health Economics Research, Inc, Waltham, Mass; Emory Univ, Atlanta, Ga; Mayo Clinic, Rochester, Minn; et al)

Stroke 27:1937–1943, 1996 4–28

Background.—Among physicians, subspecialists appear to be greater users of tests and procedures, even after adjustment for patient mix, raising concern over the large number of specialists in the United States and the costs associated with increased service intensity. Little information is available, however, describing whether treatment of stroke varies by physician specialty. The costs and outcomes of acute stroke were thus compared by physician specialty, particularly neurologist vs. nonneurologist status.

Methods.—Medicare records were examined for a random sample of 38,612 patients age 65 and older admitted for cerebral infarction during a 9-month period. The physician billing for routine hospital visits on the first 7 days of the patient's hospitalization was considered the attending physician.

Results.—When patients who had a stroke were treated by neurologists, expense was significantly greater; however, 90-day mortality rates were significantly lower. Adjustment for patient age, co-morbidity, hospital teaching status, and other characteristics did not alter these results. Neurologists were more likely than were other attending physicians to order diagnostic cerebrovascular tests, to discharge patients to inpatient rehabilitation facilities, or to prescribe warfarin.

Discussion.—Patients who have had a stroke and are treated by neurologists appear to have better outcomes, although the treatment is costlier. The differences in outcome noted between neurologists and other physicians might be because of clinical characteristics used in triage that are not reflected in the Medicare data; or, the neurologists might be better at identifying the mechanism of stroke.

Clinical Significance.—Outcome for patients who had a stroke appears better when they are treated by a neurologist. Given current pressures to substitute generalists for specialists, this topic warrants further consideration.

► This article also discusses practice variation in the treatment of patients. The analysis, based on 1991 data, concerns the differences between neurologists, internists, family practitioners, and other specialists in the treatment of acute stroke. The basis conclusion is that neurologists are more expensive but may have better outcomes. The authors rightfully recognize that there may have been differences among the patients who were referred to the various types of clinicians.

We all know from our practices that there are considerable regional variations in which types of patients who have had a stroke are seen by a neurologist. Nevertheless, this study suggests that neurologists might do things that provide better patient benefit. One could focus on imaging, but I am inclined to think that neurologists can diagnose stroke earlier, and watch for changes in the evolution of stroke better, because of their knowledge of the disease and their ability to do physical examinations, not because they order high-tech imaging.

P.J. Whitehouse, M.D., Ph.D.

Hospital Charges for Stroke Patients

Alberts MJ, Bennett CA, Rutledge VR (Duke Univ, Durham, NC; St Joseph Mercy Hosp, Ann Arbor, Mich)

Stroke 27:1825–1828, 1996 4–29

Introduction.—Stroke is a common and expensive problem. The current emphasis on managed care and cost containment could have a major impact on the delivery of care for stroke. Hospital charges and patterns of testing for stroke patients were studied, along with the ability of educational interventions to modify test utilization and related charges.

Methods.—The analysis included data on 303 stroke patients discharged from the neurology service or from other services of the department of medicine. Eighty-four percent were discharged from the department of medicine. Information on tests performed—especially radiologic and echocardiographic procedures—and on hospital charges were collected. After initial analysis, an educational intervention was performed to optimize utilization of tests in stroke patients. The effects of education on test utilization were analyzed in a group of 158 subsequent patients.

Results.—In the initial analysis, mean length of stay was 9 days for patients discharged from the neurology service vs. 10.5 days for those discharged from other services. Mean total charges per case were $13,000 vs. $16,000, respectively; however, neither of these differences was significant. Both brain CT and MRI were performed in 31% of patients on the neurology service vs. 31% on the other services. Transthoracic echocardiography was performed in 72% of patients on the neurology service vs. 54% of those on the other services. Mortality was lower for patients treated on the neurology service, 8% vs. 29%.

Education lowered the percentage of patients on the neurology service undergoing both CT and MRI to 18%. The rate of transthoracic echocardiography decreased to 60%. The educational program had no statistically significant effect on charges for stroke patients treated on the neurology service. The savings, however, were financially significant.

Conclusions.—This study shows significant differences in test utilization for stroke patients treated on the neurology service vs. other services. Educational interventions can reduce testing and associated charges for some patients with stroke. For some groups of stroke patients, a multidisciplinary case management approach may be necessary to achieve significant cost reductions.

▶ This study, conducted by a group at Duke University, compared the costs of care offered by the neurology service and medical service at that institution. It found significant differences in terms of testing and costs. An intervention was developed—educational sessions about the use of various diagnostic tests. Although overall costs did not change after the intervention, certain tests were used more selectively. The authors suggest that multidisciplinary approaches to case management, using tools such as care maps, may lead to greater cost savings in the future.

P.J. Whitehouse, M.D., Ph.D.

Stroke Rehabilitation: Are Highly Structured Units More Conducive to Physical Activity Than Less Structured Units?

Mackey F, Ada L, Heard R, et al (Illawarra Regional Hosp, Wollongong, Australia; Univ of Sydney, Australia)

Arch Phys Med Rehabil 77:1066–1070, 1996 4–30

Background.—Frequent repetition is a crucial factor in relearning motor skills, so to maximize outcome, rehabilitation units should challenge patients to repeatedly practice the skills they are unable to perform. The purpose of this study was to identify which environmental features of a stroke rehabilitation unit promote the most motor activity.

Methods.—The study compared two mixed-diagnosis rehabilitation units within general hospitals. In Unit A (15 beds), the therapy area is located about 200 m from the living area, so patients are usually transported to therapy in wheelchairs at prearranged times. In Unit B (17 beds), the therapy area is adjacent to the patient lounge and dining room, so most patients walk to therapy, and there is no formal organization of treatment time. At the time of the study, both units had 8 stroke patients. The Motor Assessment Scale for Stroke was used to document that there was no significant difference between the units in terms of the motor capability of the stroke patients.

In each unit, a researcher observed patients on three or four weekdays and on a Saturday and Sunday, from 7 AM to 7 PM. The observer recorded the location of each patient, whether other people were present, and the patient's activity. Activities were classified as exercise of the affected limb, task practice (using the affected limb in everyday activities such as walking), or activites unrelated to rehabilitation.

Results.—There was no significant difference between units in the amount of motor activity observed. Combined scores showed that patients spent most of their time (74%) in living areas, compared with only 13% of their time in therapy areas. The time spent on activities unrelated to rehabilitation (77%) was more than 4 times greater than time spent on task practice (14%) and exercise (2%) combined. On weekends, therapy areas in both units were closed, and patients were even less active.

Conclusions.—In the units studied, patients are not sufficiently challenged, physically or mentally, and the units may actually promote a culture of inactivity. The authors call for a fundamental change in the way that rehabilitation units are organized, with attention to the *process* of rehabilitation, not to individual features of the environment.

► This is a relatively small study of two rehabilitation units in Australia. One was large and structured, and the other small and more informally organized. No differences were found between the units, and the major conclusion was that individuals spent most of their time in activities thought to be largely unrelated to physical outcome. The authors stress, rightfully, that the time has come to look at rehabilitation units in a new light. They conclude, for example, that rehabilitation units are not functioning as learning environments. How can we use the principles of adult learning to assist staff and patients to develop learning goals? How can we develop more individualized approaches in which patients will take more responsibility for their own ongoing rehabilitation?

P.J. Whitehouse, M.D., Ph.D.

Age and Outcome After Aneurysmal Subarachnoid Hemorrhage: Why Do Older Patients Fare Worse?

Lanzino G, Kassell NF, Germanson TP, et al (Univ of Virginia, Charlottesville; Univ of Iowa, Iowa City)

J Neurosurg 85:410–418, 1996 4–31

Background.—Advanced age is an indicator of poor prognosis after subarachnoid hemorrhage (SAH). The relationship between age and other prognostic factors and outcome was explored.

Methods.—Data were obtained from 906 patients enrolled in a multicenter, randomized trial of nicardipine treatment conducted in 21 centers in North America. For analysis, the participants were divided into 5 age groups ranging from 40 or younger to older than age 71. In all age groups, women outnumbered men.

Findings.—Level of consciousness and World Federation of Neurologic Surgeons grade on admission worsened with increasing age. In addition, age was associated with the presence of a thick subarachnoid clot, intraventricular bleeding, and hydrocephalus on admission CT scans. The rate of rebleeding rose from 4.5% in the youngest age group to 16.4% in the oldest age group. Advanced age was also associated with pre-existing medical conditions. No age-related differences were noted in the day of admission after SAH, timing of surgery and/or location, and size of the ruptured aneurysm. During treatment, the incidence of severe complications rose with advancing age, occurring in 28% of those aged 40 years or less, 33% in 41- to 50-year-olds, 36% in 51- to 60-year-olds, 40% in 61- to 70-year-olds, and 46% in those older than 70. The reported frequency of surgical complications did not differ, nor did the overall incidence of angiographic spasm. However, symptomatic vasospasm was more common in the older patients. Overall outcome was poorer with advancing age. Adjustment for different prognostic factors did not eliminate this age effect, suggesting that the aging brain has a less optimal response to initial bleeding.

Conclusion.—These findings confirm the fact that advanced age is an important predictor of poor outcome after SAH. However, operative morbidity rates do not differ significantly among age groups, and surgical outcomes in the elderly have improved significantly in recent years. Thus, elderly patients should not be denied treatment of a ruptured aneurysm simply because of their age.

► This article identifies a number of factors that affect prognosis and need for surgery after SAH, including level of consciousness, nature of the hemorrhage, and pre-existing medical conditions. Interestingly, although the surgical risk did not differ by age, older patients did worse even when covariants were accounted for. This finding did not appear to relate to coexisting diseases, and the authors propose that this observation is the result of some lower resiliency on the part of the older brain. It is not clear whether the reduced resiliency occurs because of some mechanical problem of dealing with the excess blood or because of poorer individual neuronal reserve, but the article is useful in identifying factors for the clinician to consider.

P.J. Whitehouse, M.D., Ph.D.

Parkinson's Disease

Impact of Deprenyl and Tocopherol Treatment on Parkinson's Disease in DATATOP Patients Requiring Levodopa

Penney JB Jr, and the Parkinson Study Group (Univ of Michigan, Ann Arbor; et al)

Ann Neurol 39:37–45, 1996 4–32

Purpose.—Although levodopa provides considerable relief from the symptoms of Parkinson's disease, the underlying nigral neuron loss continues with progressive worsening of the signs and symptoms of disease. Also, years of levodopa treatment lead to motor, behavioral, and autonomic adverse effects. Previous reports have suggested that treatments to decrease oxidative stress in the substantia nigra neurons could slow the progression of Parkinson's disease and slow or prevent the development of levodopa-related adverse effects. Deprenyl and tocopherol were prospectively studied for their effects on disease progression in patients with Parkinson's disease requiring levodopa therapy.

Methods.—The analysis was part of the Deprenyl and Tocopherol Antioxidant Therapy of Parkinsonism (DATATOP) trial. This double-blind, placebo-controlled study examined the effects of treatment with deprenyl, 10 mg/day, and tocopherol, 2000 mg/day, in 800 untreated patients with Parkinson's disease. Levodopa was given to patients who required symptomatic treatment, and all patients were switched to open-label deprenyl treatment after the blinded portion of the trial. This procedure permitted an analysis of the long-term effects of deprenyl and tocopherol treatment on the subsequent development of levodopa-related side effects. Average follow-up was 35 months.

Results.—Three hundred seventy-one patients required levodopa treatment, and 352 completed the levodopa portion of the trial. Levodopa side effects were not significantly different between patients who received early vs. late treatment with deprenyl or in those who received tocopherol vs. no tocopherol. "Wearing off" was noted in approximately 50% of patients, dyskinesias in 30%, and "freezing" in 25%. By the end of the trial, all groups were comparable in their dose of levodopa and their level of disability, as measured by the Hoehn-Yahr, Schwab-England, and Unified Parkinson's Disease Rating scales. Wearing-off was more frequent in younger patients, dyskinesias were more common in women, and freezing was most likely to occur in older patients with rapidly progressive Parkinson's disease.

Conclusions.—Deprenyl and tocopherol antioxidant therapy does not reduce later levodopa-associated adverse effects in patients with Parkinson's disease. Neither does this treatment reduce the disability of Parkinson's disease nor the dose of levodopa required. (A companion article describes the effects of deprenyl treatment in Parkinson's disease patients who did not require levodopa.)

► This article from the Parkinson Study Group adds to our information concerning the value of deprenyl and vitamin E therapy in Parkinson's disease. Once touted as agents that might slow the progression of the disease, these medications are now known to have only a modest symptomatic benefit. This study now takes more of the magic away in that at the end of the study the groups were similarly disabled and took similar amounts of levodopa. The development of dyskinesias and freezing varied with sex and age. Studies of deprenyl and tocopherol are also underway in Alzheimer's disease and are reported to show some interesting positive effects on disease course.

P.J. Whitehouse, M.D., Ph.D.

Prevalence of Parkinsonism and Parkinson's Disease in Europe: The EUROPARKINSON Collaborative Study

de Rijk MC, for the EUROPARKINSON Study Group (Erasmus Univ, Rotterdam, The Netherlands)

J Neurol Neurosurg Psychiatry 62:10–15, 1997 4–33

Background.—The wide variation in prevalence estimates of Parkinson's disease across studies and countries may result from differences in methodology and diagnostic criteria. It is unclear whether a true variation exists. The prevalences of parkinsonism and Parkinson's disease in 5 European populations were assessed using similar methodology and diagnostic criteria.

Methods.—Data were obtained from 5 surveys done in Gironde, France; 8 centers in Italy; Rotterdam, The Netherlands; and Girona and Pamplona, Spain. A total of 14,636 persons 65 and older were included.

Findings.—The overall prevalences per 100 population of parkinsonism and Parkinson's disease were 2.3 and 1.6, respectively, age-adjusted to the 1991 European standard population. Overall prevalences of parkinsonism were 0.9 for 65- to 69-year-olds, 1.5 for 70- to 74-year-olds, 3.7 for 75- to 79-year-olds, 5.0 for 80- to 84-year-olds, and 5.1 for 85- to 89-year-olds. The corresponding prevalences for Parkinson's disease in these age groups were 0.6, 1.0, 2.7, 3.6, and 3.5, respectively. Prevalences did not differ significantly across surveys after adjustment for age and sex, although the prevalence was lower in the French study. Overall, men and women had similar prevalences. Twenty-four percent of the persons with Parkinson's disease were detected initially through the surveys.

Conclusion.—The prevalences of parkinsonism and Parkinson's disease increased with age, with no significant differences between men and women and with no apparent differences among the European countries studied. A high percentage of patients with Parkinson's disease in the general population had been previously unidentified.

▶ This article is of interest for several reasons. Although it confirms the increase of Parkinson's disease with age, there were no differences between men and women or across different European countries. However, the principal reason for including this paper here is to point out the large percentage of patients with Parkinson's disease who went undetected in the general population. Parkinson's disease is clearly a challenge for the generalist physician. Overdiagnosis can occur because of the existence of familial or essential tremors, which can become more apparent with age. Underdiagnosis can occur when the slowness of motor action is mistaken for normal aging.

P.J. Whitehouse, M.D., Ph.D.

Selegiline and Mortality in Parkinson's Disease

Olanow CW, Fahn S, Langston JW, et al (Mount Sinai Med Ctr, New York; Columbia Univ, New York; Parkinson Inst, Santa Clara, Calif)

Ann Neurol 40:841–845, 1996 4–34

Purpose.—Selegiline is now well accepted as an adjunct to levodopa in the treatment of Parkinson's disease (PD), although there is ongoing controversy regarding its neuroprotective effect. Selegiline has generally been regarded as a safe drug. However, a recent study by the Parkinson's Disease Research Group of the United Kingdom suggested that selegiline increases the risk of death in patients with PD treated with levodopa. This study has raised difficult questions for physicians: should they avoid selegiline because of the potential risk of early mortality or use it because of its potential neuroprotective effect? The available data on the mortality risk of selegiline are reviewed, and recommendations for its use are presented.

Mortality From Selegiline.—The UK study is the first clinical trial to link selegiline to increased mortality. In 7 controlled, long-term trials of selegiline, with or without levodopa, in patients with PD, death rates were about 5% for patients who did and did not receive selegiline. A meta-analysis confirmed the lack of difference. In contrast, the UK study found a mortality of 18% in patients assigned to levodopa alone vs. 28% in those assigned to levodopa plus selegiline. This discrepancy raises some questions regarding the UK study. The 5-year mortality rate is very high in both arms of the study, more so than in other studies. The reasons for this difference are unknown but could be related to increased disease severity.

There are also some methodological and statistical flaws with the UK study: it was open label, and many patients withdrew from their assigned treatment during the study. Under these circumstances, intention-to-treat analysis may miss differences between the treatments. Patients withdrawing from the levodopa–selegiline group had more than double the mortality of patients withdrawing from the levodopa-only group, which suggests that selegiline may actually have had a protective effect. Other problems may result from the repeated "looks" at the data and the use of *P* values appropriate for the full length of the study—rather than for the specific interim analysis—when the study was stopped. Finally, the patients in the 2 treatment arms were not receiving a comparable level of dopaminergic treatment at the beginning of the study. All of these problems suggest that the conclusion of a significant mortality difference between groups may not be valid.

Conclusions.—The UK report of increased early mortality in patients with PD treated with levodopa–selegiline must be taken seriously. However, closer examination suggests several methodological and statistical concerns with this study. The authors believe that selegiline should not be withheld from patients strictly on the basis of the UK study.

► In the article by Sano et al. (Abstract 4–21), we raised the concern that a small study of selegiline and vitamin E might lead to an inappropriately quick adoption of the use of these agents. In this article from the United Kingdom, the obverse occurs: it suggests that selegiline increases the risk of early death in patients with PD treated with levodopa. The initial report did cause concern among neurologists. However, in this paper, the authors review other studies of selegiline and PD, none of which show early mortality, and they reveal a significant number of problems with the UK study. I agree with their conclusion that, although we need to collect further data, the evidence is not persuasive that selegiline contributes to early mortality in PD.

P.J. Whitehouse, M.D., Ph.D.

Effect of Lazabemide on the Progression of Disability in Early Parkinson's Disease

Kieburtz K, and the Parkinson Study Group (Univ of Rochester, NY)

Ann Neurol 40:99–107, 1996 4–35

Objective.—Lazabemide, a competitive inhibitor of monoamine oxidase type B (MAO-B), is a safe and effective treatment for early Parkinson's disease (PD). Whether the drug can delay the progress of PD was studied in a randomized, multicenter, placebo-controlled, double-blind clinical trial over 1 year. The impact of selected dosages of lazabemide on the progression of disability in early, otherwise untreated PD was determined, and the safety and long-term tolerability was assessed.

Methods.—A total of 321 patients with Hoehn and Yahr stage I or II PD for less than 7 years were randomly allocated to received 25, 50, 100, or 200 mg/day of lazabemide or placebo for 52–54 weeks followed by placebo for 2–4 weeks to provide for a blinded, staggered withdrawal of active drug. Patients were followed up for as long as 1 year. The primary outcome variable was determination that the patient had become sufficiently disabled to begin levodopa therapy. Group results were compared statistically.

Results.—There was no relation between dosage and withdrawal for the 47 patients that withdrew from the study. Endpoint was reached by 29 placebo patients (43.9%) and 80 patients in the treatment groups (31.4%). The onset of disability was significantly reduced, by 51%, at all dosages of lazabemide compared with placebo. The proportion of adverse reactions was similar among treatment groups. The most common adverse reactions were headache, nausea, upper-respiratory infections, flu-like symptoms, insomnia, dizziness, constipation, and fatigue.

Conclusion.—Lazabemide at doses of 25–200 mg was effective in delaying disability in patients with early, untreated PD. The drug was well tolerated, with most adverse reactions being mild and not serious.

▶ More symptomatic drugs will be available for AD, Parkinson's disease, and other degenerative diseases over the next few years. The major challenge to the field has been the translation of basic science discoveries (concerning the biologic mechanisms of cell death in neurodegenerative disease) to clinical practice.

There was considerable controversy around the publication of the datatop clinical trial of selegiline for Parkinson's disease, conducted by the same group that did this study. The drug was well tolerated, and, like deprenyl, it appeared to reduce the risk of reaching the primary endpoint (the onset of the need for treatment with levodopa), compared with placebo. The mechanism behind the delay in the need for levodopa is not clear, but it may relate to the protective effects of selective MAO-B inhibitors on neurotoxicity.

As with deprenyl, studies of lazabemide are also underway in AD.

P.J. Whitehouse, M.D., Ph.D.

Miscellaneous Neurological Conditions

Usefulness of Prolonged Video-EEG Monitoring in the Elderly

Lancman ME, O'Donovan C, Dinner D, et al (Cleveland Clinic Found, Ohio)
J Neurol Sci 142:54–58, 1996 4–36

Background.—Epilepsy in the elderly is common but difficult to diagnose. The value of video-electroencephalographic (EEG) monitoring (VEEG) in diagnosing and managing elderly patients with epilepsy was investigated.

Methods.—The medical records of 20 consecutive patients older than 60 years were reviewed. These patients were selected from 1,423 patients referred during a 5-year period for VEEG assessment for epilepsy. Changes in the diagnosis and treatment of these patients before and after VEEG and assessment by the epileptologist reviewing the records before and after receiving the VEEG results were noted.

Findings.—Compared with the initial diagnosis by the referring physician, VEEG results effected a change in diagnosis and treatment in 11 patients. The epileptologist was able to correctly determine diagnosis and treatment in 16 patients without knowing the VEEG results. In the 4 remaining patients, VEEG provided additional information.

Conclusion.—Video-EEG is useful in establishing the diagnosis of epilepsy in selected elderly patients. In addition, VEEG findings may affect patient management.

► Elderly individuals are subject to a variety of causes of transient loss of consciousness, and this makes the diagnosis of epilepsy more difficult in this group. These authors report on an increasingly used technique, VEEG, and assess its value in individuals over the age of 60 years. They found a remarkably high number of individuals where use of VEEG led to a different diagnosis and, presumably, different therapy.

P.J. Whitehouse, M.D., Ph.D.

Breathing Disorders During Sleep and Cognitive Performance in an Older Community Sample: The EVA Study

Dealberto M-J, for the EVA Study Group (Institut Natl De la Santé, et de la Recherche Médicale, Paris)

J Am Geriatr Soc 44:1287–1294, 1996 4–37

Background.—Sleep apnea, characterized by loud snoring and breathing cessation during sleep, is a common disorder with a prevalence that increases with age. Severity of dementia and sleep apnea have been found to be correlated among institutionalized elderly persons. Whether poor cognitive performance was associated with the symptoms of sleep apnea syndrome (snoring and breathing cessation during sleep) in community-dwelling elderly persons was determined.

Methods.—Data were collected from 1,389 elderly residents of Nantes, France. The subjects were age 60–70 at the beginning of the 4-year cohort study. A battery of tests was administered.

Findings.—Snoring was reported by 49.5% of the subjects and breathing cessation during sleep by 10.8%. Both symptoms were significantly correlated with male sex and high body mass index. Among men, the prevalence of snoring was significantly increased when alcohol intake exceeded 40 mL per day. In women, breathing cessation during sleep was associated with depressive symptoms. In logistic regression models, both snoring and breathing cessation were associated with low scores on tests requiring visual attention skills, the Trail Making Test, and the Digit Symbol Substitution Test, after adjustment for age, sex, educational level, tobacco status, alcohol intake, depressive symptomatology, and number of medications. These associations were significant only when either snoring or breathing cessation was correlated with daytime sleepiness.

Conclusion.—In community-dwelling adults age 60–70, snoring and breathing cessation during sleep associated with daytime sleepiness appear to be risk factors for low cognitive performance on tests requiring visual attention skills. This association may be attributable to the fact that both respiratory disorders during sleep and low cognitive performance are independent consequences of brain aging. Alternatively, vascular mechanisms may be involved in this association.

▶ This article deserves wide reading because it confirms what many clinicians have long suspected: that older people have unrecognized and significant problems with sleep apnea. It confirms earlier work that male gender and high body mass index are associated with a high prevalence of snoring. It highlights the importance of daytime sleepiness as a predictor for diminished cognitive scores in association with other sleep pathology. Also of interest was the association of sleep apnea with depression in women. It is important that geriatricians learn to take a sleep history and refer patients with positive reports of sleep pathology or daytime sleepiness to appropriate specialists.

P.J. Whitehouse, M.D., Ph.D.

5 Gerontologic Research

Introduction

Even the optimists in the field have been proven wrong. The science has moved even faster than their expectations. Animal models of aging now extend from primates and rodents to worms and yeast and are adding valuable insights at a rapid pace. Programmed cell death in worms and aging in worms have their parallels in adult humans. The explosive growth of genetics, a field that traditionally has largely affected pediatrics, is now beginning to widely affect our understanding of late onset diseases. Rare single gene disorders of man and of laboratory animals, considered in the past to be of uncertain value because of their rarity, are proving to give pathophysiological insights of unexpectedly great importance for their commonly occurring cousins. Likewise, the revolution of developmental biology, which has affected our insights into disturbances of neonates and infants, is impacting on adults as well. In general, genes and proteins that are important during embryogenesis often continue to have functions in adult life, both in sustaining normal function at the adult level and in compensating during conditions of disease or injury. Again, the fundamental science is enhancing our understanding of aging and its disorders. A further trend that is very refreshing is the breakdown of barriers between fields; advances in one field are having implications in multiple fields and vice versa. The bright future is here now.

Jesse Roth, M.D.

Jay R. Shapiro, M.D.

Longevity

Heat-induced Longevity Extension in *Drosophila*: I. Heat Treatment, Mortality, and Thermotolerance
Khazaeli AA, Tatar M, Pletcher SD, et al (Univ of Minnesota, Minneapolis)
J Gerontol 52A:B48–B52, 1997 5–1

Purpose.—Previous studies have shown that brief exposure to high but nonlethal temperatures can prolong life span in experimental animals. Exposure to high temperatures can enhance thermotolerance–the ability to survive subsequent exposure to otherwise lethal levels of heat—and rapid expression of heat shock proteins, which protect against thermal stress.

The potential link between brief thermal temperature and subsequent life span at normal temperatures is unknown, however. This question was addressed in a study of fruit flies.

Methods.—Four-day-old fruit flies, *Drosophila melanogaster*, were exposed to a temperature of 36°C under saturated humidity for 70 minutes. Control populations of the same genotype received no heat treatment. Data on a total of 28,000 individuals were collected to determine the effects of thermal stress on mortality and physiologic responses. Thermotolerance was assessed by measuring lethality during and after a subsequent period of severe thermal stress.

Results.—Heat treatment extended life span by an average of 2 days. Age-specific mortality was significant reduced for several weeks after heat treatment. Heat treatment also increased subsequent thermotolerance, in most cases by a factor of 2. The heat-related extension of life span was independent of the life-prolonging effects of suppressed reproductive activity in single-sex populations.

Conclusions.—Brief exposure to nonlethal levels of heat prolongs subsequent survival at normal temperatures in fruit flies. The mechanism of this effect, including the possible contribution of heat shock proteins, is unknown. The authors plan further studies of heat-induced longevity extension.

▶ The fruit fly *Drosophila* and other selected invertebrates are proving to be valuable models of the aging process because they allow extensive genetic and molecular approaches that are impossible in vertebrates. The authors recall that two environmental treatments, dietary restriction and curtailed reproduction, extend adult longevity in animals reared at normal temperatures. Recently, brief nonlethal exposure to elevated temperatures increase the life span of the tiny worm *Caenorhabditis elegans* (or *C. elegans*, pronounced "see ĕl aganz," a favorite subject of study for many developmental biologists) by 2.7 days or 15% compared with control worms that had not been heat treated. This study in *Drosophila* shows that a brief, nonlethal heat treatment extends adult life span by an average of 2 days. This effect appears to be independent of effects on reproduction. The protection extends for many days after the treatment. Heat treatment also increases tolerance to subsequent more severe thermal stress. It will be interesting to learn whether extension of life span is related to specific known elements of the heat shock response, or to novel elements and mechanisms yet to be elucidated.

J. Roth, M.D.

Transgenic Mice Overexpressing Urokinase-type Plasminogen Activator in the Brain Exhibit Reduced Food Consumption, Body Weight and Size, and Increased Longevity

Miskin R, Masos T (Weizmann Inst of Science, Rehovot, Israel)

J Gerontol 52A:B118–B124, 1997 5–2

Background.—Plasminogen activators (PAs) are secreted serine proteases that cleave plasminogen to generate plasmin. Plasmin is a trypsin-like protease that dissolves the fibrin network of blood clots and can also cleave other extracellular proteins. This PA proteolytic cascade has a role in fibrinolysis, cell migration, ovulation, inflammation, and tissue repair and development. The 2 types of PAs in mammals, tissue-type (tPA) and urokinase-type (uPA), are encoded by different genes. The authors have generated transgenic mice (αMUPA) that overexpress murine uPA in the lens and the nerve cells of the central nervous system. These transgenic mice could be useful in understanding the effects of increased expression of uPA in the brain.

Methods.—Transgenic mice were generated from the NIH FVB/N inbred mouse line. Histologic analysis revealed no gross abnormalities. Female mice were used for all experiments. The mice were maintained under standard conditions.

Results.—Compared with the wild-type parental control mouse strain, αMUPA mice spontaneously consumed approximately 20% less food, weighed approximately 20% less, grew approximately 6% less and had an approximately 20% increase in lifespan. The transgenic mice exhibited reduced food consumption and body weight shortly after weaning and maintained these parameters throughout their lives. The transgenic mice also had approximately 9% lower blood sugar levels, approximately 14% smaller litter sizes, and approximately 10% lower birth frequency. In situ hybridization was used to localize uPA mRNA expression in the brains of the transgenic mice. This mRNA was detected in the neuronal cells of the hypothalamic paraventricular nucleus (PVN), which has been implicated in feeding behavior. Messenger RNA for uPA could not be detected in the same brain regions of wild-type mice.

Conclusions.—A line of transgenic mice, αMUPA, was created that overexpresses murine uPA in the lens and central nervous system. Increased uPA expression in the brains of these transgenic mice was associated with spontaneous reduction in food consumption, growth retardation, body weight reduction, and increased longevity. Transgenic uPA expression was localized to the hypothalamic PVN, a region implicated in the control of feeding behavior. It is possible that uPA is involved in the biochemical mechanisms of the brain that help determine food consumption, growth, weight, and longevity. The transgenic αMUPA mouse provides an excellent experimental system with which to investigate these issues.

► Calorie restriction is associated with decreased body weight and body size, as well as increased longevity. In this study, a new line of transgenic mice was created that in many ways mimics this model. Plasminogen activators are proteases secreted into body fluids that act on plasminogen, an enzyme precursor, to convert it into plasmin, the active enzyme. Plasmin, which is quite similar to trypsin, can dissolve fibrin networks and cleave peptide bonds in many other proteins, including enzyme precursors, which can be activated. Plasminogen activators have been implicated in many biologic events, including fibrinolysis, cell migration, ovulation, inflammation, tissue repair, and remodeling, as well as development of the embryo. The plasminogen activators are synthesized and released in response to many hormones and hormone-like signals. Plasminogen activators come in two types, uPA and tPA, each coded by its own gene. There also exist specific receptors for the type A uPA. Recall that thrombin, which is quite similar to both plasmin and trypsin, acts both as a protease in the clotting cascade and independently as a cell-surface–signaling agent, through a specific receptor.

In this study, the investigators created mice that overexpress uPA only in the brain. Plasminogen activators are believed normally to play some role in memory; their overproduction here is associated with some impairment of certain learning functions. I believe such impairment is always difficult to interpret because many things impair learning. Likewise, it is a little bit difficult to interpret the finding that these animals eat less and live longer because anything that will reduce food intake has the possibility of providing enhanced longevity through that mechanism.

J. Roth, M.D.

---

daf-2, an Insulin Receptor–like Gene That Regulates Longevity and Diapause in *Caenorhabditis elegans*

Kimura KD, Tissenbaum HA, Liu Y, et al (Harvard Med School, Boston)
Science 277:942–946, 1997 5–3

Background.—The metamorphosis of *Caenorhabditis elegans* is under the control of a neurosecretory signaling system that either signals the beginning of the reproductive period or arrests development in the dauer stage. The dauer stage, in which metabolic activity is greatly reduced (diapause) and longevity is greatly increased, is under the control of daf-2 genes in the metabolic pathway; daf-2 is fairly homologous with insulin receptors in humans. These investigators examine the relationship between diapause, insulin metabolism, and longevity in this nematode model, and suggest certain similarities to a mammalian model.

Findings.—A model in which daf-2 regulates metabolism, reproduction, and senescence in *C. elegans* is shown (Fig 3). This regulation is analogous to the role of insulin as a regulator of metabolism and growth in mammalian models. In *C. elegans* with mutant daf-2 genes, metabolism shifts from producing growth to producing fat. This, too, is analogous to the case of a diabetic human patient with the same insulin receptor mutation who was morbidly obese.

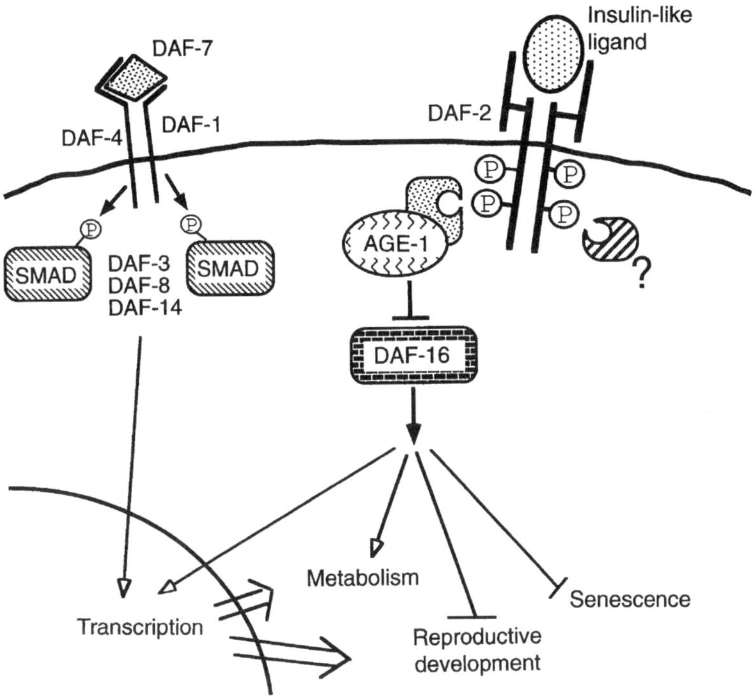

FIGURE 3.—A model of insulin-like signaling in the *C. elegans* dauer formation pathway. In the absence of dauer pheromone, an insulin-like ligand activates DAF-2, and a DAF-7 tumor growth factor-β-(TGF-β)-like signal activates the DAF-1 and DAF-4 receptors. Activated DAF-2 recruits AGE-1, which produces the second messenger PIP_3. This second messenger may regulate glucose transport, metabolic kinase cascades that include AKT and GSK-3, and transcription and translation of metabolic genes. DAF-16 acts downstream of DAF-2 and AGE-1 in this pathway and is negatively regulated by them. (Reprinted with permission from Kimura KD, Tissenbaum HA, Liu Y, et al: daf-2, an insulin receptor–like gene that regulates longevity and diapause in *Caenorhabditis elegans*. *Science* 277:942–946. Copyright 1997, American Association for the Advancement of Science.)

Conclusions.—Given the homology between daf-2 in *C. elegans* and certain insulin receptors in mammals, and the similar regulatory effects of daf-2 and insulin, the insulin signaling pathway seems to be involved in metabolic control in the dauer stage of diapause in *C. elegans*. Perhaps decreases in insulin signaling are responsible for the increased longevity in *C. elegans*. This would help bolster our understanding of how caloric restriction increases longevity in mammals. Furthermore, humans with diabetes due to obesity may have defects in their homologues of the daf-2 gene; such determinations could have research and clinical implications.

► During the life history of *C. elegans*, the family of daf genes is involved in multiple functions including reproduction and the duration of the adult life span. This article is important because of the extensive homology found between the *C. elegans* daf-2 gene and the family of human insulin receptor genes. The receptor related to the daf-2 gene is active in an intracellular signaling cascade that controls both reproductive development and normal senesence (Fig 3). Investigation of the daf-2 gene and its mutants has raised interesting questions about the evolution of the human insulin receptor family as well as its role in determining rates of aging.

Postembryonic development of *C. elegans* involves four larval stages to the adult when conditions are favorable for growth and reproduction. Under conditions of high population density and low food, *C. elegans* forms a third non-feeding larval stage, the dauer stage, which is developmentally arrested and resistant to dehydration and environmental stress.[1] The daf-2 gene controls metabolic activity in the dauer stage. The dauer larval stage in *C. elegans* is one of decreased metabolic activity (diapause) that is associated with a marked increase in longevity.[2] Also, daf-2 mutants have doubled adult life span.[3] The authors remark that this may be analogous to the decline in the rate of aging observed with caloric restriction, which is also associated with a decrease in insulin-receptor mediated signal transduction. Also remarkable is the observation that a human skeletal growth factor, bone morphogenetic factor 4 (BMP-4) can interact with the nematode daf-4 receptor and can influence the dauer larval stage.[4] Clearly, more is to be learned about the relationship between nematode and human age-related genes.

J.R. Shapiro, M.D.

References

1. Gottlieb S, Ruvkun G: daf-2, daf-16 and daf-23: genetically interacting genes controlling Dauer formation in *Caenorhabditis elegans*. *Genetics* 137:107–120, 1994.
2. Larsen PL, Albert PS, Riddle DL: Genes that regulate both development and longevity in *Caenorhabditis elegans*. *Genetics* 139:1576–1583, 1995.
3. Kenyon E, Chang J, Gensch E, et al: A *C. elegans* mutant that lives twice as long as the wild type. *Nature* 366:461–464, 1993.
4. Estevez M, Attisano L, Wrana L, et al: The daf-4 gene encodes a bone morphogenetic protein receptor controlling *C. elegans* dauer larva development. *Nature* 365:644–649, 1993.

Postmenopausal Hormone Therapy and Mortality

Grodstein F, Stampfer MJ, Colditz GA, et al (Brigham and Women's Hosp, Boston; Harvard Med School, Boston; Harvard School of Public Health, Boston)

N Engl J Med 336:1769–1775, 1997 5–4

Background.—Previous studies of the risks and benefits of postmenopausal hormone replacement therapy have not settled the question of the therapy's effect on mortality. Reports of reduced mortality may not have considered that women for whom estrogens are prescribed are often healthier initially, and the combination of current and past users into an "ever" category might also affect the validity of conclusions. The relation between postmenopausal hormones and mortality, overall and among women at high risk or at low risk for breast cancer or heart disease, was studied prospectively.

Methods.—Women studied were participants in the Nurses' Health Study. In 1976, 121,700 female registered nurses aged 30–55 years completed a mailed questionnaire on their medical history. Biennial follow-up surveys were sent through 1992 to update information on risk factors for cancer and cardiovascular disease and to identify newly diagnosed cases of major illnesses. Excluded were women who had a history of cardiovascular disease or cancer at study entry. Each of the 3,637 participants known to have died between 1976 and 1994 was matched with 10 controls alive at the time of her death. To reduce bias caused by discontinuation of hormone use between the time of diagnosis of a potentially fatal illness and death, hormone status at the last questionnaire before the diagnosis or death was defined.

Results.—Causes of death included cancer in 1,985 cases, coronary heart disease in 461, and stroke in 167. Among cancer deaths, 425 were the result of breast cancer and 58 of endometrial cancer. Current hormone use was reported by 15.8% of case subjects on the last questionnaire completed before death or the diagnosis of fatal disease; 27.8% were past users and 56.4% had never used hormones. On the same questionnaire as their matched cases, 24.5% of controls reported current use, 24.9% reported past use, and 50.6% responded that they had never used hormones. After adjustment for confounding variables, the risk of death was lower among current hormone users (relative risk, 0.63) than among those who had never taken hormones. With long-term use (10 years or more), however, the relative risk increased to 0.80 because of an increase in breast cancer deaths among long-term hormone users. The greatest reduction in mortality (relative risk, 0.51) was observed among current hormone users with coronary risk factors. Past users of hormones continued to have a decreased risk of death from all causes for 3–4 years after discontinuation of hormones, but the risk was slightly elevated after 5 years.

Conclusions.—Mortality is lower overall among postmenopausal women who use hormone replacement therapy than among nonusers, but the survival benefit is reduced with longer duration of use. The increased risk of breast cancer after 10 years of taking hormones tends to offset the advantages of reduced cardiovascular mortality, and overall survival benefits are lower for women with a low risk for coronary disease. The decision to recommend postmenopausal hormone therapy must be carefully considered in each case, taking into account a woman's existing risk factors.

► This important article and the accompanying editorial will undoubtedly influence the prescribing habits of many physicians.[1] As the availability of newer Food and Drug Administration (FDA)-approved bisphosphonates increases (alendronate) and estrogen receptor agonists now in clinical trials receive approval (raloxifene, droloxifene), there is renewed interest in the use of estrogen as the first-line treatment of osteoporosis.

This paper from the Nurses' Health Study has several conclusions. First, mortality is lower by 20% in women taking postmenopausal hormones compared with those never having taken hormones, particularly from cardiovascular disease and to a lesser extent from certain cancers including breast cancer. There was little decrease in mortality for women at low risk of heart disease. Second, there was little benefit to taking hormones past 10 years, and the protective effect was lost 5 years after therapy ceased. Finally, the risk of breast cancer mortality was elevated 43% in women taking hormone replacement for more than 10 years. This was true for even the oldest women (60–73 years) in the group, and even though cardiovascular risk was significantly diminished. One question is whether any of the cardiovascular risk factors could also be risk factors for the development of breast cancer?

The questions remain: should all women be taken off hormone replacement after 10 years, and is there a way to estimate the risks to the heart and skeleton relative to the risk of breast cancer? Age apparently does not influence this decision. Bone mass will rapidly decline when estrogen is removed. Obviously there remains a need for effective alternative therapy with limited side effects. Estrogen receptor agonists may fill the gap. Other candidates: slow release fluoride, human parathyroid hormone (hPTH) administered intermittently in low dose, and parathyroid hormone–related protein (PTHrP) now entering clinical trials.

J.R. Shapiro, M.D.

Reference

1. Brinton LA, Schairer C: Postmenopausal hormone replacement therapy: Time for a reappraisal? *N Engl J Med* 336:1821–1822, 1997.

Dehydroepiandrosterone Sulfate: A Biomarker of Primate Aging Slowed by Calorie Restriction

Lane MA, Ingram DK, Ball SS, et al (Johns Hopkins Univ, Baltimore, Md; Univ of California San Francisco—Fresno)

J Clin Endocrinol Metab 82:2093–2096, 1997 5–5

Background.—Dehydroepiandrosterone sulfate (DHEAS) levels decrease with age, and thus they may be a biomarker for aging. Increased DHEAS levels may protect against aging and its associated diseases, such as heart disease, diabetes, and cancer. Another antiaging measure, caloric restriction, has been shown to extend the life span in short-lived species. Whether caloric restriction can slow the age-related decline in DHEAS levels was investigated in a nonhuman primate model.

Methods.—Rhesus monkeys (45 male, 29 female) were involved in this 6-year longitudinal study. The control group (17 young [1–2 years], 21 young adult [3–5 years], and 18 old [older than 17 years] animals) were allowed to feed ad libitum. The test group (18 male monkeys; 8 young and 10 young adult) had been on calorie-restricted diets for 3–6 years at the start of the study. Their diet was continued at 30% less than that of control monkeys. Serum DHEAS levels were collected and assayed for all animals throughout the study.

Findings.—Serum DHEAS levels decreased for all animals with each passing year. Animals showed individual variability in DHEAS levels, yet regression analysis showed that differences within an animal were reliable from year to year. Over 4 years, DHEAS levels declined significantly (about 30%) in the control group males, but only slightly (3%) in the test group (Fig 3).

Conclusions.—Levels of DHEAS decreased with advancing age in non-human primates. Given that in humans DHEAS serum levels also show cross-sectional and longitudinal decreases with aging and, similar to these results in monkeys, individual variability in humans remains stable over time, the DHEAS level may be a useful biomarker of aging in humans. Furthermore, caloric restriction slowed the decrease in DHEAS levels with aging in these young adult male rhesus monkeys. More studies are needed

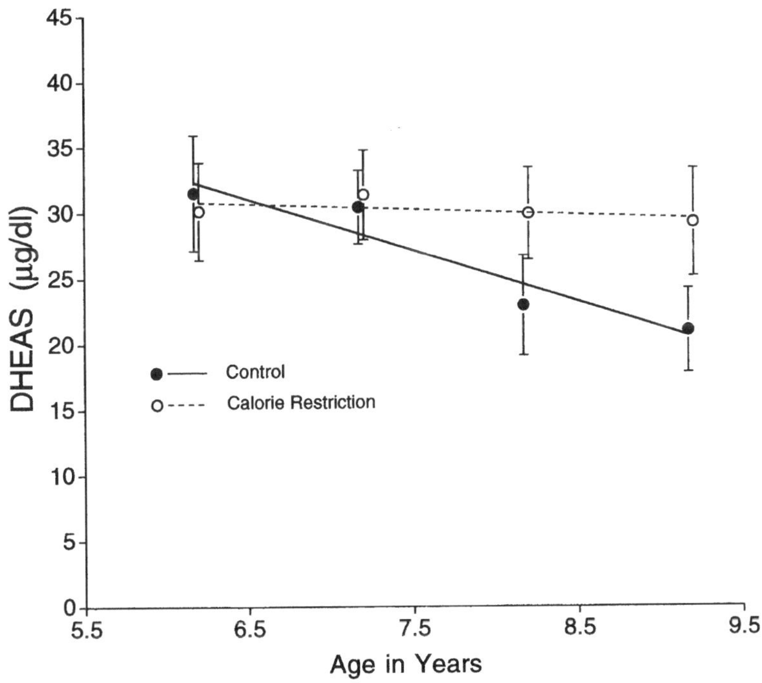

FIGURE 3.—Caloric restriction slows the rate of decline in serum deydroepiandrosterone sulfate (DHEAS). Each *point* represents the mean (±SEM) DHEAS level at a given age. Ages represent the average (±0.3 years) age of young adult male rhesus monkeys for years 3–6 of this longitudinal study. *Slopes* indicating the rate of decline were calculated from the regressions shown for each monkey group (control = −3.9 µg/dL/year and calorie restricted = −0.4 µg/dL/year). The rate of change was significantly slower in calorie-restricted monkeys ($P < 0.005$.) (Courtesy of Lane MA, Ingram DK, Ball SS, et al: Dehydroepiandrosterone sulfate: A biomarker of primate aging slowed by calorie restriction. *J Clin Endocrinol Metab* 82[7]:2093–2096, 1997. Copyright by the Endocrine Society.)

to examine the effects of calorie reduction on aging in long-lived species, especially humans.

▶ This interesting report joins 2 themes that are prominent in aging research: (1) the putative role of adrenal DHEAS as a key modulator in a variety of physiologic functions related to aging, and (2) the effects of caloric restriction on longevity in rodent studies.

Serum levels of DHEAS decline with increasing age. Conversely, elevated serum levels of DHEAS have been reported to be protective against heart disease, memory loss, depression, osteoporosis, aggressive tumors, and diabetes. Dehydroepiandosterone sulfate was observed to alter interleukin (IL) levels (to lower IL-6 and IL-10, and increase IL-2) related to the decline in immune function in the elderly and in subjects with HIV infection.[1] Not unexpectedly, many patients have found DHEAS in health food stores and are consuming the hormone in an unsupervised manner.

This report has 3 findings: (1) caloric restriction has physiologic effects in longer-lived species as previously demonstrated in shorter-lived species such as rodents; (2) caloric restriction slows the rate of decline in serum DHEAS with age; and (3) based on cross-sectional and longitudinal studies, DHEAS may be a reliable biomarker for aging. It appears that caloric restriction permits higher levels of DHEAS that are assumed to be beneficial. The question remains whether the alterations in DHEAS serum levels are merely epiphenomena (e.g., altered metabolic clearance) or whether there is physiologic significance to the observations. Although shown here for primates, a similar study could be conducted in healthy humans, perhaps using cytokine levels as biomarkers for the metabolic effect of DHEAS.

J.R. Shapiro, M.D.

Reference

1. Araghi-Niknam M, Liang B, Zhang Z, et al: Modulation of immune dysfunction during murine leukemia retrovirus infection of old mice by dehydroepiandrosterone sulfate (DHEA-S). *Immunology* 90:344–349, 1997.

Mechanisms of Aging

Molecular Identity and Cellular Distribution of Advanced Glycation End-product Receptors: Relationship of p60 to OST-48 and p90 to 80K-H Membrane Proteins

Li YM, Mitsuhashi T, Wojciechowicz D, et al (Picower Inst, Manhasset, NY; Keio Univ, Tokyo; Lindsley F Kimball Research Inst, New York)
Proc Natl Acad Sci USA 93:11047–11052, 1996 5–6

Introduction.—Advanced glycation end-products (AGEs)—produced by nonenzymatic reactions between sugars and proteins or lipids—have been linked to structural and functional changes occurring in senescence and long-term diabetes. Previous reports have described the partial sequencing of p60 and p90, 2 AGE-binding proteins isolated from rat liver membranes. Two new plasma membrane components corresponding to these AGE-binding proteins are described.

Findings.—Sequencing studies showed that the N-terminal sequence of p60 exhibited 95% identity to OST-48, a 48 kDa member of the oligosaccharyltransferase complex found in microsomal membranes. Sequence analysis of p90 demonstrated 73% identity to the N-terminal sequences and 85% identity to the internal sequences of human 80K-H, an 80 to 87 kDa protein substrate for protein kinase C. A single 50 kDa protein recognized by both anti-p60 and anti–OST-48 antibodies was produced by AGE-ligand and Western analyses of purified oligosaccharyltransferase complex, enriched rough endoplasmic reticulum, smooth endoplasmic reticulum, and plasma membranes from rat liver or RAW 264.7 macrophages. This protein also showed AGE-specific binding.

Further studies were performed with OST-48 immunoprecipitated from rat rough endoplasmic reticulum fractions, which showed AGE binding and immunoreactivity to an anti-p60 antibody. Immune IgG against recombinant OST-48 and 80 K-H showed dose-dependent inhibition of binding between AGE–bovine serum albumin and cell membranes. OST-48 and 80K-H was found by immunostaining and flow cytometry studies to be expressed on the surface of many different types of cells and tissues, including mononuclear, endothelial, renal, and brain neurons and glia.

Conclusions.—OST-48 and 80K-H are identical to the AGE receptor components p60 and p90, respectively. These 2 membrane proteins are involved in the processing of AGEs from extracellular and intracellular compartments, as well as in the associated pathogenic cellular responses. The findings will be useful in ongoing studies of AGEs in diabetic and normal tissues.

▶ Glucose and many other sugars interact to form bonds with proteins. The binding is initially reversible but becomes irreversible and then proceeds to form a series of complex products including those known as advanced glycation end-products (AGEs; pronounced āy-gee-ēz). Modification of the protein may or may not alter its behavior. For example, glycated hemoglobin biologically differs little from nonglycated hemoglobin. On the other hand, glycated low-density lipoprotein is metabolized much more slowly than the nonglycated form. Hyperglycemia and time are two key variables that produce an increase in glycation of proteins. Short-lived proteins are less affected because they are cleared quickly, whereas long-lived proteins more readily accumulate advanced glycation end-products. Receptors are present on many cells throughout the body to clear the glycated proteins. In addition to clearing the proteins, binding of the AGEs to receptors on cell surfaces can activate the receptor-bearing cells, thereby releasing cytokines and generating biologic processes such as chemotaxis, cell activation, and growth factor secretion. It is now believed that AGEs interacting with receptors for advanced glycation end-products (abbreviated RAGE; often pronounced rāyj) are an important mechanism by which aging and diabetes exert deleterious effects and promote pathologic processes. In this article, the authors—who are pioneers and leaders in this field—have shown that two of the major receptors for AGEs known temporarily as p60 and p90, are indeed two proteins that have already been characterized and known to have other functions. p60 is identical to OST-48, which is part of a complex catalyzing the transfer of oligosaccharides onto acceptor sites on glycoproteins during their biosynthesis. p90 is identical to 80K-H, which is a substrate for protein kinase C, an enzyme that is part of a major intracellular signaling pathway that links cell surface receptors to other cellular processes. How these receptors work to clear the glycated proteins and how they act as intermediaries in the activation processes promoted by AGEs is still not known, but identification of these receptors is a major step forward. Further, it is not at all clear how the known properties of these two proteins relate to their recognition of AGEs. I share with these authors the expectation that AGEs are an important intermediate in the pathologic processes associated with aging and with diabetes and that new agents that can prevent or divert these processes will be effective in slowing or preventing these pathologic processes.

J. Roth, M.D.

A Glucose-rich Diet Shortens Longevity of Mice

Mlekusch W, Lamprecht M, Öttl K, et al (Karl-Franzens-Universität-Graz, Graz, Austria)

Mech Age Dev 92:43–51, 1996 5–7

Background.—Atherogenic consequences and shortened life span result from high levels of dietary fat intake over a lifetime, combined with high levels of plasma lipids. Severe and permanent damage in many tissues has resulted from an abnormally high blood glucose level, as seen in diabetes mellitus. The genesis of diabetic complications may stem from products created from certain insulin-independent metabolic pathways for glucose. The effect of the addition of glucose to the longevity of female mice was studied.

Methods.—Seventy female mice fed a glucose-rich diet were compared with 70 mice fed a control diet. The control diet consisted of a commercial nonpurified, cereal-based pellet preparation containing an average of 223 g protein, 41 g fat, and 398 g carbohydrates per killograms. The glucose diet consisted of pure glucose pellets and control diet pellets. Per 100 g of consumed control diet pellets three were 18.5 of glucose pellets.

Results.—In the glucose group the average age of death was 511 ± 170 days, whereas in the control group the average age of death was 568 ± 139 days. The 7 oldest mice in the control group died at 890 ± 52 days, whereas the 7 oldest mice in the glucose group died at 833 ± 49 days. Body weight was not significantly affected by the diet. The risk increase of death for a glucose-diet animal was 138%, compared with a control-diet animal.

Conclusion.—A significant reduction of the average and maximal lifespan in female mice was caused by a lifelong intake of a diet with 20%

of total energy derived from glucose. Over long periods, high glucose intake has detrimental effects.

▶ The ability of reduced caloric intake to promote longevity has turned more attention to individual components of the diet. High-fat diets have been believed to be detrimental. In this study, female mice fed a high concentration of glucose showed a significant reduction of average and maximum lifespan. The glucose-fed animals ate more and weighed more than the controls. Pair-feeding would have made this experiment more meaningful.

J. Roth, M.D.

Effect of Age on In Vivo Rates of Mitochondrial Protein Synthesis in Human Skeletal Muscle

Rooyackers OE, Adey DB, Ades PA, et al (Mayo Clinic and Found, Rochester, Minn; Univ of Vermont, Burlington, Vt)

Proc Natl Acad Sci USA 93:15364–15369, 1996 5–8

Background.—The age-associated decline in muscle mass and muscle performance leads to reduced endurance capacity, increased risks for falls and fractures, and other disabilities. Mitochondrial decay appears to contribute to impaired muscle capacity in older persons. Experimental studies of mitochondria isolated from animal tissues have shown a decreased rate of protein synthesis. Using a newly developed stable-isotope technique to measure in vivo rates of mitochondrial protein synthesis in human skeletal muscle, researchers sought a potential mechanism for the age-related decline in the mitochondrial content and function of skeletal muscle.

Methods.—Study subjects were 42 healthy volunteers aged 20 to 92 years. They were divided into 3 groups according to age: young (mean, 24 years), middle-aged (mean, 54 years), and old (mean, 73 years). Body mass index, percentage of body fat, body muscle mass, and maximal rates of oxygen consumption were recorded. Plasma samples were obtained and leg muscle biopsies taken on the day of the study. Subsarcolemmal mitochondria, which appear to be more sensitive than intermyofibrillar mitochondria to contractile changes, were isolated from the needle-biopsy samples for analysis.

Results.—Aging was associated with increased body fat and decreased muscle mass. Age-related decline in skeletal muscle oxidative capacity was indicated by a decrease in cytochrome *c* oxidase and citrate synthase activity in muscle tissue (Fig 2). The decrease in mitochondrial activity of citrate synthase observed in muscle samples from older individuals was evidence of a decline in mitochondrial function. Although fractional rates of muscle mitochondrial protein synthesis were, on average, 40% lower in middle-aged than in young individuals, no further decrease was observed in the oldest group.

Conclusions.—The rate of mitochondrial protein synthesis in skeletal muscle substantially declines with age, particularly in the years between

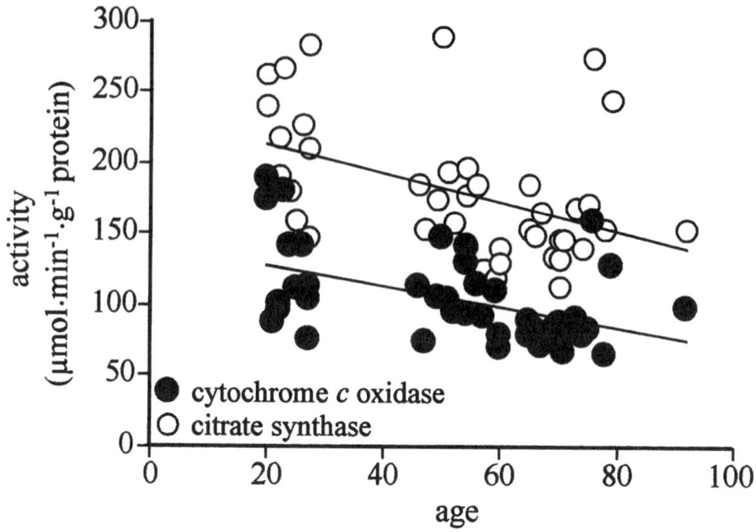

FIGURE 2.—Relationship between tissue (muscle homogenate) activities of cytochrome *c* oxidase and citrate synthase and age. Male and female subjects are presented as one group for each enzyme. Both activities of cytochrome *c* oxidase ($y = -0.72x + 142.8$; $r^2 = 0.22$) and citrate synthase ($y = -1.01x + 232.6$; $r^2 = 0.20$) decreased significantly with increasing age (respectively, $P < 0.0017$ and $P < 0.0033$). (Courtesy of Rooyackers OE, Adey DB, Ades PA, et al: Effect of age on in vivo rates of mitochondrial protein synthesis in human skeletal muscle. *Proc Natl Acad Sci USA* 93:15364–15369. Copyright 1996, the National Academy of Sciences, U.S.A.)

young adulthood and middle age. This decrease is associated with a decline in skeletal muscle oxidative capacity and mitochondrial function. The age-related decline in aerobic performance capacity may result in part from a decline in the quality of skeletal muscle, as reflected in decreased oxidative capacity.

► The loss of muscle mass and muscle strength with increasing age is a subject of considerable importance because with loss of muscle function there is a parallel loss of skeletal mass and thus increased risk of fracture, increased fatigue, and loss of muscle strength that impair daily activities of living and lead to decreased mobility. On the other hand, there is considerable interest in therapy to preserve muscle mass. Both anabolic steroids and growth hormone are under investigation for this purpose. As indicated in the abstract, an age-related decline mitochondrial function, specifically decreased mitochondrial protein synthesis related to oxidative damage, may be one manner in which mitochondrial function is affected with increasing age.[1]

This is the first in vivo study of muscle mitochondrial protein synthesis in human subjects. The investigators employed labeling with stable (nonradioactive) isotopes to demonstrate decreased rates of mitochondrial protein synthesis in women and men between the ages of 20 and 92. Fractional rates of muscle mitochondrial protein synthesis declined 40% between young and middle-aged subjects, but no further decline was apparent in specimens from the oldest subjects. However, the fractional rate of mitochondrial protein synthesis was high compared with overall tissue synthesis of mixed proteins. Interestingly, although protein synthesis showed no decline after middle age, the activity of mitochondrial oxidative enzymes continued to decline with increasing age. Of interest would be the extension of these in vivo studies to assess the effects of specific therapeutic interventions in human beings.

J.R. Shapiro, M.D.

Reference

1. Shigenaga MK, Hagen TM, Ames BN: Oxidative damage and mitochondrial decay in aging. *Proc Nat Acad Sci USA* 91:10771–10778, 1994.

Aging of the Liver: Age-associated Mitochondrial Damage in Intact Hepatocytes

Sastre J, Pallardó FV, Plá R, et al (Universidad de Valencia, Spain; Universidad de Alicante, Spain)

Hepatology 24:1199–1205, 1996 5–9

Background.—In the free radical theory of aging, oxygen-derived free radicals cause damage to cells. Because mitochondria generate high levels of oxygen radicals, mitochondrial damage may be a major cause of cellular aging. A study of intact liver cells was designed to test whether mitochondrial performance is impaired with aging. In no previous study has a correlation between age-associated changes in physiologic functions of intact cells and specific biochemical or molecular changes in mitochondria been sought.

Methods.—Hepatocytes were isolated from 3 groups of 24-hour–fasted Wistar rats: young adults (3–4 months) and old adults (22–23 months and 32–36 months). Liver mitochondria were studied by means of flow cytometric analysis and electron microscopy.

Results.—Flow cytometry studies revealed age to be associated with decreased mitochondrial membrane potential. In 3 experiments, the mean mitochondrial membrane potential of hepatocytes from old rats was 70% that of young rats. Age was associated with increased mitochondrial size, mitochondrial peroxide generation, and intracellular peroxide levels. Young and old rats did not differ in the number of mitochondria per cell or in inner mitochondrial membrane mass. Although gluconeogenesis from fructose, glycerol, or dihydroxyacetone did not change with age, the rate of gluconeogenesis from lactate plus pyruvate was 30% to 37% lower in hepatocytes from old rats than in those from younger rats.

This change in the rate of gluconeogenesis was not accompanied by changes in various hepatic parameters: phosphoenolpyruvate carboxykinase or pyruvate carboxylase activities or mitochondrial ATP/ADP or cytosolic reduced nicotinamide adenine dinucleotide/oxidized nicotinamide adenine dinucleotide ($NADH/NAD^+$) ratios. Malate content was almost 3 times higher in liver mitochondria from old rats than in those from younger rats, suggesting the likelihood of a decreased malate export from mitochondria. Hepatocytes from old rats also showed decreased ketogenesis from oleate.

Conclusions.—Experiments using intact liver cells from young adult and old rats demonstrated a correlation between age-associated impairment of cell metabolism and specific changes in mitochondrial function and structure. Although aging does not affect all mitochondrial functions, overall findings support a key role for mitochondrial damage in the process of aging.

► Results from several laboratories indicate that mitochondrial function decreases with increasing age and that oxidative damage to mitochondrial DNA may occur with aging.[1] Oxidant formation may increase the rate of proton leakage across the inner mitochondrial membrane, decrease membrane fluidity, and decrease levels of cardiolipin, supporting the function of many proteins of the inner mitochondrial membrane. In the liver, aging is associated with the accumulation of lipofuscin that may in large measure derive from injured mitochondria. The authors of this report examined whether mitochondrial function, as assessed on the basis of the parameters of gluconeogenesis and ketogenesis, is impaired with aging and whether oxidative stress affects hepatic mitochondrial function. The results indicate an increase in peroxide generation by isolated mitochondria from older animals and an increase in intracellular peroxide content. Oxidative damage may not be random; parameters related to the inner mitochondrial membrane are impaired in older animals, and previous studies indicate that high molecular weight proteins appear to be selectively damaged by oxidative stress.[2] In question is the relationship of increased peroxide generation to the abnormal mitochondrial metabolism. As summarized by Ames et al., oxidants generated by mitochondria may be a major source of the oxidative lesions that accumulate with age.[1] If so, how can this source of cell damage be contained? Caloric restriction and the administration of antioxidants such as vitamin C and E have been proposed to retard cellular damage caused by the accumulation of free radicals.[3]

J.R. Shapiro, M.D.

References

1. Ames BN, Shigenaga MK, Hagen TM: Mitochondrial decay in aging. *Biochem Biophys Acta* 1271:165–170, 1995.
2. Agarwal S, Sohal RS: Differential oxidative damage to mitochondrial proteins during aging. *Mech Ageing Dev* 85:55–63, 1995.
3. Sohal RS: Oxidative stress, caloric restriction and aging. *Science* 273:59–63, 1996.

Physiology of Aging

Relationship Between Cold-induced Thermoregulation and Spontaneous Rapid Body Weight Loss of Aging F344 Rats

McDonald RB, Florez-Duquet M, Murtagh-Mark C, et al (Univ of California, Davis)

Am J Physiol 271:R1115–R1122, 1996 5–10

Objective.—The authors have previously demonstrated attenuation of cold-induced thermoregulation in 26-month-old male Fischer 344 (F344) rats, compared with younger rats. However, not all 26-month-old rats show the same degree of hypothermia resulting from cold exposure or the same reduction of brown adipose tissue nonshivering thermogenic capacity. The variation could be related to a physiologic difference between rats that maintained stable body weight as they aged compared with those with the rapid weight loss that often occurs in aged rats. The link between cold-induced thermoregulation and rapid age-related weight loss was examined.

Methods.—Twenty-four-month-old male F344 rats underwent acute exposure to cold—4 hours at 6°C. Cold exposure took place 2 weeks in a row, then every other week as long as the animals maintained stable body weight. If there was a progressive decline in body weight over 3 to 5 days, the animal's response to cold was reassessed. If intraperitoneal temperature declined to 32.5°C or less during cold exposure, the animal was killed and the interscapular brown adipose tissue was removed for examination. Age-matched controls were also examined at each of these times.

Results.—A group of 8 rats with spontaneous rapid weight loss showed significant hypothermia in response to cold exposure, compared with none of 8 control rats with stable body weights. The weight loss occurred at 24.5 to 29 months of age. In the rats that went on to develop spontaneous weight loss, hypothermia generally did not predate the weight loss. Animals with weight loss and hypothermia had reduced levels of brown fat uncoupling protein. They also showed significant alterations of body fat and protein.

Conclusions.—Aging-related hypothermia in rats is a rapid-onset phenomenon that does not simply reflect chronologic age. The effects of aging on thermoregulation appear to have both a gradual and a rapid component, with differing physiologic states. This rat model of rapid senescence may be useful in understanding the hypothalamic changes in physiology occurring at the end of life.

► The loss of thermoregulation with old age is recorded in the biblical story of King David. A reduced ability to control temperature and other visceral functions is often found in the frail elderly. This article shows that very old rats may change from a period of steady weight to a period of sudden weight loss; this period of weight loss is associated with a serious loss of thermoregulation, followed by death in a few days. It is now well established that fat cells secrete a substrate (free fatty acids), a hormone (leptin), and a cytokine (tumor necrosis factor-α) that interact with multiple cells throughout the body, including elements of the CNS as well as liver, muscle, and fat to regulate glucose and insulin metabolism, appetite, energy expenditure and storage, and temperature regulation directly or indirectly. The changes described in the rat during old age are probably associated with major changes in some of these elements of cellular communication; I expect that the elucidation of these pathways will be most exciting.

J. Roth, M.D.

Cardiovascular Adaptation to Orthostatic Stress During Vasodilator Therapy

Lipsitz LA, Connelly CM, Kelley-Gagnon M, et al (Harvard Med School, Boston; Georgetown Univ, Washington)

Clin Pharmacol Ther 60:461–471, 1996 5–11

Objective.—The risk of orthostatic hypotension in elderly patients is often increased with the use of vasodilator therapy. Abnormal diastolic ventricular filling, impaired cardioacceleration, and stresses that reduce cardiac preload enhance the hypotensive effects. The mechanisms of postural blood pressure homeostasis in elderly patients with stable coronary artery disease in the absence of vasodilator medications and a comparison of the effects of isosorbide dinitrate and nicardipine hydrochloride on orthostatic tolerance are presented.

Methods.—After a 1-week baseline period, 20 patients, age 68–85, with stable coronary artery disease received 20 mg nicardipine 3 times a day or 20 mg isosorbide 3 times a day for 3 weeks in a double-blind, randomized, crossover study. Doppler echocardiography and tilt studies were performed at baseline and after each study arm. Heart rate, blood pressure, stroke volume, forearm blood flow, and spectral analysis of heart rate and blood pressure variability were determined before and at 3, 9, and 15 minutes during the head-up tilt. Demographic, clinical, and cardiovascular variables were compared statistically.

Results.—Patients who received isosorbide had symptoms of hypoperfusion more frequently than did patients taking nicardipine. The most frequent symptoms reported dizziness, lightheadedness, feeling faint, and postural dizziness. Nicardipine significantly reduced basal systolic and mean arterial pressure, systemic vascular resistance, and low-frequency and total systolic blood pressure variability, and increased systemic vascular resistance and heart rate compared with no drug. Isosorbide treatment and no treatment gave similar results. Nicardipine treatment significantly increased systemic vascular resistance, forearm vascular resistance and heart rate during tilt. Isosorbide treatment had no significant effect on these parameters during tilt. All treatments significantly increased low- and high-frequency systolic blood pressure power during tilt.

Conclusion.—Whereas nicardipine significantly improved cardiac output during tilt, isosorbide impaired the ability of elderly patients with stable coronary artery disease to respond to orthostatic stress.

► The authors use the knowledge gained during the last several years of the defects in cardiovascular function in the elderly with and without coronary artery disease to provide guidelines for therapy—the calcium channel blockers should be safer than nitrites. Indeed, the data support their hypothesis and should have meaningful clinical applications.

J. Roth, M.D.

The Association of Plasma IL-6 Levels With Functional Disability in Community-dwelling Elderly

Cohen HJ, Pieper CF, Harris T, et al (Duke Univ, Durham, NC; VA Med Ctr, Durham, NC; Natl Inst on Aging, Bethesda, Md)

J Gerontol 52A:M201–M208, 1997 5–12

Purpose.—Interleukin (IL)-6 is a multifunctional cytokine with a major role in inducing the acute inflammatory response as well as B-lymphocyte proliferation and differentiation. Several studies have suggested that IL-6 increases with age. Levels of IL-6 were measured in a community-based sample of elderly people and correlated with measures of functional status.

Methods.—The investigators measured IL-6 in 1,727 community-dwelling elderly participants in the Duke Established Populations for Epidemiologic Studies of the Elderly. The IL-6 measurements were made by enzyme-linked immunosorbent assay. The study included assessments of functional status and disease states, which were correlated with the plasma IL-6 measurements.

Results.—Even in subjects over age 70, IL-6 levels increase with age. For each functional status measure, IL-6 was positively correlated with functional disability. IL-6 was also correlated with the patient's self-rated health. Patients reporting cancer, heart attack, and high blood pressure had significantly higher median IL-6 levels, though those with diabetes or arthritis did not. On multivariate analysis, age and functional status continued to be associated with IL-6 even after controlling for other variables.

Conclusions.—This community-based study found that plasma IL-6 levels are significantly related to functional status in elderly people. The results suggest a link between IL-6 dysregulation and the functional disability of aging. Interleukin-6 may become a useful indicator of overall health. Also, interventions to inhibit IL-6 activity could be useful in slowing the functional decline associated with aging.

► Cytokines have been hypothesized to play an important role in aging and aging-related disorders. One exciting example is the role of estrogens in the tonic suppression of IL-6 production in bone; estrogen loss or withdrawal results in a marked elevation of IL-6 and of osteoclast activity. In the present article, the authors relate elevated IL-6 levels to functional disability, irrespective of other disease conditions. This intriguing observation suggests that functional decline in the elderly may be associated with rising levels of IL-6. I await with anticipation the pathophysiological basis for this relationship and possible therapeutic strategies.

J. Roth, M.D.

Cell Death

Apaf-1, a Human Protein Homologous to *C. elegans* CED-4, Participates in Cytochrome c-Dependent Activation of Caspase-3

Zou H, Henzel WJ, Liu X, et al (Univ of Texas, Dallas; Genentech Inc, South San Francisco)
Cell 90:405–413, 1997 5–13

Background.—One type of cell death, apoptosis, is under genetic control. In the nematode *Caenorhabditis elegans*, three controlling genes have been identified: *ced-3* and *ced-4* must be activated for apoptosis to occur, and *ced-9* inhibits such activation. Homologues of *ced-3* (caspase-3) and *ced-9* (Bcl-2) have been identified in mammalian cells, but no homologues for *ced-4* have been found—until now. These investigators isolated apoptotic protease activating factor-1 (Apaf-1), which has both CED-3 and CED-4 homologous domains.

Methods.—Caspase-3 was activated by incubation with 1 mM dATP and 1 mM magnesium chloride for 1 hour at 30°C. Apaf-1 was purified from HeLa S-100 and subjected to column spectroscopy. Apaf-1 was then electroblotted and subjected to protein sequencing. Complementary deoxyribonucleic acid (cDNA) was amplified via polymerase chain reaction, and Apaf-1 cDNA fusion proteins were produced and purified for further analysis.

Findings.—Caspase-3 activation by Apaf-1 required cytochrome c, dATP, and another factor: Apaf-1. Comparison with a protein data base revealed a sequence of 85 amino acids in the NH_2 terminal of Apaf-1 with 21% identity and 53% similarity with the same terminal of CED-3. A 320–amino acid chain of Apaf-1 after the NH_2 terminal showed 22% identity and 48% similarity with CED-4. The COOH terminal region of Apaf-1 contained 12 WD-40 repeats; such repeats are found in many regulatory proteins.

Conclusions.—After the release of cytochrome c from mitochondria, it binds to Apaf-1. Apaf-1, when combined with dATP, triggers caspase-3 activation and the resultant apoptosis. This action of Apaf-1 is similar to that of CED-4, and the sequence homology over 320 amino acids between Apaf-1 and CED-4 suggests that Apaf-1 is the mammalian homologue of CED-4.

► It appears now that every cell is continuously in Hamlet's shoes, debating whether to be or not to be; should it live or should it trigger the program of cellular suicide leading to apoptosis or apoptotic cell death, which is an essential part of the normal developmental process in humans as well as a major mechanism for pathology. It is now clear that an orderly set of signals is coming into each cell through appropriate pathways, both inside and outside the cells, which sustain life and ward off the apoptotic program while other signals promoting the apoptotic pathway are also coming in. From a biological point of view, what has been so remarkable is that the processes and molecules involved in programmed cell death are so highly conserved between humans and simple multicellular organisms such as the roundworm, *Caenorhabditis* (sē nōo răb dī tĭs) *elegans* (or *C. elegans*, as it is widely known to workers in the field); in the worm, genetic studies have identified about a dozen cell death (*ced*) genes and their corresponding (CED) proteins. (By common usage, the genes are lower case italics; the proteins are all caps.) The key crossroads in the apoptotic pathway in the worm links *ced*-3 and *ced*-4, whose gene products promote cell death, to *ced*-9 whose gene product blocks the cell death pathways. (Interestingly, *ced*-9 is the worm equivalent of the human bcl-2, a gene mutated in some forms of leukemia; bcl-2 can partially substitute for *ced*-9 in worms). All of the genes in the human pathway corresponding to the genes in the worm have been identified except *ced*-4. This paper fills in this major gap in the human pathway. This discovery also advances speculation on exactly how *ced*-3 and *ced*-9 exert their cellular tug of war on *ced*-4. (For a review of the current state of this field, see articles by Michael Hengartner[1] and David L. Vaux.[2] Apoptosis is clearly a vital mechanism for cell death in pathological situations. We can expect that an understanding of the molecular details will yield specific interventions that can be undertaken to inhibit (or enhance) the apoptotic pathway.

J. Roth, M.D.

References

1. Hengartner MO: Apoptosis: CED-4 is a stranger no more. *Nature* 388:714–715, 1997.
2. Vaux DL: CED-4: The third horseman of apoptosis. *Cell* 90:389–390, 1997.

Geometric Control of Cell Life and Death

Chen CS, Mrksich M, Huang S, et al (Harvard Med School, Boston)
Science 276:1425–1428, 1997 5–14

Objective.—Pharmacologic or genetic disruption of the extracellular membrane (ECM) leads to apoptosis, or programmed cell death, within adjacent cells. It has been assumed that changes in integrin signaling are responsible for mediating adhesion-dependent control of apoptosis. However, recent evidence suggests that apoptosis could be initiated by cell foreshortening caused by ECM dissolution. The role of cell shape vs. integrin binding in controlling cell life and death was studied.

Methods and Results.—In initial experiments, human capillary endothelial cells were more likely to undergo apoptosis when they were adherent to large fibronectin-coated beads than when they were nonadherent or adherent to smaller beads. Capillary cells were then plated on fibronectin-coated islands of different shapes and size. Square-shaped islands produced square-shaped cells that closely matched the shape of the island. As island size increased, apoptosis declined progressively. Measures to promote cell and nuclear spreading switched on DNA synthesis. When cell spreading was increased without changing the total cell–ECM contact area, DNA synthesis changed in accordance with projected cell area, not with cell–ECM contact area. Cell spreading switched off apoptosis, even at a constant cell–ECM contact area.

Conclusions.—Although the mechanism is unclear, cell shape appears to be the major influence in switching cells between life and death and between proliferation and quiescence. Membrane-associated focal adhesions and their kinase enzymes may be responsible for integration of shape-related mechanical signals and chemical signals may be elicited directly by integrin binding. The findings suggest the possibility that adhesive substrates could prevent cell death and promote cell growth via resistance of contractile forces transmitted across integrins. The results also show that local mechanical deformation can cause cells to produce different functional outputs in response to the same chemical inputs—in this case, growth or apoptosis as a result of integrin activation and growth factor receptor signaling. Loss of shape-dependent regulation could play a role in cell survival during malignant transformation.

▶ This study provides a remarkable view of how cell survival is affected when cells are influenced by the extracellular matrix to undergo changes in shape. Cell adhesion is mediated by a family of heterodimeric cell membrane receptors, the integrins. Integrins with both extracellular and intracellular extensions are connected to the intracellular signal-transducing cascade through specialized membrane structures, termed *focal adhesions*. Focal adhesions act as the membrane attachment site for actin fibrils inside the cell.[1] In this study, the authors have questioned whether cell viability is altered through integrin binding per se, or whether it is dependent on a variation in cell shape in response to the altered architecture of the extracellular matrix. Their studies indicate that cell shape rather than integrin binding to specific matrix proteins governs whether cells survive or undergo apoptosis. There are several consequences of this observation: local deformation of the cell in response to integrin binding or cytokine–growth factor stimulation can direct the cell to a growth mode or can initiate apoptosis. Cell overgrowth or crowding can initiate the death of members of that community, but the loss of cell-shape–dependent regulation may play an important role in permitting malignant overgrowth of cells.

J.R. Shapiro, M.D.

Reference

1. Ruoslahti E: Stretching is good for a cell. *Science* 276: 1345–1346, 1997.

Interaction of CED-4 With CED-3 and CED-9: A Molecular Framework for Cell Death

Chinnaiyan AM, O'Rourke K, Lane BR, et al (Univ of Michigan, Ann Arbor)

Science 275:1122–1126, 1997 5–15

Background.—Programmed cell death, or apoptosis, is essential for the health of multicellular organisms. This process is both evolutionarily conserved and genetically regulated. Core components in the apoptosis cascade have been identified in *Caenorhabditis elegans: ced-3, ced-4, ced-9*. The CED-3 protein is a cellular death effector that is homologous to the mammalian protein ICE, or caspase-1. A nematode inhibitor of cell death, CED-9 is homologous to the mammalian Bcl-2. Although CED-4 is an activator of cell death, no mammalian homologue has been identified yet. The interaction of these components of the apoptosis cascade is not well understood. Genetic analysis in the nematode suggests that CED-9 functions upstream of CED-3 and -4 and that CED-4 functions upstream of CED-3. To examine the biochemical interactions between the nematode components of the apoptosis cascade and some of their mammalian homologues, mammalian cells were used.

Methods and Results.—Ectopic expression of CED-4 in 293T human embryonic kidney cells or MCF7 breast carcinoma cells induced rapid apoptosis. Expression of mutated forms of CED-4 failed to induce programmed cell death in these cells. Cell death induced by expression of CED-4 in mammalian cells was blocked by CED-9, Bcl-X_L, caspase inhibitors, and an inactive mutant of CED-3. To investigate the interaction of CED-4 and CED-9 in vivo, 293T cells were transiently transfected with plasmids that directed the synthesis of AU1–tagged CED-9 and HA-tagged CED-4. Immunoprecipitation of AU1–CED-9 quantitatively coprecipitated HA–CED-4 and immunoprecipitation of HA–CED-4 quantitatively coprecipitated AU1–CED-9, confirming their interaction. Truncation of the CED-4 protein interfered with its ability to interact with CED-9. Also, CED-4 interacted with the mammalian CED-9 homologue, Bcl-X_L, in immunoprecipitation assays. Immunoprecipitation assays also detected an interaction between CED-4 and CED-3. Coprecipitation assays also showed that CED-4 interacted with the large prodomain caspases, ICE and FLICE, but not the small prodomain caspases, YAMA and Mch2. Also, CED-4 was able to simultaneously coprecipitate CED-3 and CED-9, suggesting that CED-4 can biochemically link and interact with both.

Conclusions.—The interactions of core components of the nematode programmed cell death cascade were investigated in mammalian cells as a model of mammalian programmed cell death. It was found that CED-4 can interact with and activate caspases, such as CED-3. The interaction of

CED-4 and CED-9 (Bcl-X_L, Bcl-2) could interfere with this activation and thereby block apoptosis. The mammalian homologoue of CED-4 has not yet been identified. If the mammalian CED-4 homologue were identified, it would be a potential target for therapy in disease of dysregulated programmed cell death.

▶ This article is 1 of 4 recent *Science* publications (Feb 21, 1997)[1-3] that describe the molecular basis for critical steps in the highly orderly cascade leading to programmed cell death. As discussed by Golstein,[4] programmed cell death is genetically determined and dependent upon several steps leading from damaging extracellular events to activation of a central control mechanism and ultimately to the cell execution stage. Studies in the nematode *C. elegans* have shown that cell death occurring during development involves the molecules CED-3 and CED-4, which facilitate cell death, and CED-9, which inhibits CED-4 to prevent the cell death activity of CED-3.[5] Thus, CED-4 appears to play a pivotal role as the molecular "death switch" promoting activation of CED-3. The CED-3 proteins are cysteine proteases now termed caspases, CED-9 corresponds to the protein Bcl-2, a cell-death supressor found in the mitochondrial membrane, and the equivalent of CED-4 in mammals is not known.[4] In this cascade, CED-9 functions upstream of CED 4, which functions upstream of CED-3 (caspase). Caspase activation leads to the structural changes characteristic of apoptosis, e.g., cytoplasmic and chromatin condensation and DNA fragmentation.

This study used mammalian cells to evaluate biochemical interactions between the *C. elegans* death proteins and their known mammalian analogues. The investigators have conducted a series of experiments using nematode CED-9, CED-4, and CED-3 and mutants of these proteins interacting with mammalian analogues Bcl-2 and Bcl-x_L and their mutants, as well as various capsases transfected into mammalian cells to plot the interactions among these proteins that ultimately control the apoptotic cascade. As the authors indicate, identification of the human CED-4 homologue would permit therapeutic modification of diseases of "dysregulated apoptosis."

J.R. Shapiro, M.D.

References

1. Wu D, Wallen HO, Nunez G: Interaction and regulation of subcellular localization of CED-4 by CED-9. *Science* 275:1126–1129, 1997.
2. Yang J, Liu X, Bhalla K, et al: Prevention of apoptosis by Bcl-2 release of cytochrome c from mitochondria blocked. *Science* 275:1129–1132, 1997.
3. Kluck RM, Bossy-Wetzel E, Green DR, et al: The release of cytochrome c from mitochondria: A primary site for Bcl-2 regulation of apoptosis. *Science* 275:1132–1136, 1997.
4. Golstein P: Controlling cell death. *Science* 275:1081–1082, 1997.
5. Hengartner MO: Programmed cell death in invertebrates. *Curr Opin Genet Dev* 6:34, 1996.

DNA Damage and Repair

Oxidative Thymine Dimer Repair in the DNA Helix
Dandliker PJ, Holmlin RE, Barton JK (California Inst of Technology, Pasadena)
Science 275:1465–1468, 1997 5–16

Background.—Ultraviolet radiation damages DNA, which can lead to mutations and cancer. The most studied of these light-induced DNA lesions is the cyclobutyl thymine dimer. Eukaryotic cells usually eliminate this dimer by excision, but work with model compounds has indicated that lesion repair also can occur through photo-induced oxidation with ultraviolet light. Intercalating complexes of rhodium(III), which bind to DNA and are strong photo-oxidants, might promote the repair of thymine dimers. The effect of intercalated rhodamine complexes on photo-induced thymine dimer repair was investigated in model DNA oligonucleotide duplexes.

Methods.—The metallointercalator $Rh(phi)_2DMB^{3+}$ was intercalated at varying sites in a 16–base pair DNA duplex. A thymine dimer was site-specifically incorporated into this model oligonucleotide. Visible light was used to trigger the repair mechanism.

Results.—Excitation of the rhodium complex at 400 nm in the presence of the dimer-containing duplex resulted in disappearance of dimer-containing DNA in a first-order kinetic process, with simultaneous appearance of the repaired DNA strand. Because the DNA π-stack can mediate long-range electron transfer reactions, remote repair was investigated. Dimer-containing 16–base pair duplexes were prepared with the Rh(III) intercalator covalently tethered to 1 end, where it could not come in direct contact with the dimer. These complexes were irradiated with 400-nm light, under conditions where duplex dimerization was insignificant. High-performance liquid chromatography showed the continuous disappearance of the dimer-containing strand and the appearance of the repaired strand as a function of irradiation. Repair occurred in an intraduplex reaction from a remote position. A series of duplexes was prepared containing a thymine dimer and a covalently bound rhodium intercalator to test the sensitivity of this repair reaction to both distance and helix destacking. The results indicated that repair was sensitive to stacking of both donor and acceptor into the helix and to the stacking of the intervening bases. Repair was not sensitive to distance or to the 3' or 5' position of the intercalator. The DNA helix mediated this long-range oxidative repair reaction.

Conclusions.—These results show how a synthetic catalyst may be used to repair thymine dimers in DNA using visible light. The repair process can occur over at least 26 A and illustrates long-range DNA-mediated electron transfer. The repair process was sensitive to disruption of the intervening π-stack.

► This article on DNA repair, although seemingly complex, is important because it shows that the DNA helix can perform what the authors term "chemistry at a distance."[1] The basic mechanisms involve whether DNA is considered to transfer electrons in a protein-like manner, e.g., functioning as a "resistor" of electron transfer, or whether it is akin to a "wire" as an electron-conducting complex. The authors conclude that electrons can flow freely through a channel that runs through the DNA molecule. How this happens is not clear. Nevertheless, this property appears to be related to the ability of electron transfer to mediate a chemical change in a distal portion of the helix, leading to the repair of a patch of damaged DNA. Here, the model was DNA damage induced by solar radiation that may facilitate the development of skin cancer.

In previous studies, the authors have used a photo-oxidant agent, rhodium (III), bound to DNA. When activated by light, the rhodium appears to facilitate the repair, e.g., excision, of thymine dimers previously incorporated at specific sites in synthetic oligonucleotide strands. The repair can be accomplished over a distance of 16–26 A. Moreover, the DNA helix that facilitates long-range electron transfer also mediates the long-range repair of the thymine dimer.

The potential applications of this DNA repair process cannot be overstated. First, it points to important long-range chemical reactions within the DNA helix, and second, it opens the field to the development of other synthetic agents that could facilitate repair after specific types of DNA damage.

J.R. Shapiro, M.D.

Reference

1. Taubes G: Double helix does chemistry at a distance—but how? *Science* 275:1420–1421, 1997.

Metabolic Regulation

Prevention of Vascular and Neural Dysfunction in Diabetic Rats by C-Peptide

Ido Y, Vindigni A, Chang K, et al (Washington Univ, St Louis)
Science 277:563–566, 1997 5–17

Background.—C-peptide is a cleavage product (from proinsulin to insulin) believed to have little, if any, biological activity of its own. C-peptide levels are decreased in insulin-dependent diabetes, and glucose stimulates its secretion. To evaluate whether C-peptide has a biological effect, vascular dysfunction and impaired nerve conduction (decreased Na^+,K^+, adenosine triphosphatase activity) were studied in 4 models of insulin-dependent diabetes.

Methods.—To examine its preventive effects, C-peptide was injected twice a day for 5 weeks in control rats and in rats with diabetes. Vascular (albumin permeation and blood flow) and neural function (nerve conduction velocity) were evaluated. To examine the effects of C-peptide on vascular function after established (8 weeks) untreated diabetes, rats received either neutral protamine Hagedorn (NPH) insulin, C-peptide, both, or neither compound for 4 weeks. Vascular and neurologic parameters were again measured.

In a skin chamber granulation model, the effects of high C-peptide levels on glucose-induced increases in blood flow and albumin permeation were examined. Finally, a reverse (retro) human C-peptide was synthesized to determine any biological differences compared to native C-peptide.

Findings.—In the prevention study, C-peptide significantly lessened blood flow in the anterior uvea, retina, and sciatic nerve in diabetic rats. It also prevented albumin permeation in these tissues and in the aorta of diabetic rats. Caudal motor nerve conduction velocity was improved by C-peptide in the diabetic rats. C-peptide showed no effects in control rats or in tissues not directly affected by diabetes. In rats with established diabetes, C-peptide plus NPH insulin significantly decreased albumin permeation in the aorta, anterior uvea, and retina and nerves.

In the skin chamber model, 100 nmol C-peptide prevented glucose-induced increases in blood flow and albumin permeation. Finally, the synthesized C-peptide was almost as effective as the native compound.

Conclusions.—C-peptide had preventive effects on diabetes-induced vascular and permeability changes. In established diabetes, the combination of C-peptide and NPH insulin significantly reduced vascular dysfunction. Supraphysiologic levels of C-peptide improved vascular function in diabetic rats when administered after a glucose bolus. Data indicate that C-peptide activity is dependent on nonchiral interactions rather than binding sites or stereospecific receptors.

▶ This is an important and biologically intriguing report. The general suggestion that protein propeptides, products of cellular protein processing, or in the case of insulin, the C-peptide cleavage product, could have metabolic activity is not unique. It has been known that the N-propeptide extension of type I collagen, normally cleaved in the extracellular space, is capable of regulating collagen synthesis by its parent cell. Other reports have cited biological activity for the C-peptide in insulin-dependent diabetes, including decreased glomerular hyperfiltration, augmented glucose utilization, and improved autonomic nervous function. Furthermore, the C-peptide may regulate insulin secretion by stimulating Na^+, K^+-adenosine triphosphatase activity.[1, 2] The authors speculate that the C-peptide in some manner not related to the sorbitol pathway inhibits metabolic "imbalance caused by hyperglycemia-induced reductive stress," e.g., altered intracellular redox potential. They draw an analogy to certain antibiotic peptides that induce membrane ion channels and inhibit phospholipase A2 activity.

The action of C-peptide administration to increase Na^+, K^+-adenosine triphosphatase activity may also underlie the improvement in nerve conduction, the decrease in vascular permeability, and increase in blood flow. It is remarkable that reversal of these mechanisms so crucial to the development of diabetes complications occurs without an effect of the C-peptide on hyperglycemia. Certainly the possibility that C-peptide therapy may be beneficial in patients with insulin-dependent diabetes mellitus should be evaluated.

J.R. Shapiro, M.D.

References

1. Steiner, DF, Rubenstein AH: Proinsulin C-peptide–biological activity? *Science* 277: 531–532, 1977.
2. Wahren J, Johansson BL, Wallenberg-Henriksson H, et al: C-peptide revisited: New physiological effects and therapeutic implications. *J Intern Med* 240:115–124, 1996.

Insulin Receptor mRNA Splicing and Altered Metabolic Control in Aged and Mildly Insulin-Deficient Rats

Wiersma MML, Auboeuf D, Nieuwenhuizen-Bakker IM, et al (Univ Hosp Leiden, The Netherlands; Institut National de la Santé et de la Recherche Médicale, Lyon Cedex, France)
Am J Physiol 272:E607–E615, 1997 5–18

Introduction.—The molecular basis of insulin resistance in noninsulin–dependent diabetes mellitus remains unclear. One line of evidence suggests that alterations in insulin receptor isoform expression could play a role. There are few data on the expression of insulin receptor isoforms in animal models of insulin resistance. The authors have recently developed a reverse transcription-competitive polymerase chain reaction assay to quantitate the mRNAs encoding the 2 insulin receptor isoforms in rat tissue. This assay was used to study the association between insulin receptor isoform expression and insulin action under different circumstances of altered metabolic control in rats.

Methods.—Mild insulin deficiency was induced in male Wistar rats using a low-dose of streptozocin during the neonatal period. Insulin-resistant 12-month-old rats were also studied. The animals were fitted with long-term right jugular vein and left carotid artery cannulas for IV glucose tolerance testing (IVGTT) and a euglycemic hyperinsulinemic clamp. One week after these tests, the animals were killed and tissues were obtained for measurement of insulin receptor mRNA variants.

Results.—During the IVGTT, the return to baseline glucose values was significantly inhibited both in the older control rats and in rats treated with streptozocin. The streptozocin-treated rats showed a reduced plasma insulin response to glucose, whereas the older control rats had a slight but nonsignificant reduction in plasma insulin levels. Both groups of mice showed a reduction in the relative abundance of the mRNA with exon 11 ($Ex11^{+}$) in liver, heart, and adipose tissue and in tibialis muscle. The level of Ex11$^+$ mRNA was slightly increased in the extensor digitorum longus muscle and unchanged in the soleus muscle. The mRNA without exon 11 (Ex11$^-$) was predominant in the 3 muscle tissues tested. Control rats showed similar expression of the 2 Ex11 isoforms in heart and adipose tissues. In these 2 tissues, the streptozocin-treated rats showed an increase in the Ex11$^-$ form, whereas the older control rats showed a decrease in the absolute level of the Ex11$^+$ form. A significant correlation was noted between decreased levels of the Ex11$^+$ variant and insulin resistance of whole body glucose uptake. However, the changes in expression of insulin receptor variants appeared to be caused by rather than the cause of insulin resistance.

Conclusions.—Rats with altered glucose tolerance show a reduction in the relative abundance of the Ex11$^+$ form of insulin receptor mRNA. However, the reported changes in isoform expression appear to be secondary in nature rather than the cause of changes in glucose metabolism and insulin sensitivity. The alterations in insulin receptor isoform expression could still take part in regulating some specific receptor function.

► Insulin resistance is a central problem in the cause of hyperglycemia in individuals with type II (non–insulin-dependent) diabetes mellitus (NIDDM). The question explored by this study is whether the recently described alterations in the expression of insulin receptor isoforms play a role in insulin receptor resistance in patients with NIDDM. Insulin receptor isoforms are the result of alternative mRNA splicing of exon 11. Alternative splicing, which reflects the interaction of hormones and metabolic substrates at the tissue level, plays a role in the variable expression of many other genes and is, in part, the basis for differences in tissue sensitivity to various hormones. Aging, per se, is associated with a decrease in the isoform Ex11$^+$ in liver and heart tissue and skeletal muscle. Here, both control and streptozotocin-treated rats were compared for receptor expression, and this was related to parameters of glucose regulation. There was no correlation between total insulin receptor mRNA and different parameters of glucose metabolism. A decrease in Ex11$^+$ was confirmed for 12-month-old rats and also for neonatally streptozocin-treated (nSTZ) animals in heart and adipose tissue and tibialis muscle. In several skeletal muscles, significant variation in receptor isoform abundance was seen, but no reciprocal alteration in Ex11$^-$ was found. Thus, the expression of different isoforms is dependent on the type of muscle studied. The reasons for the alterations of receptor expression in various muscle groups remains unexplained. The mRNA for Ex11$^-$ was increased in heart and adipose tissue in nSTZ rats. The authors conclude that altered glucose tolerance in rats is associated with a decrease in the relative abundance of Ex11$^+$ mRNA. However, this may be a relatively minor event and not the primary cause for insulin resistance.

J.R. Shapiro, M.D.

Uncoupling Protein-2: A Novel Gene Linked to Obesity and Hyperinsulinemia

Fleury C, Neverova M, Collins S, et al (CNRS/CEREMOD, Meudon, France; UC Davis, Calif; Duke Univ, Durham, NC)

Nature Genet 15:269–272, 1997 5–19

Background.—Uncoupling protein 1 (UCP1) has been implicated in thermoregulation and the regulation of body composition and glucose metabolism. A second entity, uncoupling protein 2 (UCP2), has been discovered that has 59% amino acid identity to UCP1. The effects of UCP2 were compared with those of UCP1 to see which was more effective in the control of body temperature and composition and glucose metabolism.

Methods.—Four studies were performed. In the first study, yeast was transfected with UCP1 or UCP2 and its growth in medium supplemented with galactose was determined. In the second study, yeast was transfected with UCP1 or UCP2 and the associated decrease in membrane potential (uncoupling of respiration) was evaluated by flow cytometry. The third experiment involved northern blot analysis to determine whether tissue distribution of the 2 uncoupling proteins differed. Finally, the fourth study examined the chromosomal location of UCP2.

Findings.—In the first study, yeast transfected with UCP2 grew significantly more slowly than samples transfected with either UCP1 or a control vector. The second study revealed that both UCP1 and UCP2 significantly decreased the mitochondrial potential. However, flow cytometry of UCP2 revealed 2 peaks, one corresponding with that of UCP1 and another corresponding with a very low mitochondrial potential. In the third study, tissue distribution of the 2 uncoupling proteins differed significantly, with high UCP2 levels in the spleen, thymus, leukocytes, macrophages, bone marrow, and stomach. The fourth study showed that the gene encoding UCP2 maps to chromosomes 11 and 7, which are involved in obesity and diabetes.

Conclusions.—UCP2 functions at least partially like UCP1 in that both decrease yeast growth and both affect the mitochondrial membrane potential. The distribution of UCP2 in tissues involved with immunity and thermoregulation suggests that it may play a role in the development of the inflammatory response. Furthermore, the gene encoding UCP2 maps to the same chromosomal regions involved with obesity and hyperinsulinemia. Thus, UCP2 may be a key regulator of energy balance.

► Peter Mitchell won a Nobel Prize for elucidating the mechanism by which oxidation is linked to phosphorylation and the synthesis of adenosine triphosphate in mitochondria. As substrates are oxidized, there is an orderly flow of electrons and protons. The generation of a gradient of protons across the mitochondrial membrane is the driving force that leads to the production of ATP. Some years ago, a protein had been found in brown adipose tissue of rodents that is capable of allowing the protons to leak out of the mitochondria without generating ATP; because it uncoupled oxidation from phosphorylation, it was named "uncoupling protein." This waste of chemical energy turned up as heat, i.e., thermogenesis, and was believed to be an important mechanism for regulation of heat production. Recently, a second uncoupling protein (UCP2) has been found which is more widely distributed in cells including white fat and macrophages. A thoughtful and stimulating editorial accompanies it.[1] Shortly thereafter, two laboratories reported a third uncoupling protein (UCP3), again with a broader cellular distribution including skeletal muscle.[2, 3] Others in the family are anticipated and high levels of regulation are starting to emerge. Thus, we can expect new insights on how thyroid hormones and fever regulate heat production. The subject of obesity and cachexia from now on will be discussed in the context of uncoupling proteins, where they are and how they are affecting energy balance. In essence, these proteins provide a mechanism for generating heat as well as wasting energy. Our ability to control the function of these proteins may have a profound effect on our ability to help patients achieve a body composition more to their benefit than now occurs. (That similar proteins have now been found in plants suggests these proteins are evolutionarily ancient and widespread.)

J. Roth, M.D.

References

1. Flier JS, Lowell BB: Obesity research springs a proton leak (news; comment). *Nat Genet* 15:223–224, 1997.
2. Boss O, Samec S, Paoloni-Giacobino A, et al: Uncoupling protein-3: A new member of the mitochondrial carrier family with tissue-specific expression. *FEBS Lett* 408:39–42, 1997.
3. Vidal-Puig A, Solanes G, Grujic D, et al: UCP3: An uncoupling protein homologue expressed preferentially and abundantly in skeletal muscle and brown adipose tissue. *Biochem Biophys Res Commun* 235:79–82, 1997.

Hormones—Fundamental Science

Cloning and Characterization of a Specific Coactivator, ARA_{70}, for the Androgen Receptor in Human Prostate Cells
Yeh S, Chang C (Univ of Wisconsin, Madison)
Proc Natl Acad Sci USA 93:5517–5521, 1996 5–20

Introduction.—The androgen receptor (AR), a member of the steroid receptor superfamily based on structural similarity, can up- or down-regulate expression of androgen target genes through a complex process that may involve other adaptors or coactivators. The shift from androgen-dependent to androgen-independent prostate cancer may involve mutations or abnormal expression of AR. The specificity of AR target gene activation may depend on selective interaction between the AR and accessory factors. Experiments were performed in an attempt to identify associated factors involved in the activation of AR.

Methods and Findings.—The study used a yeast 2–hybrid system to investigate the mechanism of androgen-AR function. A ligand-dependent AR-associated protein was identified and designated ARA_{70}. In human prostate cancer cells, ARA_{70} produced a 10-fold increase in AR transcriptional activity in the presence of 10^{-10} M dihydrotestosterone or 10^{-9} M testosterone, but not in the presence of 10^{-6} M hydroxyflutamide. Other steroid receptors—including estrogen receptor, glucocorticoid receptor, and progesterone receptor—showed only a slight increase in transcriptional activity in response to ARA_{70}.

Conclusions.—ARA_{70} is identified as the first ligand-dependent AR-associated protein. In prostate cancer cells, ARA_{70} may serve as a specific coactivator to increase transcriptional activity of AR. Further research may offer new insights into the molecular mechanisms of androgen activity.

▶ The traditional steroid hormone receptors are part of a large superfamily of transcriptional factors that have very similar structures. The ligand binds to its specific binding site near the C-terminus of the receptor and thereby changes the conformation of the receptor so that a DNA binding domain in the middle of the molecule can now bind to specific DNA sequences, typically found in multiple loci throughout the genome. There is obviously specificity in the ligand binding site. There is also specificity in the DNA binding region. In this study, the authors have found an androgen receptor–associated protein that they designate ARA_{70}, which only binds well to an androgen receptor that has a biologically active hormone bound to it but not when it is lacking a ligand or when it has an antagonist such as hydroxyflutamide. Binding of the ARA_{70} to the androgen receptor markedly enhances the DNA-activating properties of the androgen receptor. It has much less effect on other hormone receptors. Thus, the power of the androgen receptor to activate transcription of DNA depends on the presence of additional factors. In trying to understand the androgen sensitivity and resistance of prostate cancer, factors such as these will prove of great interest. There is suddenly an explosion of new data relating to the importance of accessory factors, including co-activators and co-repressors, for the steroid type receptor. They modify the specificity of the hormones and synthetic analogs, as well as modify the magnitude of each response in one target cell. Expect lots more data soon.

J. Roth, M.D.

Differential Ligand Activation of Estrogen Receptors ERα and ERβ at AP1 Sites

Paech K, Webb P, Kuiper GGJM, et al (Univ of California, San Francisco; Karolinska Inst, Novum, Sweden)

Science 277:1508–1510, 1997 5–21

Background.—Antiestrogens are often used to treat and perhaps prevent breast cancer. Differences in their actions may be related to their different effects on two estrogen receptors, ERα and ERβ, and on the response element, such as estrogen or an AP1 enhancer element (Fig 1). These authors evaluated the transactivation properties of ERα and ERβ on 2 estrogens and 3 antiestrogens with 2 different response elements (estrogen and AP1).

Methods.—HeLa cells were transfected with an ERα or an ERβ plasmid and a luciferase gene whose transcription was controlled by an estrogen response element or the AP1 element. Transcription induction by 2 estrogens (E_2 and diethylstilbestrol) and 3 antiestrogens (ICI 164384, tamoxifen, and raloxifene) was measured in each of the different experiments

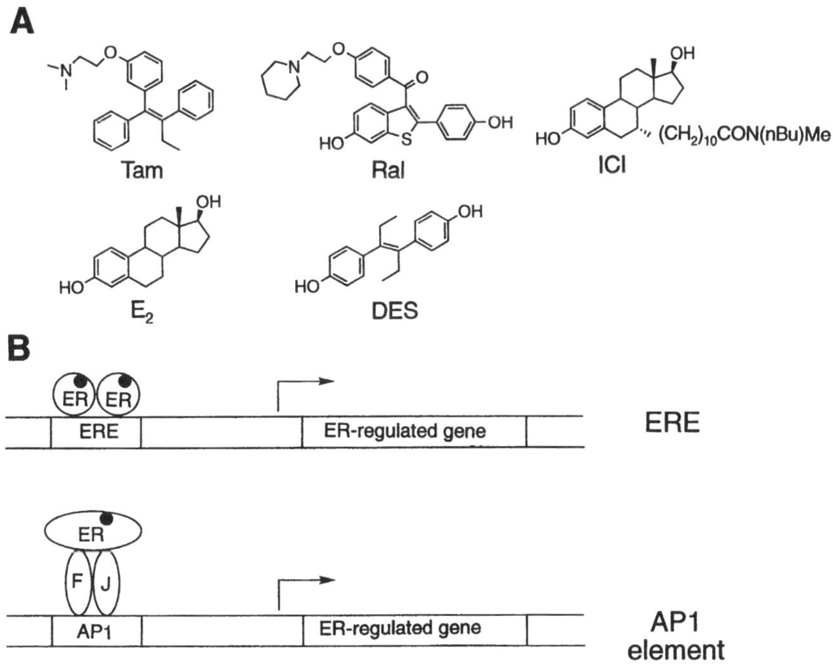

FIGURE 1.—A, Structures of ER ligands. The estrogens E_2 and diethylstilbestrol (DES) and the antiestrogens tamoxifen (*Tam*), raloxifene (*Ral*), and ICI 164384 (*ICI*) are shown. *Bu*, butyl; *Me*, methyl. B, models of ER action at a classical estrogen response element (*ERE*) and an ER-dependent AP1 response element. The *filled circles* represent the ligand bound to the ER. The AP1 proteins Jun and Fos are labeled J and F, respectively. (Reprinted with permission from Paech K, Webb K, Kuiper GGJM, et al: Differential ligand activation of estrogen receptors ERα and ERβ at AP1 sites. *Science* 277:1508–1510. Copyright 1997, American Association for the Advancement of Science.)

and was compared among these 5 ligands and against a control with no ligand added.

Findings.—With an estrogen response element, ERα and ERβ showed the same transactivation profiles. In this model, the 2 estrogens showed substantially more luciferase production than the 3 antiestrogens (Fig 2). With an AP1 response element, however, ERα and ERβ showed different transcription profiles. With ERα, all 5 ligands stimulated luciferase production (Fig 3), while with ERβ the 3 antiestrogens actually stimulated luciferase production (Fig 4).

Conclusions.—In an estrogen response element, the 2 estrogens stimulated transcription and the 3 antiestrogens inhibited transcription. But in an AP1 response element, ERα stimulated transcription with all 5 ligands, and ERβ actually reversed the effects found in the estrogen response element model (i.e., estrogens inhibited transcription and antiestrogens stimulated transcription). These differences in transcription indicate differ-

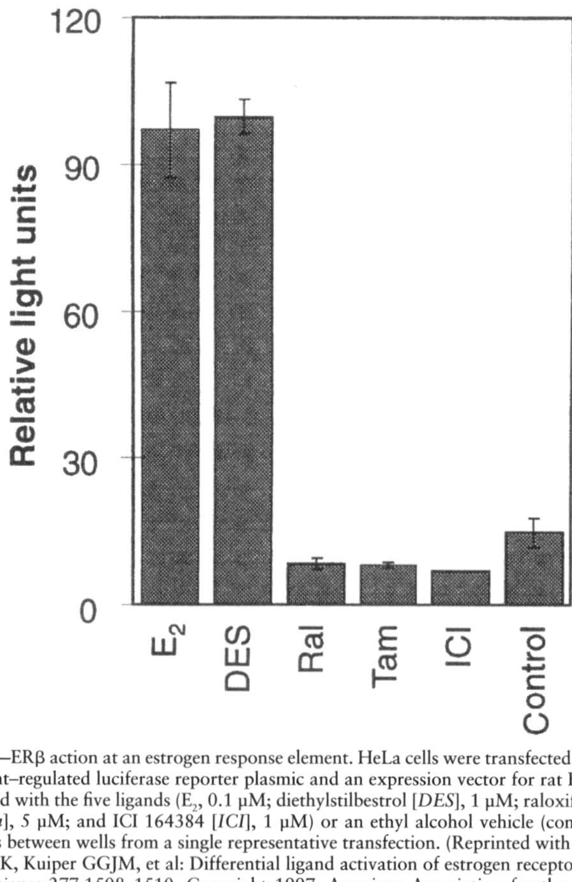

FIGURE 2.—ERβ action at an estrogen response element. HeLa cells were transfected with an estrogen response element–regulated luciferase reporter plasmic and an expression vector for rat ERβ. Transfected cells were treated with the five ligands (E_2, 0.1 μM; diethylstilbestrol [*DES*], 1 μM; raloxifene [*Ral*], 1 μM; tamoxifen [*Tam*], 5 μM; and ICI 164384 [*ICI*], 1 μM) or an ethyl alcohol vehicle (control). *Error bars* show deviations between wells from a single representative transfection. (Reprinted with permission from Paech K, Webb K, Kuiper GGJM, et al: Differential ligand activation of estrogen receptors ERα and ERβ at AP1 sites. *Science* 277:1508–1510. Copyright 1997, American Association for the Advancement of Science.)

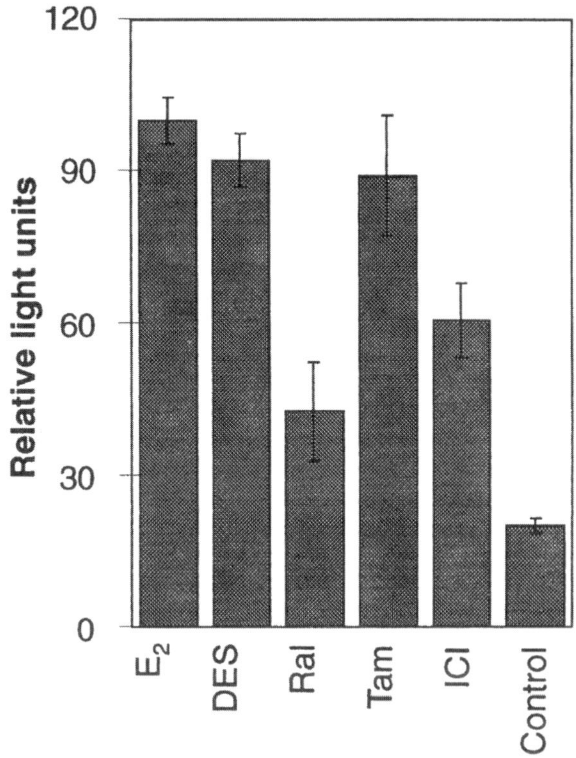

FIGURE 3.—ERα action at an AP1 element. HeLa cells were transfected with an AP1 reporter plasmic and an ERα expression plasmid and treated with the 5 ligands. Ligand concentrations were E_2, 0.1 μM; diethylstilbestrol (*DES*), 1 μM; raloxifene (*Ral*), 1 μM; tamoxifen (*Tam,*), 5 μM; and ICI 164384 (*ICI*), 1 μM. (Reprinted with permission from Paech K, Webb K, Kuiper GGJM, et al: Differential ligand activation of estrogen receptors ERα and ERβ at AP1 sites. *Science* 277:1508–1510. Copyright 1997, American Association for the Advancement of Science.)

ences in estrogen receptor subtypes α and β depending on the response element. This, in turn, suggests that estrogen-like drugs with specific target tissue effects at specific response element sites can be developed.

► With tamoxifen as the forbearer (it blocks estrogen action at the breast but simulates estrogen at the uterus and bone), there has recently been a proliferation of molecules that act as mimics of estrogen in some tissues and as inhibitors in others. Raloxifene is in the vanguard of what appears to be an expanding number of compounds coming to market that appear to stimulate some of the desirable effects of estrogen (on bone) while blocking some of the undesirable effects of the hormone (on breast and uterus). Until recently, it was believed that estrogen exerted its effects solely in the nucleus through a single class of nuclear receptors. As noted elsewhere in this section, estrogens can also bind to the sex hormone binding globulin in blood, which in turn can activate its cell surface receptors to produce biological effects we associate with sex steroids. It is now clear that there

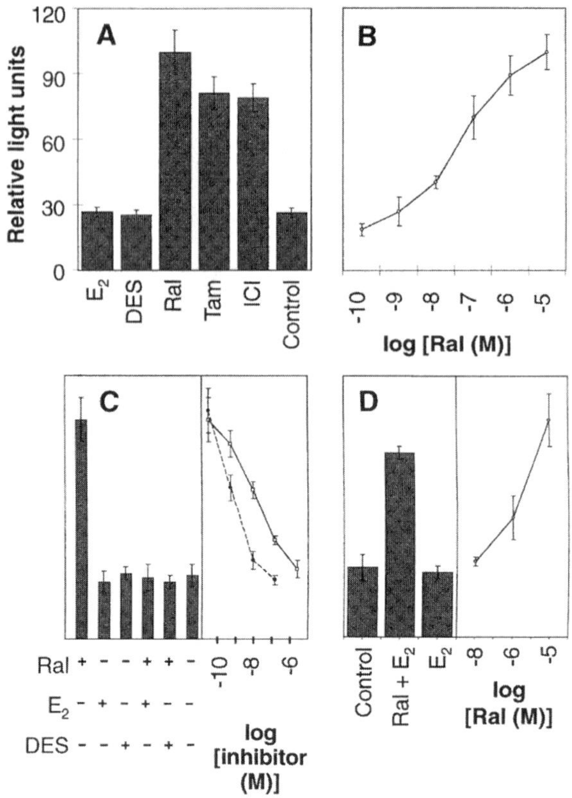

FIGURE 4.—**A**, ERβ action at an AP1 response element. HeLa cells were transfected with an AP1 reporter plasmid and a rat ERβ expression plasmid. Transfected cells were treated with the following ligand concentrations: E_2, 0.1 μM; diethylstilbestrol (*DES*), 1 μM; raloxifene (*Ral*), 1 μM; tamoxifen (*Tam*), 5 μM; and ICI 164384 (*ICI*), 1 μM. **B**, dose response of raloxifene induction with ERβ at an AP1 element. HeLa cells transfected as described for **A** were treated with the indicated range of raloxifene concentrations. **C**, competitive inhibition of raloxifene induction by E_2 and DES. HeLa cells were transfected as described for **A** and treated with ligands. The *left panel* shows transactivation induction by raloxifene (1 μM), the lack of induction by E_2 (0.1 μM) and DES (1 μM), and the ability of E_2 (0.1 μM) and DES (1 μM) to inhibit competitively raloxifene (1 μM) induction to the amount observed with the control (no ligand added). The *right panel* shows the dose dependence of inhibition of raloxifene (1 μM) induction by DES (*solid line*) and E_2 (*dashed line*). **D**, raloxifene overriding E_2 inhibition. HeLa cells were transfected as described for **A** and treated with ligands. The *left panel* shows the transcription induction resulting from the vehicle control (ethyl alcohol), raloxifene (*Ral*) (10 μM) plus E_2 (10 nM), and E_2 (10 nM) alone. The *right panel* shows the dose dependence of raloxifene induction in the presence of E_2 (10 nM). (Reprinted with permission from Paech K, Webb K, Kuiper GGJM, et al: Differential ligand activation of estrogen receptors ERα and ERβ at AP1 sites. *Science* 277:1508–1510. Copyright 1997, American Association for the Advancement of Science.)

are at least two nuclear estrogen receptors, the α and the β, each with its own gene. Further, each estrogen receptor, when linked to an agonist, can act as an estrogen response element on DNA, or as an AP1 enhancer site. This article highlights the importance of that difference in conferring unique spectra of activity on each of the estrogen-like analogues. It is now also clear that the effects of the α and β receptors are modulated substantially by a new and growing list of co-activators and co-repressors that bind to the activated forms of the receptors. While this complexity is daunting, it affords an extraordinary opportunity to generate estrogen analogues with narrow specificity at the level of target cell or gene. It is no longer a pipe dream to consider the possibility that estrogen analogues will be developed for individual clinical situations that will give an exactly tailored package of events while avoiding all of the undesired effects of estrogen. This unbundling of estrogen effects heralds the possibility that other steroid hormones and their cousins may also be joined by narrowly specific analogues in the future as well. (An entertaining and lucid survey of the cutting edge of the nuclear receptor field, based on a meeting in May 1997, by Perlmann and Evans[1] appears in *Cell* including up-to-date references.) One disconcerting consequence of the new data is that each new compound may have a quite unpredictable profile of effects; this uncertainty would push me to recommend only estrogens and estrogen analogues whose composition and/or effects are very well studied. The newly popular plant estrogens would not pass this test.

J. Roth, M.D.*

*This reviewer is a consultant for Eli Lilly, the manufacturer of raloxifene.

Reference

1. Perlmann T, Evans RM: Nuclear receptors in Sicily: All in the famiglia. *Cell* 90:391–397, 1997.

Hormonal Changes of Aging

Potentially Predictive and Manipulable Blood Serum Correlates of Aging in the Healthy Human Male: Progressive Decreases in Bioavailable Testosterone, Dehydroepiandrosterone Sulfate, and the Ratio of Insulin-like Growth Factor 1 to Growth Hormone

Morley JE, Kaiser F, Raum WJ, et al (VA Med Ctr, St Louis; St Louis Univ; Harbor-Univ of California, Los Angeles; et al)

Proc Natl Acad Sci USA 94:7537–7542, 1997 5–22

Objective.—This study sought to obtain a broad view of key rate-limiting variables affecting the uncomplicated aging process in men. It started by looking at neuroendocrine markers measurable in the serum—including bioavailable testosterone (BT), dehydroepiandrosterone sulfate (DHEAS), and the ratio of insulin-like growth factor 1 (IGF-1) to growth hormone (GH)—and related these to cognitive and physical tests that can be affected by aging.

Methods.—The cross-sectional survey included 56 men, age 21–84, with no evidence of acute or chronic disease. A wide range of steroidal components and peptide hormones were measured in serum. Blood tests were also performed in two middle-aged men after oral ingestion of a 175 mg pregnenolone (P) capsule. Cognitive tests included the Rey Visual Design Learning and Auditory Verbal Tests, the animal naming test, and the Mini-Mental Status Examination. Physical tests included measurement of the waist/hip ratio, a balance test, and handgrip strength measurement.

Results.—A number of androgen-related steroids plus pregnenolone sulfate showed a high negative correlation with age ($r > -0.6$). For all of these substances, the mean serum value declined with increasing median cohort age. The ratio of IGF-1 to GH met both of these criteria, and BT, DHEAS, and IGF-1/GH all showed progressive patterns of age-related change. Functional variables were more closely correlated with age than with any of the biochemical variables, except for BT. The findings suggested that testosterone played a direct role in the rate-limiting processes of the functions measured, while DHEAS played a more indirect role. The IGF-1/GH ratio had a highly negative correlation with age and a relatively low correlation with BT. These findings, along with the correlations of IGF-1/GH and functional measures, suggested that the GH-IGF-1 axis and BT had independent effects on function.

Findings in the men studied after P ingestion suggested that oral P may be a precursor of glucocorticoids, mineralocorticoids, and sex steroids. The steroid with the greatest increase after P ingestion was pregnenolone sulfate, which was 3 times slower to clear than P. Other measures showing a prolonged increase over control values were DHEA, total estrogens, 17α-OH progesterone, and progesterone. The IGF-1/GH ratio showed the closest pattern of elevation to that of PS, largely because of reductions in GH level after PS ingestion.

Conclusions.—The hormonal marker that is best correlated with aging and with indicators of age-related cognitive and physical function is BT. Serum DHEAS appears to be a limiting factor on the level of total serum testosterone. The ratio of IGF-1 to GH shows a much better correlation with age than either measure alone, and is consistent with the pattern of age-related reduction in BT and DHEAS. The functional variables that correlate best with the biochemical findings are those related to learning, memory, and vestibular function. The findings suggest that giving small doses of DHEA and testosterone to aging men might restore serum BT, IGF-1/GH, and DHEAS to normal young adult levels.

▶ The exciting results of this study provide considerable insight about the relevance of various hormonal levels to patient well being and functionality in men with increasing age. The authors have examined the age relationship of commonly assessed hormones in healthy men and have related these to a series of functional parameters, both physical and cognitive. Although other clinical trials involving the administration of DHEAS, testosterone, and growth hormone/IGF-1 are in progress, the potential importance of this study rests in: (1) developing a matrix of standards against which dysregulation relative to age can be assessed, and (2) as indicated in the title, defining parameters that are potentially manipulable. Thus, it should be possible to return reduced serum levels of these hormones to young adult levels with the goal of improving a specific cognitive or physical function.

The take-away messages are these: (1) bioavailable testosterone (BT) was the variable that correlated best with chronological age and age-related cognitive and physical deficits, (2) the availability of serum DHEAS appeared to be limiting in determining the level of total serum testosterone (T). Also, of great interest was the finding that the molar ratio of BT to DHEA appeared fixed at all levels of DHEAS, (3) DHEAS raised serum IGF-I levels, (4) the ration of IGF-I/GH correlated best with balance measures and less with cognitive measures, pointing to the potentially prominent role IGF-I plays in the maintenance of neural function (see Abstract 5–23 by Sonntag et al. for a discussion of IGF-I and cerebral blood flow).

The importance of DHEAS continues to be explored with interesting results.

J.R. Shapiro, M.D.

Decreases in Cerebral Microvasculature With Age Are Associated With the Decline in Growth Hormone and Insulin-like Growth Factor 1

Sonntag WE, Lynch CD, Cooney PT, et al (Wake Forest Univ, Winston-Salem, NC)

Endocrinology 138:3515–3520, 1997 5–23

Introduction.—Age-related reduction of cerebral blood flow is thought to contribute to neurodegenerative changes in aging animals and humans. Vascular maintenance and remodeling are influenced by growth hormone (GH) and insulin-like growth factor 1 (IGF-1), which also decrease with age. This raises the possibility that declining GH and IGF-1 may cause rarefaction of the cerebral blood vessels, in association with reduced cerebral blood flow. This hypothesis was tested in a study of rats.

Methods.—Experiments were performed in Brown-Norway and Fisher 344/Brown-Norway male rats. Each animal had a chronic cranial window implanted to permit observation of the arterioles and venules of the cortical surface. Microvascular mapping was performed using a printout of a video photograph of the cortical microvasculature. Each arteriole was assessed for length, average diameter, and tortuosity. The number of vessels, normalized to cortical surface area, was assessed as well. At the same time vascular mapping was performed, blood samples were obtained for measurement of IGF-1. The vascular measures were also assessed in young and aged animals after 35 days of treatment with bovine GH, 0.35 μg/kg twice daily.

Results.—Comparison of young and aged rats clearly demonstrated age-related rarefaction of the cerebral vascular circulation. Compared with 5-month-old rats, cortical surface arterioles per cortical surface area decreased by 15% at 13 months of age and 40% by 29 months. A significant reduction in arteriole-to-arteriole anastomoses per area of cortical surface was noted as well. In aged rats, the ratio of arteriolar anastomoses to arterioles increased as a result of a greater loss of arteriolar anastomoses, compared with the number of arterioles. The number of venules per cortical surface area decreased as well, but not significantly. There were no age-related differences in average diameter, tortuosity, or

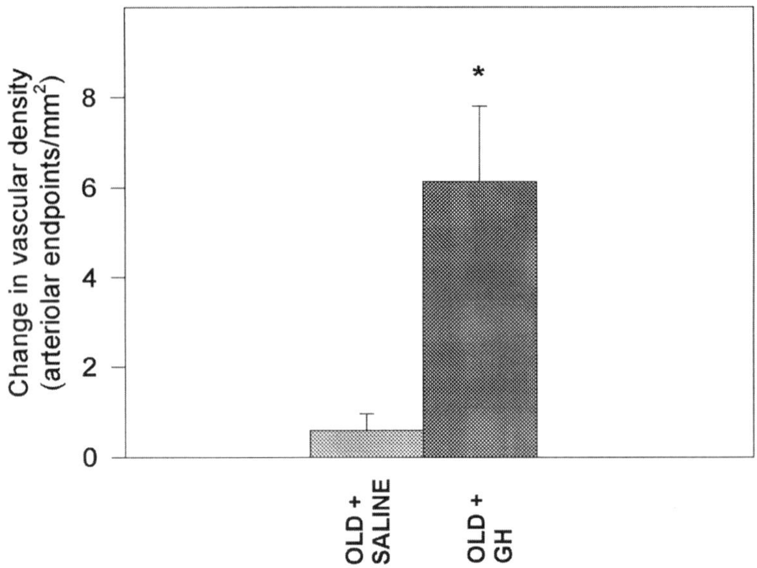

FIGURE 4.—Effects of bovine GH (25 μg/kg, twice daily) or vehicle administration for 35 days on changes in arteriolar density in 30-month-old F344/BN rats. Data are expressed as the percent increase in arteriolar density from baseline and represent the mean ± SEM of 10 (GH-treated) and 7 (saline-treated) animals/group. No vascular growth was observed in 8- (data not shown) or 30-month-old saline-treated animals. (Courtesy of Sonntag WE, Lynch CD, Cooney PT, et al: Decreases in cerebral microvasculature with age are associated with the decline in growth hormone and insulin-like growth factor 1. *Endocrinology* 138:3515–3520. Copyright 1997, the Endocrine Society.)

length of arterioles and venules. The 2 strains or rats showed similar reductions in arteriolar density.

Cortical arteriolar density was highly correlated with plasma IGF-1 levels. Treatment with bovine GH that increased IGF-1 levels was associated with a significant increase in arteriolar density among 30-month-old rats (Fig 4). Growth hormone treatment increased the number of arteriolar endpoints by 6.05/mm², whereas aged rats treated with saline showed minimal growth.

Conclusions.—As they age, rats show decreasing numbers of arterioles and arteriolar anastomotic connections per cortical surface area. Arteriolar number is significantly correlated with plasma IGF-1 level, and treatment with GH increases cortical vascular density in aged animals. The age-related decline in vascular density appears to result at least partly from age-related reductions in plasma GH and IGF-1. This study provides the first in vivo evidence linking reduced secretion of these hormones to the vascular deficiency of aging.

► Blood flow to the central nervous system is regulated mainly by the density of arterioles and arteriolar anastomoses. An alteration in arteriolar density with age could decrease cerebral blood flow and increase the risk of ischemic disease. This important study provides data relating: (1) the density of cerebral arterioles and arteriolar anastomoses, (2) growth hormone (GH) and insulin-like growth factor-1 (IGF-1) levels and their effects on the maintenance of the microvasculature, and (3) increasing age. Of considerable importance is the fact that growth hormone and IGF-1 also have a major role to play in the maintenance of neural integrity. IGF-1 binds throughout the brain with the greatest amount of binding in cortical gray matter. In tissue culture, IGF-1 is a potent inducer of astrocyte and oligodendrocyte development.[1]

IGF-1 has been administered to humans during treatment for a variety of disorders including amyotropic lateral sclerosis, diabetes type II, and osteoporosis. A problem recognized early in these trials was the expression of a number of side effects, including headaches and significant peripheral edema that limited its continued administration to many patients. Nevetheless, understanding the interaction between GH/IGF-I and cerebral arteriolar density may have significant implications for affecting cerebral function as well as the treatment of cerebral ischemic disease.

J.R. Shapiro, M.D.

Reference

1. McMorris FA, Smith TM, DeSalvo S, et al: Insulin-like growth factor-1/somatomedin C: A potent inducer of oligodendrocyte development. *Proc Nat Acad Sci USA* 83: 822–826, 1986.

Aging and Glucocorticoids: Effects on Cell Signaling Mediated Through Adenylyl Cyclase

Slotkin TA, Thai L, McCook EC, et al (Duke Univ, Durham, NC)
J Pharmacol Exp Ther 279:478–491, 1996 5–24

Background.—Increased glucocorticoids have been implicated in age-related loss of neural function. Aging also affects the transduction of neuronal signals by target cells, and damage to cell signaling capabilities may be of particular importance in aging. This experimental study addressed 3 issues in the role of cell signaling defects in the aged rat: the mechanisms underlying the loss of responsiveness to neurotransmitters in the aged brain, the effect on cell signaling of long-term administration of dexamethasone to young rats; and the effects of glucocorticoids on cell signaling in brain and peripheral tissues in old vs. younger animals.

Methods.—Six groups of Sprague-Dawley rats were studied in a 2 (age) × 3 (treatment) design. Each age group (9 weeks and 19 months) was infused with vehicle or 2 different regimens of dexamethasone (10 or 50 μg/kg/day) for 26 days. At the end of the infusion period the animals were decapitated and the temporal/occipital cortex, corpus striatum, heart, and 1 lobe of the liver dissected.

Results.—Compared with young rats, aged control rats showed significant deficits in total adenylyl cyclase activity in the brain and heart. The striatum and heart exhibited interference, with the response mediated either at the level of G-protein coupling to cyclase (striatum) or neurotransmitter receptor coupling to G-proteins (heart). Infusions of dexamethasone resulted in nearly equivalent plasma concentrations in young and aged rats and in similar dose-related losses of body weight. Although a higher dose of dexamethasone produced cushingoid effects in young rats, dexamethasone did not reproduce the effects of aging on any measures of adenylyl cyclase. In aged rats, however, dexamethasone altered G-protein coupling mechanisms in the cortex and in serotonergic-mediated cyclase responses in the striatum and decreased basal enzyme activity in the heart. In contrast to the effect seen in the heart, dexamethasone treatment led to a significant decline in both age groups in total enzymatic activity in the liver.

Conclusions.—Although results of these experiments do not indicate a specific role for glucocorticoids in the loss of cell function during aging, support is provided for the view that aging is associated with loss of activity and reactivity of adenylyl cyclase in the central nervous system and heart. The specific coupling of receptors to adenylyl cyclase by way of the G-proteins appears to be targeted by aging.

► One of the significant alterations in endocrine function in older people is an excessive response of the hypothalamic-adrenal-pituitary axis (HPA) to stress. This excessive response is reported to involve cortisol responsive regions of the hippocampus that normally exert an inhibitory effect on the HPA. Prolonged or repeated exposure to increased cortisol levels, either endogenous or exogenous, has been considered to contribute to hypertension, diabetes, and, at times, personality changes in older people. Hypercortisolism is also a feature of depression in older people, in whom dexamethasone supression of the HPA may be abnormal and in whom an increased cortisol level may match that of subjects with Cushing's disease. Under investigation is whether glucocorticoids contribute to neuronal degeneration in older people by directly altering second messenger activity in the brain or by indirectly altering cell-signaling mechanisms coupled to adenyl cyclase.

The results indicate that chronic dexamethasone administration did not directly affect adenyl cyclase activity in the brains of young animals. In older animals there were hormone-induced changes in G-protein coupling not found in the young. Thus, although the evidence does not support a direct role of glucocorticoids in the neuronal decay that occurs with age, it appears that in older animals, glucocorticoids do alter cell-signaling mechanisms in specific regions of the brain. This is worth considering in the evaluation of older people exposed to excessive glucocorticoid during treatment for such common conditions as polymyalgia rheumatica and chronic obstructive pulmonary disease.

J.R. Shapiro, M.D.

The Zona Reticularis Is the Site of Biosynthesis of Dehydroepiandrosterone and Dehydroepiandrosterone Sulfate in the Adult Human Adrenal Cortex Resulting From Its Low Expression of 3β-Hydroxysteroid Dehydrogenase

Endoh A, Kristiansen SB, Casson PR, et al (Baylor College of Medicine, Houston)

J Clin Endocrinol Metab 81:3558–3565, 1996 5–25

Purpose.—The zona reticularis of the adrenal cortex is commonly assumed to be the source of the steroids dehydroepiandrosterone (DHEA) and DHEA sulfate (DHEAS) in adult humans. However, few studies have directly addressed this issue. Compared with adult zonal cells, fetal zonal cells have low expression of 3β-hydroxysteroid dehydrogenase (3βHSD) and secrete large amounts of DHEA(S). Northern blotting and radioimmunoassay were used to compare the properties of adult and fetal zona reticularis cells.

Methods.—Experiments were performed using 9 adrenal glands from subjects of varying age. Zona fasciculata and zona reticularis cells were separated and cultured. Five days later, the serum was washed out of the medium by 24-hour incubation in defined, serum-free medium. This was followed by another 24 hours in serum-free medium, with the addition of cyclic adenosine monophosphate analogues and optional insulin. Experiments were performed to test the zonal separation of DHEA(S) and cortisol (F) biosynthesis in primary human adrenocortical cells.

Results.—Production of DHEA(S)/F production differed greatly between the separated fasciculata and reticularis cells from pregnenolone precursor. The results suggested that fasciculata cells produced only F and little or no DHEA(S), whereas reticularis and fetal zone cells produced mostly DHEA(S) but little or no F. The reticularis cells expressed a much lower level of type II 3βHSD, similar to that observed in fetal zone cells. For other genes, regulation by cyclic adenosine monophosphate and insulin was similar in the 2 adult zones and the fetal zone. In both types of cells, the response of messenger RNA levels for 17α-hydroxylase, cholesterol side-chain cleavage enzyme, 21-hydroxylase, and 11β-hydroxylase to cyclic adenosine monophosphate and insulin was similar to that observed in fasciculata cells. When 3βHSD in fasciculata cells was inhibited with trilostane, the cells increased their DHEA/F production ratio to a level even higher than that seen in fetal zone cells. This demonstrated the importance of limited 3βHSD expression in the DHEA(S)-synthesizing properties of reticularis cells.

Conclusions.—The age-related decrease in adrenal reticularis and fasciculata cells is not related to any change in gene expression. The more likely cause is an age-related reduction in the number of functional reticularis cells, unaccompanied by changes in the differentiated properties of the zonal cells.

► Dehydroepiandrosterone is an adrenal androgen whose concentration in vivo progressively falls with age. There has been tantalizing but not yet widely agreed upon data to suggest that DHEA replacement may improve some features of aging. The authors of this article give further evidence to show that the cells of the adrenal zona reticularis are the unique source for dehydroepiandrosterone production. Low in vivo expression of one enzyme, 3β-hydroxysteroid dehydrogenase, is responsible for the elevated DHEA/cortisol ratio in the zona reticularis. To account for the loss of DHEA production with age, the authors postulate a progressive loss in the number of DHEA-producing cells.

J. Roth, M.D.

Growth Hormone-induced Nuclear Translocation of Stat-3 Decreases With Age: Modulation by Caloric Restriction

Xu X, Sonntag WE (Wake Forest Univ, Winston-Salem, NC)

Am J Physiol 271:E903–E909, 1996 5–26

Background.—Previous studies have shown that growth hormone-induced phosphorylation of Janus-activated kinase (JAK-2) and growth hormone receptor (GHR) in liver decrease with age. Expression of insulin-like growth factor I (IGF-I) mRNA also decreases with age. These changes can be reversed by moderate restriction of calories. This study attempted to determine whether signal transducer and activator of transcription (Stat-3) and mitogen-activated protein (MAP) kinase are involved in GHR signal transduction, and whether either of these pathways are implicated in age-related deficiencies.

Methods and Results.—Liver tissues from B6D2 mice were analyzed to compare basal levels of JAK-2, Stat-3, and MAP kinase, as well as growth hormone-induced nuclear translocation of Stat-2 and MAP kinase. The goal was to determine how specific signaling pathways are affected by age and moderate caloric restriction. In animals fed ad libitum, age had no effect on basal JAK-2, Stat-3, or MAP kinase levels. However, JAK-2 levels were increased 3-fold in calorie-restricted animals. After treatment with growth hormone, nuclear translocation of Stat-3 was more than 3-fold greater in 7-month-old mice than in 36-month-old mice fed ad libitum. Mice with caloric restriction did not show an age-related reduction in Stat-3 activation. Mice of all ages fed ad libitum showed similar growth hormone-induced nuclear MAP kinase. This measure was slightly but not significantly increased in calorie-restricted mice.

Conclusions.—This study shows a specific decrease in growth hormone-induced Stat-3 activation in mice. This change may play a role in the age-related decline in GHR signal transduction and IGF-I gene expression. All of these changes are reversed by moderate caloric restriction, which leads to an enhanced tissue response to growth hormone and increased secretion of IGF-I.

► Recently, a great deal of attention has been paid to the decline in growth hormone levels associated with aging. Independently, there is an age-dependent decline in IGF-I levels. Both have been hypothesized to contribute to the decline in muscle mass and the increase in fat mass (as well as other deteriorations) associated with aging. Treatments with growth hormone or of IGF-I (or growth hormone–releasing hormone to stimulate growth hormone production) have been promising but fall short of the ideal in many ways. In this article, the authors show that a major intracellular pathway by which growth hormone activates its target cells is diminished with aging and that caloric restriction, a widely touted universal ameliorator of the effects of aging, also restores this pathway towards normal. JAK (pronounced "jack") and Stat (pronounced "stat") each represent a family of specific proteins that act in sequence to link activation of a cell surface receptor (for growth hormone, prolactin, and a myriad of cytokines) to intracellular events, such as activation of MAP kinase (pronounce "map"). These intriguing observations add new insights and raises new questions: is the diminution in growth hormone effects in vivo due to both a diminution in growth hormone and growth hormone-related hormones as well as a diminution in sensitivity to growth hormone? Can this diminution in sensitivity be overcome in an easy safe way?

J. Roth, M.D.

Essential Role of Growth Hormone in Ischemia-induced Retinal Neovascularization

Smith LEH, Kopchick JJ, Chen W, et al (Harvard Med School, Boston; Ohio Univ, Athens; Merck Research Labs, Rahway, NJ)

Science 276:1706–1709, 1997 5–27

Introduction.—The most frequent cause of blindness is retinal neovascularization, a condition present in diabetic retinopathy, retinopathy of prematurity, and age-related macular degeneration. Several lines of evidence suggest a role for growth hormone (GH) in diabetic retinopathy. By using transgenic mice expressing a GH antagonist gene and normal mice given an inhibitor of GH secretion (MK678), the role of GH in ischemia-associated retinal neovascularization was examined.

Methods and Results.—Neovascularization was induced in 2 transgenic mouse lines, the first (G119K) expressing a GH antagonist that results in a dwarf phenotype and the second (E117L) expressing a GH antagonist and exhibiting a giant phenotype. Compared with nontransgenic littermates, the GH antagonist mice exhibited a 34% decrease in neovascularization at postnatal day 17. Transgenic mice expressing the GH agonist E117L had no increase in retinal neovascularization relative to controls.

The G119K retinas showed no abnormal retinal or vascular development or toxicity when examined by light microscopy.

Nontransgenic mice treated with MK678, a long-acting somatostatin analogue that potently inhibits GH release, reduced retinal neovascularization up to 44% compared with untreated controls. The reduction was dose related. In both G119K transgenic and MK678–treated mice, there was an inverse correlation between extent of neovascularization and GH and insulin-like growth factor-1 (IGF-I) levels. Inhibition of retinal neovascularization was reversed with exogenous IGF-I administration. Neither hypoxia-stimulated retinal vascular endothelial growth factor (VEGF) or VEGF receptor expression was diminished by GH inhibition.

Conclusions.—In the early 1950s, a role for a pituitary-associated factor in diabetic retinopathy was hypothesized when a diabetic patient exhibited regression of retinal neovascularization after pituitary infarction. For a decade thereafter, pituitary ablation was used to treat many diabetic patients. Data from this experimental study suggest that some forms of retinopathy may be prevented by systemic inhibition of GH and/or IGF-I.

▶ This article is another example of the remarkable utility of transgenic animal models in the study of disease processes and potential therapies. Here, 2 mouse models, one expressing a GH antagonist and the other a GH agonist, were used to study the role of GH in ischemic retinal neovascularization. Neovascularization is a feature of several common disorders associated with blindness including diabetes and age-related macular degeneration. The positive relationship of neovascularization to GH and IGF-I levels was confirmed in the mice expressing the GH antagonist. The results suggest, as seen in several organ systems, that the GH effect is mediated through IGF-I. A somatostatin analogue, MK678, also blocked neovascularization, again pointing to a critical role for GH/IGF-I. Overexpression of GH or administration of IGF-I did not increase the incidence of neovascularization. However, neovascularization was only partly suppressed in the GH antagonist model, raising the possibility that other factors may be important in the retinal response to ischemia. Retinal vascular endothelial growth factor could be one factor, but these studies demonstrate its independence from the GH/IGF-I mediated neovascularization. Several other factors could be working in concert with GH/IGF-I including 2 groups of mitogenic peptides, the fibroblast growth factors (FGFs) and the transforming growth factors (TGFs), as well as locally produced TNF-α (tumor necrosis factors).[1, 2] In addition, the inhibition of cell membrane integrin receptors may also inhibit retinal angiogenesis.[3] Targeting local cytokine/growth factor production may prove of therapeutic value in the control of this major cause of blindness in the geriatric population.

J.R. Shapiro, M.D.

References

1. Agata N, Yamamoto C, Niyashiro M, et al: Expression of transforming growth factor beta mRNA in experimental choroidal neovascularization. *Curr Eye Res* 16:9–18, 1997.
2. Spranger J, Meyer Schwikerath R, Klein M, et al: TNF-α in the vitreous body: Increase in neovascular eye diseases and proliferative diabetic retinopathy. *Mediz Klin 90:134–137, 1995.*
3. Luna J, Tobe T, Mausa SA, et al: Antagonists of integrin alpha v beta 3 inhibit retinal neovascularization in a murine model. *Lab Invest* 75:563–573, 1996.

Suggested Reading

Wang Y, Perfetti R, Greig NH, et al: Glucagon-like peptide-1 can reverse the age-related decline in glucose tolerance in rats. *J Clin Invest* 99:2883–2889, 1997.

▶ In selecting this paper for review and introducing it, I should note that I was a major collaborator on the studies that form the foundation upon which this study rests, and that many of the authors are my colleagues. Previously, we (and another group) had shown that GLP-1, a hormone secreted by cells of the gastrointestinal tract in response to ingested glucose—which is important in enhancing glucose-stimulated insulin release acutely—can act chronically in a trophic fashion. Here, the authors demonstrate another aspect of this trophic effect on GLP-1 on islets, reversal of some of the reduced insulin secretion associated with aging in the rat. This study extends in vivo the group's observations in vitro with islets of older rats where GLP-1 corrected age-associated abnormalities of glucose-stimulated insulin release. That some of the effects on islets can be reversed effectively by a single agent is heartening and encourages other simple approaches to losses that occur with aging. These studies also point out that agents that act acutely may in other settings act as trophic agents: e.g., to maintain or restore advanced states of specialized function, promote differentiation, or recruit replacement cells.

J. Roth, M.D.

Hormone Replacement

Effects of Hormone-Replacement Therapy on Fibrinolysis in Postmenopausal Women

Koh KK, Mincemoyer R, Bui MN, et al (Natl Heart, Lung, and Blood Inst, Bethesda, Md; NIH, Bethesda, Md)

N Engl J Med 336:683–690, 1997 5–28

Objective.—Postmenopausal women taking equine-derived conjugated estrogens appear to have a lower risk of cardiovascular events than untreated women because the oral estrogen replacement produces a lipid profile similar to that of premenopausal women. Plasminogen-activator inhibitor type 1 (PAI-1), a fibrinolysis inhibitor known to increase the risk of atherosclerosis, is found at higher levels in postmenopausal women. In a randomized, crossover study, the effects on PAI-1 levels of estrogen alone and in combination with a progestin were examined in postmenopausal women.

Methods.—After a 2-month washout period, 30 postmenopausal women received daily either 0.625 mg of conjugated estrogen or the conjugated estrogen plus 2.5 mg of medroxyprogesterone acetate for 1 month. After a 1-month washout period, the groups were crossed over to the opposite regimen for 1 month. Fasting PAI-1 levels and serum D-dimer levels were determined before and after each treatment arm by "blinded" investigators. Data were compared statistically before and after each treatment.

Results.—There were no significant differences between baseline values in either treatment phase. Conjugated estrogens alone and in combination with a progestin significantly increased plasma levels of estrone, 17β-estradiol, and high-density lipoprotein (HDL) cholesterol. Plasma low-density lipoprotein (LDL) cholesterol and PAI-1 levels were significantly lowered. The extent of reduction in PAI-1 levels was significantly inversely related to pretreatment levels of PAI-1 in both treatment arms. Levels of PAI-1 were significantly inversely correlated with D-dimer levels. Conjugated estrogen was more effective than transdermal estrogen in lowering PAI-1 levels. Addition of progestin does not significantly alter the effects of conjugated estrogen.

Conclusions.—Conjugated estrogens alone and in combination with a progestin significantly lowered PAI-1 levels and probably account at least in part for the cardioprotective effects of hormone replacement therapy in postmenopausal women. Hormone replacement therapy had little effect on women with relatively low pretreatment levels of PAI-1.

▶ The issue of postmenopausal estrogen replacement remains clouded...both for patients and their physicians. The question of benefit vs. risk has not been decided, nor is there agreement on the appropriate age at which to start hormone replacement. Of considerable importance is the proposed extension of hormone replacement treatment to individuals in their late 70s and older. This may be of value in limiting osteoporotic bone loss even in the elderly and may lessen the risk of heart disease. Several studies have shown a relationship between coronary artery disease and plasma fibrinolytic activity.[1, 2] This report confirms the role of estrogen in 1 mechanism by which hormone replacement may lessen the risk of cardiovascular disease: a decrease in the inhibitor of a ubiquitous fibrinolytic enzyme, PAI-1. There are several messages to be gleaned from the study. First, that conjugated estrogen is more effective in lowering PAI-1 than is transdermal estradiol. Second, that adding progestin (2.5 mg) to conjugated estrogen does not alter (i.e., lessen) the effects of conjugated estrogen. Third, transdermal estradiol, with or without added progestin, does not change lipoprotein or PAI-1 levels.

Estrogen agonists with site-specific activity are now in clinical trials. A current study involves 1 agent (raloxifene, Lilly) that has trophic effects on bone and not on other tissues. This prototype could perhaps be applied to the development of agents that exert beneficial effects on the clotting/fibrinolytic system and lipoprotein system (without involving other organ systems) in those women with elevated PAI-1 levels.

J.R. Shapiro, M.D.

References

1. Olofsson BO, Dahlen G, Nilsson TK: Evidence for increased levels of plasminogen activator inhibitor and tissue plasminogen activator in plasma of patients with angiographically verified coronary artery disease. *Eur Heart J* 10:77–82, 1989.
2. Ridker PM, Vaughan DE, Stampfer MJ, et al: Endogenous tissue-type plasminogen activator and risk of myocardial infarction. *Lancet* 342:1165–1168, 1993.

Estrogen Inhibits the Vascular Injury Response in Estrogen Receptor α-Deficient Mice

Iafrati MD, Karas RH, Aronovitz M, et al (Tupper Research Inst, Boston; Univ of Missouri, Columbia; Natl Inst of Environmental Health Sciences, Research Triangle Park, NC)
Nature Med 3:545–548, 1997 5–29

Background.—The authors have demonstrated that physiologic levels of estrogen can suppress the carotid response to injury in ovariectomized mice. The investigators have developed estrogen receptor-α knockout (ERKO) mice, which lack functional ERα. Although they have abnormal reproductive function, the ERKO mice are otherwise normal and have no apparent cardiovascular abnormalities. The role of ER-α in mediating estrogen's effects on the vascular injury response was studied using ERKO mice.

Methods and Findings.—Normocholesterolemic, ovariectomized female mice, including ERKO mice and their wild-type littermates, were studied. They were randomized to receive either estrogen replacement with 17β-estradiol or subcutaneous vehicle alone. In response to endothelial denudation injury in the carotid artery, both types of mice showed a significant increase in medial area. Surprisingly, estrogen replacement inhibited this response to a similar extent in both wild-type and ERKO mice. Suppression of the carotid artery injury response by estrogen was also demonstrated by other methods of assessing vascular injury, including immunostaining and measurement of medial vascular smooth muscle proliferation.

Conclusions.—The findings to date suggest that the vasoprotective effects of estrogen are mediated by a novel estrogen signaling pathway, independent of ERα. This mechanism appears to be involved in estrogen-induced inhibition of vascular smooth muscle cell growth, protection against atherosclerosis and vascular injury, and regulation of gene expression in vascular cells. The novel mechanism could involve the newly discovered ERβ, which is expressed in the vasculature of ERKO mice. Further study is needed to test this hypothesis.

► This is a very interesting and important article that dissects, through the use of gene knockout mice, certain of the recognized functions of 2 different ERs, the α and β receptors, and helps explain different sensitivities of various tissues to estrogen and estrogen antagonists.[1] The novel β receptor was recently discovered in prostate, uterus, ovary, and bladder tissue.[2] Although ERα and ERβ share similarities in terms of substrate and antagonist binding affinities, there exist differences in gene transcriptional activities and the tissue localization of the 2. The development of an ERKO mouse (i.e., one with a disrupted gene) permitted an evaluation of the role of ERα, here, examined by virtue of its role in regulating the beneficial effects of estrogen on damaged vascular tissues. The vascular protective effects of 17β-estradiol were present in both the wild-type and knockout mice. Thus, it appears that the vascular protective effects of estradiol must be mediated through ERβ rather than through the classic ERα. Although the vascular effects of estrogen may be independent of both receptors, a more reasonable hypothesis is that either the vascular protective actions are specific for the β-receptor, or the α- and β-receptors interact in some manner to exert this action on arterial tissues.[3] Also, the relative tissue abundance of the 2 receptors remains undefined. Note the emerging development of tissue-specific estrogen *agonist* compounds, some of which are being used in clinical trials for the treatment of osteoporosis, i.e., these provide an estrogen effect on bone but not on other tissues such as those from the breast and the uterus.

J.R. Shapiro, M.D.

References

1. Katzenellenbogen BS, Montano MM, Le Goff P, et al: Antiestrogens: Mechanisms and actions in target cells. *J Steroid Biochem Mol Biol* 53:1–6, 387–393, 1995.
2. Kilper GGM Jr, Carlsson B, Grandien K, et al: Comparison of the ligand binding specificity and transcript tissue distribution of estrogen receptor α and β *Endocrinology* 138:863–870, 1997.
3. Gustafsson JA: Estrogen receptor β: Getting in on the action. *Nature Med* 3:493–494, 1997.

Comparison of Dietary Calcium With Supplemental Calcium and Other Nutrients as Factors Affecting the Risk for Kidney Stones in Women

Curhan GC, Willett WC, Speizer FE, et al (Brigham and Women's Hosp, Boston; Harvard Med School, Boston; Massachusetts Gen Hosp, Boston)
Ann Intern Med 126:497–504, 1997 5–30

Background.—Calcium intake is thought to play an important role in kidney stone formation. However, little is known about the risk factors for stone formation in women. The association of dietary and supplemental calcium intake and the risk for kidney stones in women was studied.

Methods.—A prospective cohort study included 91,731 female participants in the Nurses' Health Study I, with a 12-year follow-up. The women were between the ages of 34 and 59 at study enrollment in 1980, with no history of kidney stones. Self-administered food-frequency questionnaires were completed in 1980, 1984, 1986, and 1990.

Findings.—Eight hundred sixty-four cases of kidney stones occurred during 903,849 person-years of follow-up. After potential risk factors were controlled, dietary calcium intake was found to be inversely associated with the risk for kidney stones, and supplemental calcium intake was associated positively with risk. Women in the highest quintile of dietary calcium intake had a 0.65 relative risk for stone formation compared with women in the lowest quintile. Women taking supplemental calcium had a relative risk of 1.2 compared with women who did not. Sixty-seven percent of the women taking supplemental calcium either did not take it with a meal or took it with meals with an oxalate content that was probably low. In addition, compared with women in the lowest quintile, women in the highest quintile of sucrose intake had a relative risk of 1.52; of fluid intake, 0.61; and of potassium intake, 0.65.

Conclusions.—High dietary calcium intake apparently reduces the risk for symptomatic kidney stones in women. Taking supplemental calcium may increase this risk. This apparent difference may be associated with the timing of calcium ingestion relative to the amount of oxalate consumed. However, other factors in dairy products, the main source of dietary calcium, could be responsible for the reduction in risk associated with dietary calcium.

► This article is of note because it addresses one of the poorly researched questions related to the effects of dietary calcium supplements in women (and men) with osteoporosis. Not only are women who have had menopause advised to increase their calcium intake to 1,500 mg/day, but the same recommendation also was made by an NIH Consensus Conference in 1994 for men older than 65 years.[1] At issue is whether increasing calcium supplements can increase the incidence of kidney stones.

These authors have reported that in men, supplemental calcium *decreases* kidney stone formation.[2] The mechanism is related to calcium decreasing oxalate excretion, particularly when taken with food. This study suggests a difference between dietary and supplemental calcium on stone formation in women.

Increased dietary calcium was associated with a *decrease* in stone risk. Increased supplemental calcium was associated with an increased relative risk (1.26) up to an extra 100 mg/day, but *no increase* in risk was observed with intakes higher than 100 mg/day. Of note is that increased sucrose and increased sodium, which increase calcium clearance, were associated with an increase in relative risk. The authors comment that increased phosphorus intake in dairy foods may have a protective effect for stone formation.

The real issue may be when the supplemental calcium is consumed. Taking calcium with meals both decreases oxalate absorption and facilitates calcium absorption from the upper small intestine. When not taken at mealtimes, the supplemental calcium will not decrease oxalate absorption and may only provide a burst of absorbed calcium that is excreted.

The lack of a dose response is unsettling and raises the question of the role of other factors not revealed in the questionnaires. Finally, it has been taught that increased diet protein increases calcium loss and potentially, kidney stones. This seems not to be the case. The pros and cons of this subject are discussed in an accompanying editorial.[3]

J.R. Shapiro, M.D.

References

1. Anonymous: NIH Consensus conference. Optimal calcium intake. NIH Consensus Development Panel on Optimal Calcium Intake (see comments). *JAMA* 272:1942–1948, 1994.
2. Curhan GC, Willett WC, Rimm EB, et al: A prospective study of dietary calcium and other nutrients and the risk of symptomatic kidney stones. *N Engl J Med* 328:833–838, 1993.
3. Coe FL, Parks JH, Favus MJ: Diet and calcium: The end of an era? (editorial) *Ann Intern Med* 126:553–555, 1997.

►With each new advance in pharmacologic treatment, there is always some concern about possible adverse effects associated with the therapy. Such is the case with calcium, which has emerged as an important component of osteoporosis prevention and treatment. In the short run, the major problems with calcium have been dyspepsia and constipation. However, in the long run, renal stones are also a concern. In this analysis, the investigators found that those who had the highest dietary intake of calcium had the lowest risk for symptomatic kidney stones. In contrast, those who took calcium supplements had slightly increased risk. These data support the hypothesis that the greater consumption of dairy products decreases the risk of symptomatic kidney stones, perhaps by its effect on oxalate absorption. The authors also suggest that the problem with supplements may be related to the timing of the supplemental calcium and might be reduced if it is taken with meals. The take-home message is that the safest method of providing sufficient calcium intake is through the adequate ingestion of dairy products.

D.B. Reuben, M.D.

Intermittent Etidronate Therapy to Prevent Corticosteroid-induced Osteoporosis

Adachi JD, Bensen WG, Brown J, et al (McMaster Univ, Hamilton, Ont; Centre Hospitalier de l'Université Laval, Ste-Foy, Quebec; Univ of Calgary, Alta; et al)

N Engl J Med 337:382–387, 1997 5–31

Background.—Corticosteroid treatment commonly causes osteoporosis, suggesting the need for preventive therapy for patients who will be taking corticosteroids for more than a few weeks. There is some evidence that intermittent cyclic therapy with etidronate can prevent corticosteroid-induced osteoporosis. The ability of etidronate to prevent corticosteroid-induced osteoporosis was assessed in a randomized, controlled trial.

Methods.—The study included 141 adult patients who had started high-dose corticosteroid therapy. All were expected to receive at least 1 year of treatment with prednisone or its equivalent, with a mean daily dose of 7.5 mg for 90 days followed by a mean daily dose of 2.5 mg or greater. They were randomized to receive cycles of intermittent etidronate, 400 mg/day for 14 days, or placebo. Both treatments were followed by 76 days of treatment with calcium carbonate, 500 mg. Over a 1-year treatment

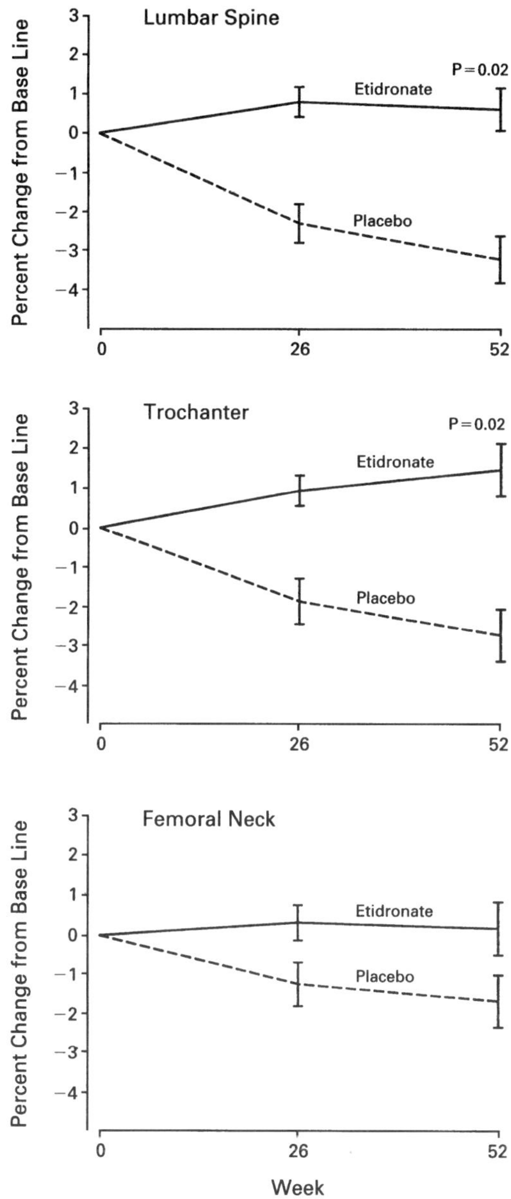

FIGURE 1.—Mean (±SE) change in the bone density of the lumbar spine (top panel), trochanter (middle panel), and femoral neck (bottom panel) between base line (week 0) and weeks 36 and 52 in the etidronate and placebo groups. The P values indicate significant differences between treatment groups. (Reprinted by permission of *The New England Journal of Medicine* from Adachi JD, Bensen WG, Brown J, et al: Intermittent etidronate therapy to prevent corticosteroid-induced osteoporosis. *N Engl J Med* 337:382–387. Copyright 1997, Massachusetts Medical Society. All rights reserved.)

period, the cycle was repeated 3 times. The main outcome measure at 1 year was the mean percent change in lumbar spine bone density. Bone density was measured in other sites as well, and the incidence of vertebral fractures was compared.

Results.—One hundred seventeen patients completed the study. The 2 groups had comparable mean daily corticosteroid doses throughout the study: 14 mg/day in the placebo group and 13 mg/day in the etidronate group at 26 weeks, and 11 mg/day in both groups at 52 weeks. Cumulative corticosteroid dose was 4,119 mg and 3,911 mg, respectively. One-way analysis of variance showed no significant difference in lumbar spine and trochanter density in the etidronate group but a significant decline in the placebo group (Fig 1). The difference in mean percentage change from baseline was 3.72% in the lumbar spine, 4.14% in the trochanter, and 1.88% in the femoral neck. Etidronate was associated with a smaller decrease in lumbar spine density for men, premenopausal women, and postmenopausal women; mean differences between groups were 2.50%, 4.47%, and 4.56%, respectively. A response to treatment—i.e., slope of the bone density of the spine greater than zero, as determined by linear regression analysis—was present in 59% of the etidronate group vs. 23% of the placebo group.

Vertebral fractures occurred in 15% of the placebo group versus 9% of the etidronate group, for a relative risk of 0.6. For postmenopausal women, etidronate treatment reduced the proportion of vertebral fractures by 85%. At 26 weeks, serum bone-specific alkaline phosphatase was reduced by 18% in the etidronate group. By 52 weeks, this marker of bone turnover was no different between groups.

Conclusions.—Intermittent etidronate therapy prevents bone loss and vertebral fractures in patients receiving long-term corticosteroid therapy. For postmenopausal women receiving corticosteroids, etidronate reduces risk of new vertebral fractures by 40%. Etidronate is generally well tolerated.

► Corticosteroids have marked effects on bone metabolism leading to osteoporosis and an increased risk of fracture. The threshold is at approximately the dose equivalent of 7.5–10 mg of prednisone daily. Glucocorticoids significantly impair every step in bone formation including decreasing calcium absorption and increasing renal calcium loss, to blocking the effect of multiple growth factors (IGF-I, IGF-I binding proteins, TGF-) on osteoblastic bone formation.[1] Osteoclastic resorptive activity is increased. Bisphosphonates counter the effect of glucocorticoids by decreasing osteoclastic bone resorption.

Etidronate, widely used in the therapy of postmenopausal osteoporosis, is a "first generation" bisphosphonate. Although previous studies have demonstrated the effectiveness of bisphosphonates in lessening glucocorticoid-related bone loss, this paper reports a randomized, double-blind, placebo-controlled, multicenter trial.[2] As such, it establishes a baseline against which the use of more potent third-generation bisphosphonates can be assessed.

Of interest is the observation that bone density of the lumbar spine and trochanter did not change significantly in the etidronate group, but it decreased in the placebo group. Nevertheless, the vertebral fracture rate declined 85% in the etidronate-treated women. As noted in the paper by Dawson Hughes and reviewed here (Abstract 1–26), there exists a disparity between the modest effects of treatment on bone density vs. the prominent effect in diminishing fracture rate.

Unlike several earlier studies, a vitamin D compound was not provided along with the bisphosphonate: the subjects received an additional 500 mg of calcium carbonate during the period when the etidronate was not consumed. Usually, the addition of vitamin D is advisable because of the negative glucocorticoid action on calcium absorption. Also, we advise that daily calcium intake be adjusted to a minimum of 1200 mg daily.

Not addressed is the question of when bisphosphonates should be started in glucocorticoid-treated patients. Bone density should be assessed at the start of treatment and during treatment so that the glucocorticoid effect is minimized before bone loss becomes a significant factor.

J.R. Shapiro, M.D.

References

1. Canalis E: Clinical review 83: Mechanisms of glucocorticoid action in bone—Implications to glucocorticoid-induced osteoporosis. *J Clin Endocrinol Metab* 81:3441–3447, 1996.
2. Diamond T, McGuigan L, Barbagallo S, et al: Cyclical etidronate plus ergocalciferol prevents glucocorticoid-induced bone loss in postmenopausal women. *Am J Med* 98:459–463, 1995.

Testosterone Replacement in Older Hypogonadal Men: A 12-month Randomized Controlled Trial

Sih R, Morley JE, Kaiser FE, et al (St Louis Univ; St Louis VA Med Ctr)

J Clin Endocrinol Metab 82:1661–1667, 1997 5–32

Background.—Older men typically experience declining levels of testosterone. Replacement therapy in older hypogonadal men may attenuate the age-related changes associated with declining testosterone levels. Whether testosterone replacement therapy increased upper extremity strength and what side effects would occur after 1 year of therapy were investigated.

Methods.—All subjects were 50 or older and were healthy. In the test group, 15 men received 200 mg of IM testosterone cypionate every 14–17 days for 1 year. In the control group, 17 men received IM saline according to the same schedule. Tests at baseline included a memory test, a depression scale, measurements of grip strength, body fat levels, laboratory tests, and a physical examination.

Findings.—Grip strength increased significantly in the group receiving testosterone. Hemoglobin levels were also significantly higher in the treat-

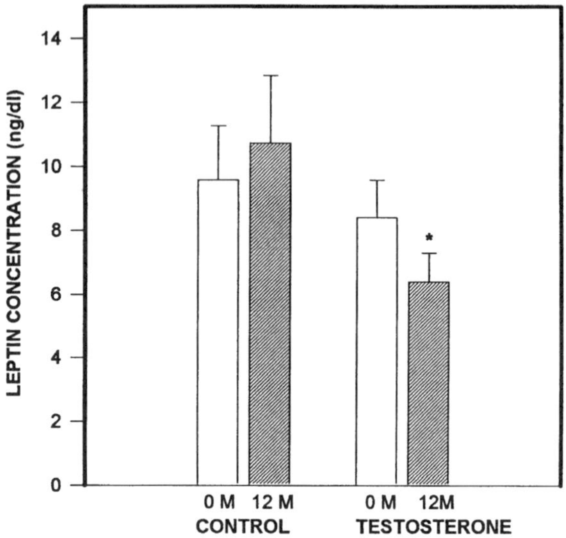

FIGURE 2.—Effects of testosterone administration on leptin concentrations at baseline (*OM*) and 12 months (*12M*) in control and testosterone-treated groups. $*P < 0.02$ for differences from baseline (δ) as determined by Student's *t* test. (Courtesy of Sih R, Morley JE, Kaiser FE, et al: Testosterone replacement in older hypogonadal men: A 12-month randomized controlled trial. *J Clin Endocrinol Metab* 82[6]:1661–1667, 1997. Copyright the Endocrine Society.)

ment group; 4 test subjects had elevations in hematocrit greater than 52%. Significantly lower leptin levels were found in the testosterone group (Fig 2), and leptin levels correlated significantly with body mass index, body fat, and triglyceride levels. Prostate-specific antigen levels and cognitive test results did not differ between the 2 groups. On chemistry panels, the only significant decreases with testosterone were for luteinizing hormone and 1,25–dihydroxyvitamin D levels.

Conclusions.—Testosterone replacement therapy improves grip strength and hemoglobin concentrations in hypogonadal older men. Leptin concentrations decreased, which may indicate a mechanism whereby steroid hormones affect body fat. These beneficial changes occurred with no changes in prostate-specific antigen levels or cognition. The decreased levels of 1,25–dihydroxyvitamin D levels in the testosterone group may have been an aberrant finding because it is not consistent with other studies in the literature.

► This article provides additional information pointing to a beneficial effect of testosterone replacement in older hypogonadal men. The diagnosis of hypogonadism was based on a bioavailable testosterone (BT) (non-sex hormone binding globulin-bound) level of less than 60 ng/dL (normal = 7z–250 ng/dL). Although subject to individual variability, half of healthy men between ages 50 and 70 will have a BT level below the lowest level seen in men ages 20–40.[1]

J.R. Shapiro, M.D.

Reference

1. Korenman SG, Morley JE, Mooradian AD, et al: Secondary hypogonadism in older men. *J Clin Endo Metab* 71:963–969, 1990.

Developmental Biology

Osf2/Cbfa1: A Transcriptional Activator of Osteoblast Differentiation

Ducy P, Zhang R, Geoffroy V, et al (M.D. Anderson Cancer Ctr, Houston; Univ of Texas, Houston)
Cell 89:747–754, 1997 5–33

Introduction.—There are no data on the molecular mechanism of osteoblast-specific gene expression and differentiation. The presence of an osteoblast-specific *cis*-acting element, designated OSE2, in the *Osteocalcin* promoter was previously reported. The cDNA encoding Osf2/Cbfa1, the protein that binds to OSE2, has now been cloned.

Methods and Findings.—Osf2/Cbfa1 was identified by Northern blot analysis using poly(A)$^+$ RNA from mouse thymus and spleen and from primary osteoblasts. In adult mice, Osf2/Cbfa1 transcripts were detected only in bone and osteoblasts, not in other tissues. When C3H10T1/2 fibroblasts were treated with BMP7, which induces osteoblast differentiation, Osf2/Cbfa1 expression occurred before expression of any osteoblast-specific gene. In primary mouse osteoblasts, Osf2/Cbfa1 expression was abolished by treatment with 1,25$(OH)_2D_3$. Analysis of DNA-binding ability identified a core sequence in which mutations affected His-Osf2/Cbfa1 binding to DNA. A 2-bp mutation in OSE2 abolished binding of His-Osf2/Cbfa1. In mouse embryos, peak expression of Osf2/Cbfa1 occurred 2 days before the first ossification centers appeared. Study of the ossification centers showed high levels of Osf2/Cbfa1 expression before the bones had become mineralized. Expression was restricted to the cells of the mesenchymal condensations and of the osteoblast lineage. Studies of the effects of Osf2/Cbfa1 on expression of genes expressed in osteoblasts suggested that Osf2/Cbfa1 could induce osteoblast differentiation of nonosteoblastic cells. This was confirmed by studies in calvarial cells committed to the osteoblast lineage and in mouse skin fibroblasts.

Conclusions.—Osf2/Cbfa1 is an osteoblast-specific transcription factor and a regulator of osteoblast differentiation. It plays an essential function during bone development in vivo. Its contribution to osteoblast differentiation, compared with that of other factors, will be clarified when the cDNAs for those factors become available.

► This report, one of 4 papers published in this issue of the journal *Cell*, describes one of the major biological findings of the year related to the role of osteoblast function in skeletal disorders (see references) . The identification of the transcription factor Cbfa 1 as the "master gene for bone growth" promises to provide crucial insight into the pathogenesis and treatment of osteoporosis and other skeletal disorders.[1] As reported by Komori and colleagues, targeted disruption of the Cfba 1 gene results in a complete lack of bone formation because of maturational arrest of osteoblasts.[2] The mutation induced a complete lack of ossification in mice, who died shortly after birth without breathing. Two related papers describe mutations in Cbfa 1 as causative in cleidocranial dysplasia, which involves defective endochrondral and membranous bone formation.[3, 4]

Several experiments point to the central role this transcription factor plays in osteoblast differentiation. In situ hybridization showed that Cbfa 1 expression occurs early in skeletal development and is restricted to cells of the osteoblast lineage. Remarkable is the ability of Cbfa 1 when transfected into several nonosteoblastic cell strains to induce production of osteoblast-specific proteins such as osteocalcin. In pluripotential fibroblasts, Cbfa 1 induced expression of bone sialoprotein, collagen type I, and osteocalcin genes.

The report by the Komori group demonstrates that homozygous transgenic mice generated with a mutation in Cbfa 1 have no skeletal ossification, i.e., membranous and endochrondral ossification was blocked. Heterozygous expression of this mutation as reported by Otto et al. and Mundlos et al. is associated with cleidocranial dysplasia, a syndrome of hypoplasia of clavicles, patent fontanelles, short stature, and dysplastic pubic bones.

Together, these papers present a remarkable story, critical for understanding osteoblast development, but also significant for the development of therapies to promote bone formation in the elderly.

J.R. Shapiro, M.D.

References

1. Dickman S: No bones about a genetic switch for bone growth. *Science* 276:1502, 1997.
2. Komori T, Yagi H, Nomura S, et al: Targeted disruption of CBFA 1 results in a complete lack of bone formation owing to maturational arrest of osteoblasts. *Cell* 89:755–764, 1997.
3. Mundlos S, Otto F, Mundlos C, et al: Mutations involving the transcription factor CBFA 1 cause cleidocranial dysplasia. *Cell* 89:773–779, 1997.
4. Otto F, Thornell AP, Crompton T, et al: Cbfa 1 a candidate gene for cleidocranial dysplasia syndrome is essential for osteoblast differentiation and bone development. *Cell* 89:765–771, 1997.

Central Nervous System and Its Disorders

Preserved Neuron Number in the Hippocampus of Aged Rats With Spatial Learning Deficits

Rapp PR, Gallagher M (Univ at Stony Brook, NY; Univ of North Carolina, Chapel Hill)

Proc Natl Acad Sci USA 93:9926–9930, 1996 5–34

Objective.—Hippocampal neuron loss is part of the normal aging process and is thought to be responsible for problems with hippocampal-based learning and memory in aging. Using stereologic sampling techniques, hippocampal neuron loss in the CA3 and CA1 pyramidal cell fields of aged rats with severe spatial learning impairments was quantified.

Methods.—Hippocampal learning was evaluated in young and old male Long-Evans rats with the Morris water maze. The total number of neurons in each principal cell layer of the hippocampus was estimated by the optical fractionator method.

Results.—The aged rats demonstrated significantly impaired spatial searching behavior, although there was substantial variability among individuals. There were no differences between groups with regard to nonspatial learning. The packing density of pyramidal cells was similar in the brains of young, age-impaired, and age-unimpaired rats. Neuron number was not related to age, cognitive status, or spatial learning ability.

Conclusion.—Hippocampal neuron loss is not a function of aging in rats. Other neurobiologic processes are responsible for functional learning deficits that result from hippocampal aging.

► Loss of neurons in the hippocampus has long been thought to be typical of normal aging and that these losses in neurons are associated with deficits in cognition. In this article, the authors used substantially improved methods to show that there is no loss of neurons in the hippocampus in the regions that have been specifically thought to be responsible. They found no correlation to account for age-dependent learning defects. Back to square one!

J. Roth, M.D.

Is Metabolic Evidence for Vitamin B-12 and Folate Deficiency More Frequent in Elderly Patients With Alzheimer's Disease?

Joosten E, Lesaffre E, Riezler R, et al (Univ Hosp K.U. Leuven, Belgium; Severi Med, Münster, Germany)

J Gerontol 52A:M76–M79, 1997 5–35

Background.—An association between vitamin B_{12} deficiency and mental impairment has been reported in older people. Measurement of serum methylmalonic acid (MMA) and total homocysteine (tHcy) levels are useful for the interpretation of serum vitamin B_{12} and folate levels. A prospective study was conducted to compare the vitamin B_{12} and folate status of older hospitalized Alzheimer's disease (AD) patients, older nondemented inpatients, and healthy older community dwellers.

Methods.—The study group included 52 AD patients, 50 nondemented older inpatient controls matched for age and sex, and 49 healthy older people living independently in the community. The patients were evaluated by means of radiography, serum folate and vitamin B_{12} concentrations, MMA, tHcy and routine laboratory tests.

Results.—Serum vitamin B_{12} and folate levels were not significantly different among the 3 groups. The AD patients had the highest serum tHcy levels. Both AD patients and hospitalized controls had significantly higher MMA levels than community dwellers.

Conclusions.—In this comparison of older AD patients, older nondemented inpatients, and older community dwellers, no significant differences were found in serum B_{12} and folate levels. Both AD and nondemented older inpatients had higher MMA levels than older community dwellers. Total Hcy levels were significantly higher in AD patients than in the other 2 groups. These results indicate that the interpretation of vitamin B_{12} and folate status in older patients depends on methodology and control group, as well as other factors. The possible association between impaired tHcy metabolism and AD merits further investigation.

▶ Deficiencies of vitamin B_{12} and folate have been considered in a wide range of disorders, especially those of old age. Although susceptibility to severe cardiovascular disorders has dominated recently, neuropsychiatric disorders have also been given much attention over the years. In the early years of this century, vitamin deficiencies were usually defined in terms of dietary intake necessary to prevent extreme clinical forms of the vitamin-deficiency diseases. As methods for measuring the levels of vitamins in body fluids improved in sensitivity and specificity, vitamin deficiencies were defined in those terms. As we have come to understand in detail the biochemical and cellular pathways that require these vitamins, scientists have worked to devise more direct measures of whether the body has adequate amounts of these micronutrients in appropriately activated forms at the biochemical sites of action. In this study, the authors show that the levels of vitamin B_{12} and folate in blood are similar in patients with Alzheimer's disease and in two sets of control subjects but that the serum levels of methylmalonic acid and homocysteine are increased. These two metabolites accumulate under conditions of vitamin B_{12} and folate deficiency; the authors speculate that the increases in metabolite levels may be caused by deficiencies. Although these tests are more sensitive, the authors also make it clear that other conditions unrelated to vitamin deficiency can cause increases in metabolite concentrations. The proof will come with the demonstration that the abnormal levels of metabolites are restored to normal levels by the addition of vitamin supplements and, even more impressively, if the clinical symptoms attributed to them can be ameliorated substantially.

J. Roth, M.D.

Monoclonal Antibodies to a 100-kd Protein Reveal Abundant Aβ-Negative Plaques Throughout Gray Matter of Alzheimer's Disease Brains

Schmidt ML, Lee VM-Y, Forman M, et al (Univ of Pennsylvania, Philadelphia)

Am J Pathol 151:69–80, 1997 5–36

Background.—Recent findings in the study of Alzheimer's disease (AD)—including the presence of cortical Lewy bodies and "diffuse" β-amyloid (Aβ) deposits in the brains of AD patients—underscore the need for clarification of the molecular and cellular neuropathology of AD. In studies using monoclonal antibodies to immunogens isolated from AD brains, the authors have identified a 100 kd protein and numerous plaquelike lesions, distinct from all Aβ deposits. The initial characterization of the 100 kd protein and the new plaquelike lesions are reported.

Methods.—Four of 59 antibodies studied recognized the 100 kd protein. The antibodies did not recognize hyperphosphorlyated tau in Western blots, nor neurofibrillary lesions by immunohistochemistry. One of the antibodies, designated AMY117, was used in a detailed study of the plaquelike lesions.

Results.—The plaquelike lesions were positive for AMY117 but did not appear on amyloid stains and were not colocalized with Aβ deposits. Lesions positive for AMY117 and Aβ did commonly appear in the same cortical and subcortical gray matter regions, however. Of 32 patients with sporadic AD and 6 elderly people with Down's syndrome, all showed abundant AMY117-positive plaques. These plaques also occurred in the brains of patients without dementia but with numerous Aβ deposits. However, other elderly controls or patients with other neurodegenerative or neuropsychiatric disorders showed few or no AMY117-positive plaques.

Conclusions.—The newly described AMY117-positive plaques appear to be major lesions of the brain in Alzheimer's disease. Their widespread occurrence suggests that they may play a key function in the onset or progression of AD. Future research will lend insight into the etiologic and pathogenetic roles of the 100 kd protein and the AMY117-positive plaques.

► Neurodegenerative disorders of old age are characterized by abnormal deposits of protein including amyloid (Aβ peptide) in the extracellular plaques and hyperphosphorylated tau in the intracellular tangles of patients with Alzheimer's disease. (Recent studies indicate that Huntington's disease is associated with intranuclear deposits of a characteristic protein linked to ubiquitin and that Parkinson's disease, at least in one of its rare familial forms, is associated with deposits of synuclein, another neuron-related protein.) In this article, the authors show that monoclonal antibodies derived by immunization with extracts of brain from patients with Alzheimer's disease recognize plaque-like structures that are distinct from the amyloid plaques previously described in Alzheimer's disease. They are present in all patients with Alzheimer's disease, raising the possibility that these deposits may play an important role in the pathogenesis of the disease. How these deposits are formed and how they relate to the pathological process are quite unknown; it is still not known how the other proteinaceous deposits (even those that are well characterized) relate to the neurodegeneration. This exciting finding heightens the mystery associated with the pathological degeneration of neurons in Alzheimer's disease. The knowledge that other proteins (apo E, synuclein, and possibly an anti-chymotrypsin) are often associated with the amyloid protein in the typical plaques, and that there are other plaque-like structures with other proteins, deepens the mystery.

J. Roth, M.D.

Mutation in the α-Synuclein Gene Identified in Families With Parkinson's Disease

Polymeropoulos MH, Lavedan C, Leroy E, et al (NIH, Bethesda, Md; Univ of Medicine and Dentistry of New Jersey, Piscataway; Seconda Università degli Studi di Napoli, Italy; et al)

Science 276:2045–2047, 1997 5–37

Background.—In some cases, heritable factors may predispose a person to develop Parkinson's disease. These researchers have previously shown cosegregation of gene markers on chromosome 4q21–q23 with the Parkinson's disease phenotype in a large Italian kindred. These gene markers map to the same region as α-synuclein, a presynaptic nerve terminal protein believed to influence neural plasticity. This study investigated the molecular association of α-synuclein with the Parkinson's disease phenotype in the same Italian kindred and in a group of unrelated Greek families.

Methods.—Genotype analysis in the Italian kindred revealed that the α-synuclein gene completely segregated with the Parkinson's disease phenotype, with one mutation in α-synuclein at position 209 from G to A. Comparison with a selection of 314 chromosomes from other people indicated that none of them carried this G209A mutation. Once cosegregation was thus confirmed in the Italian kindred, Greek patients with the Parkinson's disease phenotype were identified and examined for this G209A mutation.

Findings.—The G209A mutation was found in three of the Greek kindreds. As in the original Italian kindred, this mutation cosegregated with the Parkinson's disease phenotype. The α-synuclein mutation was found in all 4 families with the Parkinson's disease phenotype, but not in any of 314 control chromosomes studied.

Conclusions.—A mutation in the α-synuclein gene may account for the development of Parkinson's disease in families with a highly penetrant, autosomal dominant inheritance. Although this mutation may account for only a few percent of cases of Parkinson's disease, its further study may give insights into the pathogenesis of this disease.

► In trying to track down genes and proteins that are important in complex disorders of the elderly, investigators try to find families where the disease is highly familial, with a mendelian pattern of transmission, and where the onset is earlier than usual. This approach can lead to patients where single genes are responsible for the disorder. While single-gene defects typically account for only a small minority of affected patients (e.g., Alzheimer's or diabetes mellitus), these single genes provide important new insights into pathophysiologic and molecular mechanisms of disease. This group, studying an Italian family, successfully combined both major genetic approaches that are used to uncover disease-related genes, first positional cloning, and then the candidate gene approach. They found that a mutation in the α-synuclein gene was associated with the disease in this family and that several Greek families also suffer the same mutation. While these familial forms of Parkinson's represent only a minority of the total, they represent an interesting advance (also see Vogel[1] in *Science*, June 27, 1997). Synuclein, first discovered in electric organs of sting rays, has previously been found as a minor component of plaques in Alzheimer's disease. A recent report[2] also shows that α-synuclein is present in "Lewy bodies, a defining pathological characteristic of Parkinson's disease and dementia with Lewy bodies." Goedert[3] reviews α-synuclein (and speculates about its possible functions) as well as other members of the synuclein family; these proteins will probably attract a lot of attention from investigators who study Parkinson's, Alzheimer's, and other neurodegenerative disorders.

J. Roth, M.D.

References

1. Vogel G: Gene discovery offers tentative clues to Parkinson's (comment). *Science* 276:1973, 1997.
2. Spillantini MG, Schmidt ML, Lee VM, et al: Alpha-synuclein in Lewy bodies (letter). *Nature* 388:839–840, 1997.
3. Goedert M: Familial Parkinson's disease: The awakening of alpha-synuclein. *Nature* 388:232–233, 1997.

Suggested Reading

LaFerla FM, Troncoso JC, Strickland DK, et al: Neuronal cell death in Alzheimer's disease correlates with apoE uptake and intracellular Aβ stabilization. *J Clin Invest* 100:310–320, 1997.

► Alzheimer's disease is characterized by extracellular plaques that contain deposits of the β-amyloid peptide (Aβ) as well as apolipoprotein (apo) E and other proteins. The authors studied nerve cells that were dying, using DNA labeling to detect the precise form of DNA fragmentation that is typically associated with the apoptotic form of cell death. Their finding of Aβ immunoactivity and apoE in increased amounts in the same cytoplasmic granules in the dying cells suggests to them that the proteins intracellularly are there in high concentrations and probably causing the neurotoxicity; their findings suggest that the extracellular plaques, the hallmarks of Alzheimer's, are a later event. The molecular mechanism of the neurotoxicity in Alzheimer's disease will be very important; that will become the target for pharmacological intervention.

J. Roth, M.D.

Cancer

Stimulation of Prostate Cancer Growth by Androgens and Estrogens Through the Intermediacy of Sex Hormone-binding Globulin

Nakhla AM, Rosner W (St Luke's/Roosevelt Hosp, New York; Columbia Univ, New York)

Endocrinology 137:4126–4129, 1996 5–38

Objective.—The downstream consequences of the increase in cyclic adenosine monophosphate (AMP) as a result of activation of the receptor–sex hormone binding globulin (SHBG) complex are not known. The effect of the R_{SHBG} system on the growth of ALVA-41 cells, a line derived from a bony metastasis from a human prostate cancer, is reported.

Methods.—Using cell membranes from ALVA-41 cells, generation of dihydrotestosterone (DHT)-stimulated cyclic AMP during the presence and absence of SHBG was measured. The effect on cell growth of dihydrotestosterone and estradiol was examined.

Results.—Whereas neither DHT nor estradiol alone increased the production of cyclic AMP in serum-free medium, in the presence of the receptor-SHBG complex, both DHT and estradiol stimulated a dose-dependent increase in cyclic AMP. The growth-enhancing effect of the receptor complex was potentiated by addition of the protein phosphatase inhibitor okadaic acid.

Conclusion.—Cyclic AMP has a growth-enhancing effect on ALVA-41 prostate cancer cells. That growth is potentiated by addition of SHBG-estradiol and SHBG-DHT, particularly in the presence of protein phosphatase inhibitors.

▶ Traditionally, peptide hormones (and other water-soluble hormones such as epinephrine) bind to and activate cell surface receptors; the activated receptors in turn generate intracellular messengers such as cyclic AMP. This is in contradistinction to the lipid-soluble hormones, including all of the steroid hormones and thyroid hormones, which enter the cells, and then link to and activate their specific receptors. The hormone-activated receptors, translocated to the nucleus, bind to specific sites on DNA and thereby regulate the production of messenger RNAs for proteins in the cell and thereby help to regulate their rates of synthesis. The lipid-soluble hormones typically have specific binding proteins; sex hormone-binding globulin SHBG is the circulating transporter for both androgens (testosterone and dihydrotestosterone [DHT]) and estrogens. In addition to contributing to the regulation of the concentrations of free estrogens and free androgens in plasma, the SHBG bind to a specific receptor on the plasma membrane of prostatic cells. When SHBG is occupied by a hormone, the triplex of hormone, SHBG, and its cell surface receptor causes activation of the receptor and the generation of cyclic AMP as well as other events in the cytoplasm that are quite rapid and resemble those of a water-soluble hormone (e.g., epinephrine). This increase in cyclic AMP does not involve the classic steroid receptors of the nucleus. Well-characterized hormone analogues that do or do not bind to the nuclear receptors or to SHBG have been used to implicate the cell surface receptor and to exonerate the nuclear receptor in a group of these cellular activities. The authors show that the growth-stimulating effects of DHT and estradiol on prostate cancer cells in culture occur in the absence of serum, but in the presence of SHBG. Elevation of cyclic AMP by the hormone bound to SHBG or by other mechanisms produces cell growth. This approach provides a whole new possible strategy for controlling the growth of prostatic cancers. More important, it opens up a whole new avenue for discussing hormone actions in target cells that previously have been associated with nuclear receptors only. Indeed, the pioneers who have labored for several decades to try to show that cell surface receptors are an additional pathway by which steroidlike hormones can operate are now being vindicated, and some effects of thyroid hormones, vitamin D, as well as other steroidlike hormones are being shown now to have additional pathways via cell surface receptors.

J. Roth, M.D.

Human Prostate Carcinoma Cells Express Enzymatic Activity That Converts Human Plasminogen to the Angiogenesis Inhibitor, Angiostatin

Gately S, Twardowski P, Stack MS, et al (Children's Mem Hosp, Chicago; Northwestern Univ, Chicago; Duke Univ, Durham, NC)

Cancer Res 56:4887–4890, 1996 5–39

Objective.—The mechanism for generating angiostatin, an angiogenesis and metastasis inhibitor, is not known, although recent studies of antimetastatic factors suggest they are also angiogenesis inhibitors. Results of a study of PC-3 human prostate carcinoma cells demonstrate that these cells secrete enzymatic activity capable of cleaving plasminogen to bioactive angiostatin.

Methods.—Culture medium, collected from human prostate cancer cell lines PC-3, DU-145, and LN-CaP, was used to cleave plasminogen or plasmin in the presence of various proteinase inhibitors. The angiostatin produced was purified and sequenced. The ability of the purified angiostatin to inhibit human endothelial cell proliferation, basic fibroblast growth factor–induced migration, endothelial cell tube formation, and basic fibroblast growth factor–induced corneal angiogenesis was studied.

Results.—Both plasmin, a serine proteinase, and plasminogen generated angiostatin. Only serine proteinase inhibitors were completely effective at blocking angiostatin generation. PC-3–derived angiostatin inhibited endothelial cell proliferation and migration, blocked basic fibroblast growth factor–induced corneal angiogenesis, and inhibited human endothelial cell tube formation. Affinity chromatography established that PC-3–derived angiostatin was an internal fragment of plasminogen and an inhibitor of angiogenesis.

Conclusion.—PC-3–derived angiostatin may be responsible for inhibiting angiogenesis and therefore the slow progress of human primary prostate cancer and related metastases.

► It is now clear that the development of tumors requires the production of angiogenesis factors that then allow access of nutrients for the growing cancer cells. In addition, it appears that angiogenesis and cell growth are closely linked. This article describes mechanisms for converting plasminogen, an enzyme precursor, and plasmin, a natural anticoagulant closely related to trypsin, into angiostatin, an inhibitor of angiogenesis and growth. Presumably, the experimental tumor cells produce angiostatin, which acts to keep the cell growth controlled. It is exciting to speculate how angiostatic agents might vie with the angiogenesis agents to control cell growth.

J. Roth, M.D.

Genetic Alterations in Untreated Metastases and Androgen-independent Prostate Cancer Detected by Comparative Genomic Hybridization and Allelotyping

Cher ML, Bova GS, Moore DH, et al (Univ of California, San Francisco; San Francisco/Mt Zion Med Ctr; Johns Hopkins Univ, Baltimore)

Cancer Res 56:3091–3102, 1996 5–40

Introduction.—Studies of the molecular genetic mechanisms responsible for the development and progression of prostate cancer have narrowed the regions of common deletion on chromosomes 8p and 16q, but there is yet no overall view of regional chromosomal alterations in the disease. Investigators applied a newly developed technique of comparative genomic hybridization (CGH) to DNA isolated from a set of prostate cancer lymphatic and bony metatases. The technique was also performed with DNA extracted from a set of prostate tumors from patients with androgen-independent metastatic disease.

Methods.—Tissue was obtained from 31 patients with metastatic prostate cancer. Twenty patients (group I) had not been exposed to long-term androgen deprivation or other therapies, and 11 (group II) had clinical disease progression after long-term androgen deprivation therapy. Eighteen group I metastatic tissue samples were from pelvic lymph nodes and 2 were from bone metastases. For group II, genetic analysis was performed on primary tumors in 4 cases, persistent or recurrent primary tumor in 6 cases, and metastatic tumor in 1 case. Multiple CGH analyses were obtained for each chromosome in each tumor. On all tumor DNA samples, t thresholds of +1.6 were used for gains and −1.6 for deletions.

Results.—All tumors in both groups I and II displayed some DNA alterations. Group I averaged 15% of genome gained and 14% lost; group II averaged 16% gained and 11% lost. Analysis of group I tumor samples yielded the highest reported rate of alterations in several chromosomal regions: 8q gain (85%), 8p loss (80%), 13q loss (75%), 16q loss (55%),

17p loss (50%), and 10q loss (50%). Chromosomal alterations observed in group II samples were very similar to those in group I, particularly in a loss in chromosome 8p, a gain in chromosome 8q, and a loss in chromosome 13q. Similarities between the 2 groups suggest that most chromosomal alterations occur without androgen-deprivation therapy.

Discussion.—Several new regions of frequent deletion or gain of DNA copy numbers have been identified in prostate cancer by means of CGH. The malignant behavior of prostate cancer may result from modified function of genes contained within the most frequently altered regions. Although the pattern of genetic alterations was largely the same for tumors from African-Americans and caucasians, gains were more frequent in the region 4q25–q28 in African-Americans.

▶ The advances in understanding of the molecular biology of cancer continue to progress substantially. Although some cancers are caused by a single-point mutation in a single gene, it appears now that most of the common cancers are associated with multiple genetic defects. Indeed, often there is the deletion (or addition) of a substantial piece of DNA. In an attempt to understand the molecular mechanisms responsible for the development and progression of prostate cancer, the authors have used a new technique by which deletions or additions all over the genome of the cancer cells can be detected. In doing so, they detected a remarkably large number of gains and losses both in metastases and in primary tumors that have not yet metastasized. This will help greatly in characterizing and identifying the tumors. Also, areas with gains and deletions that recur from tumor to tumor suggest common mechanisms. Examination of these regions in great detail to determine which specific genes have been gained or lost when these chunks of DNA have been added or lost will add greatly to our understanding of the disease and provide a rational strategy for counteracting these abnormalities.

J. Roth, M.D.

Specific Accumulation of Tumor-derived Adhesion Factor in Tumor Blood Vessels and in Capillary Tube-like Structures of Cultured Vascular Endothelial Cells

Akaogi K, Okabe Y, Sato J, et al (Yokohama City Univ, Japan; Kobe Pharmaceutical Univ, Japan)

Proc Natl Acad Sci USA 93:8384–8389, 1996 5–41

Objective.—Angiogenesis—formation of new blood vessels—is necessary for tumor growth and metastasis, as well as for normal physiologic processes. Previous studies in the human bladder carcinoma cell line EJ-1 identified a 30 kDa cell adhesion protein designated tumor-derived adhesion factor (TAF). In in vitro studies, TAF stimulated direct adhesion of human vascular endothelial cells and other types of cells to plastic plates.

This study sought to gain insight into the physiologic function of TAF by studying its distribution in human tumors and normal tissues.

Methods.—Immunohistochemical studies were performed with a monoclonal anti-TAF antibody. Expression of TAF was assessed in various cancer tissues and in cultured vascular endothelial cells.

Results.—Studies showed accumulation of TAF in small blood vessels and capillaries in the area of tumor nests, but not around normal tissues. Specific staining for TAF was noted in blood vessels associated esophageal, brain, lung, stomach, and other human cancers. Tumor-derived adhesion factor and type IV collagen were found to be colocalized in the vascular basement membrane on double immunofluorescent staining. Further experiments showed that TAF bound preferentially to type IV collagen, and not to the other extracellular matrix components studied. Tumor-derived adhesions factor induced morphologic change of cultured human umbilical vein endothelial cells, as well as their adhesion to type IV collagen substrate. After type I collagen caused the endothelial cells to form capillary tubelike structures, TAF and type IV collagen were found only on these structures. Heparin inhibited TAF binding to endothelial cells and prevented formation of the capillary tubes.

Conclusions.—Tumor adhesion factor is expressed by tumor blood vessels, as well as by capillary tubelike structures formed by cultured endothelial cells. The finding suggest that TAF likely plays a role in new blood vessel development in tumor tissues by modulating the interaction between endothelial cells and type IV collagen. The authors propose the functional name angiomodulin for this new vascular protein.

▶ Angiogenesis or development of new vessels is critical for embryonic development and for wound repair. In pathologic states, tumors are particularly dependent on new vessel growth. Angiogenesis by tumor cells is known to be stimulated by vascular endothelial cell growth factor and basic fibroblast growth factor, two soluble ligands with specific receptors that are known to stimulate the production of new endothelial cells. We also know that intercellular matrix molecules play an important role in cell signaling as well as cell differentiation. A new cell adhesion protein, named tumor-derived adhesion factor, appears to be produced by many cancer cells and appears to play an important role in linking endothelial cells to the intercellular matrix molecules like type IV collagen. The absolutely vital role of angiogenesis in tumor growth is supported by findings that specific inhibition of vessel growth results in regression of tumors. Elucidation of each of the individual molecules in this process provides new targets for therapy.

J. Roth, M.D.

Gene Expression Profiles in Normal and Cancer Cells

Zhang L, Zhou W, Velculescu VE, et al (Johns Hopkins Univ, Baltimore, Md)
Science 276:1268–1272, 1997 5–42

Introduction.—Most cancer research in the past 5 decades has focused on analyzing genes that are expressed differently in tumor cells. Hundreds of investigations have reported differences in the expression of 1 or more genes, but there are no comprehensive reports of gene expression in cancer cells. Serial analysis of gene expression (SAGE) was used to identify and quantify RNA transcripts from genes derived from human colorectal (CR) epithelium, CR cancers, or pancreatic cancers.

Findings.—There were 303,706 RNA transcripts derived from approximately 49,000 different genes that ranged from 1 to 5,300 copies per cell. About 75% of the messenger RNA (mRNA) mass consisted of transcripts expressed at an average of more than 5 copies per cell. Eighty-six percent of transcripts were expressed at less than 5 copies per cell; in aggregate, this low-abundance class consisted of only 25% of the mRNA mass. Many SAGE tags (expressed gene sequences) seemed to represent previously undescribed transcripts. Only 54% of tags matched GenBank entries; the likelihood of a tag being present in databases was associated with abundance. Ninety-eight percent of GenBank matches were expressed at greater than 500 copies per cell. Only 51% of transcripts were expressed at 5 or less copies per cell. Most transcripts were expressed at similar levels in normal colon epithelium and primary colon cancers, but 289 transcripts were expressed at significantly different levels. A comparison of the expression pattern of CR cancer cells and normal colon cells showed 548 differently expressed transcripts. Genes expressed at higher levels in normal colon epithelium than in CR tumors were frequently related to differentiation. Most genes identified by SAGE as being higher in CR cancers and pancreatic cancers could be reproducibly expressed in many cancers evaluated by Northern blot analysis.

Conclusion.—Hundreds of specific genes were expressed at different levels in colorectal cancers. Some of these were expressed differentially in pancreatic cancers.

▶ Technology has progressed to the point at which, with relative efficiency, gene expression or mutational analysis can be accomplished for many cell strains in a short time. Two general types of analyses are used: 1 based on positional cloning in which nucleotide sequence markers, dinucleotide repeats, and trinucleotide repeats are used to assign DNA patterns to previously mapped regions of a chromosome and, thus, to the "position" of a gene, and the second, based on the analysis of different patterns of mRNA expression by the specific cell types in question. Differential display methodology (of RNA patterns) is an example of the latter. Here, the SAGE method was used to identify large numbers of RNA transcripts from genes in normal and cancer cells.[1]

Serial analysis of gene expression is based on 2 principles: first, a short nucleotide sequence tag (9–10 base pairs) contains sufficient information to uniquely identify an RNA transcript provided it is isolated from a defined position in the transcript; and, second, short sequence tags permit an efficient analysis of transcripts in a serial manner that can be accomplished within a short time by sequencing of multiple tags linked end to end within a single clone.

More than 500 transcripts were expressed at different levels by normal and neoplastic cells. The goal is identification of genes of primary importance to cancer genesis, as contrasted with the numerous genes activated in a secondary manner by the basic neoplastic mechanism. Here, multiple genes related to cell differentiation or neoplastic growth patterns and previously identified in cancer cells were confirmed. Not all the transcripts have been identified, but the technique is representative of methods that are finding increasing use in defining the cause of the disease as well as opening the door for the development of new therapies.

J.R. Shapiro, M.D.

Reference

1. Velculescu VE, Zhang L, Vogelstein B, et al: Serial analysis of gene expression. *Science* 270: 484–487, 1995.

Switch From Monoallelic to Biallelic Human *IGF2* Promoter Methylation During Aging and Carcinogenesis

Issa J-PJ, Vertino PM, Boehm CD, et al (Johns Hopkins Univ, Baltimore, Md; Univ of California, San Diego, La Jolla, Calif)

Proc Natl Acad Sci USA 93:11757–11762, 1996 5–43

Background.—In humans, about 60% of gene promoters contain a CpG-rich stretch of DNA called a CpG island. These islands are usually unmethylated, whereas methylation is associated with irreversible inhibition of gene expression from that promoter. Methylation has been observed to increase with aging and to be associated with neoplasia. The insulin-like growth factor II (*IGF2*) protein is a fetal growth promoter that is transcribed from 4 promoters, P1 through P4. These promoters, P2 to P4, are contained within a CpG island and only the paternal copy is expressed. The P1 promoter is upstream and differently regulated. The dynamics of methylation during aging and neoplasia were investigated in the promoter of the *IGF2* gene.

Methods and Results.—When methylation was examined in normal tissues by DNA digestion with methylation-sensitive restriction enzymes, partial methylation was always present, at the silent maternal allele. This methylation was more extensive in the liver, which expresses high levels of *IGF2* through the P1 promoter. When normal human fibroblasts were cultured, *IGF2* promoter methylation increased with the number of cell passages. To study aging-related methylation in vivo, a panel of normal colon tissues from 34 individuals 8- to 90-years-old was examined. The extent of promoter methylation at this locus increased with age. This increase resulted at least partially from methylation of the original unmethylated paternal allele. Methylation also was increased in 31 cells derived from human tumors. Most human tumors expressed *IGF2* from the P1 promoter.

Conclusions.—The *IGF2* promoter-associated CpG island is methylated at the silent maternal allele in young individuals. With age, this methylation is extended to the paternal allele. Biallelic methylation also appears in tumor cells. This high methylation level is associated with loss of expression from P2 to P4 but preserved biallelic expression from P1. Age-related methylation increases and the resulting changes in gene expression may explain some of the physiologic changes observed during normal aging and also may be involved in tumorigenesis.

▶ This article presents fascinating insight into the regulation of gene expression as affected by age and in carcinogenesis. Methylation of portions of a gene leads to its inactivation: gene expression is associated with demethylation. Previous studies by this group have shown an age-related increase in methylation of portions of the estrogen receptor gene in the colon and an association of this with neoplasia.[1]

This report is about the role of de novo methylation of the promoter region of the *IGF2* gene and its effect on expression of the gene with increasing age and various tumors. Insulin-like growth factor II is not increased by growth hormone (as is IGF1). However, it is a growth factor for the fetus but with less well defined growth-related actions in adult tissues. The results of *IGF2* gene analysis indicate increased methylation of specific promotor regions involving both paternal and maternal alleles in an age-dependent manner. As with the estrogen receptor in colon tumors, increased *IGF2* methylation also occurs in a variety of tumors.

Several intriguing questions arise from these important data. First, why is age a factor in sequential methylation and expression of both the inactive (the paternally imprinted *IGF2* allele) and active alleles? Second, does methylation-induced suppression of specific promoters permit other promoter regions to facilitate the development of cancer? Third, is this a general mechanism involving other growth factor genes, and what is its overall effect on aging of certain organs?

J.R. Shapiro, M.D.

Reference

1. Issa JP, Ottaviano YL, Celano P, et al: Methylation of the oestrogen receptor CpG island links aging and neoplasia in human colon. *Nat Genet* 7:536–540, 1994.

Novel Therapy—Now and Future

Amyloid Deposition is Delayed in Mice With Targeted Deletion of the Serum Amyloid P Component Gene

Botto M, Hawkins PN, Bickerstaff MCM, et al (Hammersmith Hosp, London)

Nature Med 3:855–859, 1997 5–44

Background.—Tissue amyloid deposits are found in many diseases, including Alzheimer's disease. Such deposits always contain serum amyloid P component (SAP), and it is believed that SAP stabilizes the amyloid fibrils. Perhaps disruption of the SAP could lead to destabilization of the amyloid deposits and, thus, attenuate the development of amyloidosis. In this study, the SAP gene in mice was manipulated to determine whether its absence would affect the development of amyloidosis.

Methods.—The SAP gene was eliminated in mice by use of a homologous recombination vector. Three types of mice were used: homozygotes for the deleted gene ($SAP^{-/-}$), heterozygotes ($SAP^{+/-}$), and wild-type controls ($SAP^{+/+}$). Casein was injected in $SAP^{-/-}$ and $SAP^{+/-}$ mice to induce systemic amyloid AA amyloidosis. In another experiment, amyloid-enhancing factor (AEF) depleted of SAP was injected, followed by casein injection, to see if AEF would have its usual effect of accelerating amyloid deposition.

Findings.—Casein induced significantly less and significantly later amyloid deposition in the $SAP^{-/-}$ mice compared with the $SAP^{+/-}$ mice. However, concentrations of the precursor for systemic amyloid AA were similar in both groups. Although the SAP-depleted AEF did induce amyloid deposition in all three groups of animals, deposition was significantly less in the $SAP^{-/-}$ mice.

Conclusions.—Deletion of the SAP gene blocked deposition of amyloid even when AEF was used to enhance deposition. Therefore, drug therapies aimed at inhibiting SAP binding should reduce or eliminate the deposition of amyloid and would be useful in treating diseases involving such deposits.

Restoration of the Growth Suppression Function of Mutant *p53* by a Synthetic Peptide Derived From the p53 C-Terminal Domain

Selivanova G, Iotsova V, Okan I, et al (Karolinska Inst, Stockholm, Sweden; Tumor Biology Ctr, Breisacherstrasse, Freiburg, Germany)

Nature Med 3:632–638, 1997 5–45

Background.—The *p53* gene is a tumor suppressor that is mutated in many human tumors. Typically, a mutated *p53* gene has a single amino acid substitution that weakens its specific binding to DNA. This study examined whether mutant *p53* genes that have lost their ability to suppress cell growth in tumors could be "rescued" by the addition of a gene fragment that contained the correct amino acid sequence.

Methods.—Human wild-type p53 fusion protein was purified; peptide 46 showed the most efficiency in activating *p53* specific DNA binding and was used in the study. Then, various cancer cell lines (HeLa, SW480, others) were grown as models for examining the effects of peptide 46 on cell growth and apoptosis.

Findings.—Cell growth was significantly inhibited by peptide 46 in cells with mutant p53 proteins. In cells without the mutant p53 proteins, however, the addition of peptide 46 had no effect. Apoptosis was significantly increased by peptide 46 in cell lines with either mutant or wild-type *p53*, whereas tumor cells devoid of *p53* showed no effect from peptide 46.

Conclusions.—Peptide 46, a C-terminal peptide, restored the growth suppression function of endogenous mutant p53 proteins. Restoring this protein's ability to induce apoptosis would have implications for anticancer therapy.

▶ The repair of many molecular defects in vivo appears to be so complex that practical therapy seems far off. These articles (Abstracts 5–44 and 5–45) are two examples where relatively simple solutions appear to have promise for complex problems. In the first, the authors target serum amyloid P component, an important constituent of several forms of amyloid. They show that when the gene for the serum amyloid P component is deleted in mice, formation of amyloid fibrils is markedly inhibited. Thus, this circulating protein may well be an attractive focus for prophylaxis or early intervention, a much less daunting prospect than targeting intracellular proteins.

In the second paper, *p53*, a normal suppressor of abnormal cell growth, which is mutated (and thereby inactivated) in a very high fraction of human cancers, can have its function restored by a 22–amino acid peptide. Again, the whole protein need not be replaced, only a well-defined sub-piece. This may be a much more achievable task than replacing the entire defective protein. The principle here is that a complex protein in its final functioning form is really a series of stretches of peptide acting in concert. Pieces that are defective in the native protein can be replaced by modular pieces. In effect, we may be able to use a protein patch in place of replacing the whole protein—analogous to patching a tire rather than replacing it. In addition to simplicity and economy, the "peptide patch" may have the advantage of having no activity at all except in cells that have the defective protein with which it can interact specifically. Further, its concentration in a cell would need to be above some minimum level but not neatly regulated; the system would have a major element of functional self-regulation. This level of regulatory control in theory exceeds by far that typically achievable by many conventional gene therapy techniques.

Another example[1] focuses on nephrogenic (i.e., vasopressin-resistant) diabetes insipidus due to a mutant vasopressin receptor. Although this seven transmembrane domain protein has a very complex structure, its function can be restored by the expression of a relatively small peptide corresponding to the region that is defective. This experiment is based on a body of observations that a complex protein, formed in nature as a single continuous chain of amino acids, actually functions in its folded state as a cluster of small peptide chains. This cluster of peptides can interact with one another even when they are no longer connected covalently. To the protein chemist pioneers whose work is the foundation of this project, it is probably no surprise and a great joy.

Taken together, these 3 studies provide optimism for simple approaches to the correction of complex defects.

J. Roth, M.D.

Reference

1. Schöneberg T, Sandig V, Wees J, et al: Reconstruction of mutant V2 vasopressin receptors by adenovirus-mediated gene transfer: Molecular basis and clinical implication. *J Clin Invest* 100:1547–1556, 1997.

Transmissible Diseases

Molecular Analysis of Prion Strain Variation and the Aetiology of 'New Variant' CJD

Collinge J, Sidle KCL, Meads J, et al (Imperial College, London; Western Gen Hosp, Edinburgh, Scotland; St Mary's Hosp, London)

Nature 383:685–690, 1996 5–46

Background.—The transmissible spongiform encephalopathies are neurodegenerative diseases associated with the accumulation of an abnormal isoform of a host-encoded glycoprotein, the prion protein (PrP), in the brain. The disease-related isoform, PrP^{Sc}, can be distinguished from the normal cellular isoform, PrP^{C}, by its insolubility and partial protease resistance. The current model of prion disease propagation involves direct protein-to-protein interaction, with PrP^{Sc} converting PrP^{C} in an autocatalytic process. Public interest in these unusual diseases has recently increased because of an outbreak of bovine spongiform encephalopathy (BSE) in the United Kingdom, which may represent a significant public health threat through the ingestion of BSE-infected tissue. The pathogenicity of bovine prions for humans is not known. There are several known strains of human prion disease, Creutzfeldt-Jakob disease (CJD), that can be distinguished by different incubation times and patterns of neuropathology when passaged in mice. Recently, a new form of human prion disease was reported in the United Kingdom, with a unique clinicopathologic pattern. All patients with this new variant CJD who have been studied are homozygous for methionine at residue 129 of PrP and have no history of iatrogenic exposure to human prions. This suggests that there is a new risk factor for prion disease in the United Kingdom, dietary exposure to bovine offal. A wide range of cases of CJD have been examined and compared with the new variant CJD to determine whether it represents a new strain.

Methods.—The study was conducted on brain tissue samples from 26 neuropathologically confirmed sporadic cases of CJD, including all 3 codon 129 genotypes; 7 neuropathologically confirmed iatrogenic CJD cases, and 10 neuropathologically confirmed new variant CJD cases from the National CJD Surveillance Unit or the Prion Disease Group. Brain samples were from the cerebral cortex. DNA was extracted from blood or brain and analyzed for mutations in the PrP gene.

Results.—Both sporadic and iatrogenic CJD were associated with 3 distinct patterns of protease-resistant PrP on Western blots. The new variant of CJD was associated with its own unique and consistent pattern in this assay. Transmission to inbred mice of the established CJD variants produced a glycosylation pattern characteristic of the inoculated CJD; transmission of BSE produced a pattern identical to new variant CJD. Experimental BSE in macaques and naturally acquired BSE in cats had a glycoform pattern indistinguishable from experimental murine BSE and new variant CJD.

Conclusions.—New variant CJD can be distinguished from the established strains of CJD by its characteristic pattern on Western blots and is a distinct new strain of prion disease. The spontaneous occurrence of a novel human prion disease in multiple individuals in the United Kingdom seems an unlikely explanation. It is more likely that these cases arose from a common source of exposure to an animal strain of prion disease. That the glycoform of the new strain is identical to that of BSE is consistent with the hypothesis that the new variant of CJD is a result of the transmission of BSE to humans.

► The emerging understanding of CJD and the other transmissible spongiform encephalopathies, a group of neurodegenerative diseases of humans and other mammals, is one of the most extraordinary stories in contemporary medicine. (The Nobel Prize for Physiology or Medicine for 1997 to Dr. Stan Prusiner is a highly deserved recognition of this achievement.) These diseases are caused by accumulation of PrP^{Sc}, a disease-related form of the normal prion (pronounced Prē′ on) protein, designated PrP^{Sc}. The abnormal protein, PrP^{Sc}, can be coded in the genome and lead to an inherited form of CJD, which constitutes about 15% of the total cases. Most amazingly, abnormal protein by an autocatalytic process can cause the conversion of normal protein into abnormal protein that leads to disease. The abnormal protein template can be introduced by iatrogenic routes, including derived pituitary hormones (growth hormone or gonadotropin), by grafting of dura mater or corneas, or by the use of inadequately sterilized neurosurgical instruments. Most patients have a sporadic form of the disease in which neither genetic or iatrogenic routes can be implicated.

How the abnormal protein converts normal protein into its abnormal form is quite unknown, but how the abnormal form causes pathology is starting to emerge. It appears that the abnormal proteins are less soluble and less susceptible to proteases, causing their accumulation, followed by cellular abnormalities that lead to the neurodegeneration characteristic of these diseases. Clinical variations are now appearing that depend on both the route of entry and the specific difference in structure between the pathological and normal forms of the protein. Creutzfeldt-Jakob disease of humans is related to kuru, the affliction that was widespread among the natives of New Guinea when they engaged in ritual cannibalism. It also is related to bovine spongiform encephalopathy, or mad cow disease, as well as scrapie in sheep and mink encephalopathy. It is believed that material derived from infected cattle, especially neural tissue, can be a source of transmission to other species. Whether this is an important source of abnormal prions for human diseases is under study. It is hoped that examination of the minute details of the structure of the abnormal proteins will yield clues to the sources of the abnormal variants and their role in human diseases.

J. Roth, M.D.

Essential Roles of the Fas Ligand in the Development of Hepatitis

Kondo T, Suda T, Fukuyama H, et al (Osaka Bioscience Inst, Japan; Osaka Univ, Japan)

Nature Med 3:409–413, 1997 5–47

Background.—The Fas ligand (FasL) is expressed on the surface of activated T cells and functions as an effector for cytotoxic T lymphocyte (CTL)-induced toxicity. Binding of FasL to Fas causes apoptosis in Fas-containing cells. Administration of anti-Fas antibody causes apoptosis in murine hepatocytes leading to acute liver failure and death. This process is similar to that seen in human fulminant hepatitis, suggesting an involvement of the Fas/FasL system in this disease. A mouse model system was used to investigate the role of the Fas/FasL system in the development of this disease.

Methods and Results.—The cell line, 6C2, is a hepatitis-B surface antigen (HBsAg)-specific CTL clone, which expresses high levels of FasL when activated. When activated 6C2 cells were administered to transgenic mice expressing the hepatitis-B virus (HBV) large envelope protein on their liver cells, hepatitis was induced. When liver tissue sections from transgenic mice injected with 6C2 cells were examined, apoptotic hepatocytes were detected. The 6C2 cells were cytotoxic to primary hepatocytes from HBV transgenic mice, but not from wild-type mice. Injecting 6C2 cells into HBsAg-transgenic mice significantly increased the level of serum glutamic pyruvic transaminase (GPT). When mFas-Fc, a soluble form of Fas, was co-injected with 6C2 cells into transgenic mice, serum GPT levels were not elevated and the mice did not die of hepatitis.

Conclusions.—A murine model of hepatitis was used to demonstrate that the Fas/FasL system plays an important role in the pathogenesis of this disease. The FasL expressed on the surface of HBV-specific CTLs was responsible for inducing apoptosis in hepatocytes expressing HBV surface antigen and initiating the process leading to hepatitis. If the involvement of the Fas/FasL system in human fulminant hepatitis can be demonstrated, it is possible that a soluble form of Fas, anti-Fas antibodies or inhibitors of Fas-mediated apoptosis would have therapeutic value in this disease.

► This report involves an emerging area of major importance to geriatric medicine. It appears that several diseases of disordered immune function are related to the Fas system that is one factor regulating apoptosis. Papers by Giordano[1] and French and Tschopp[2] are related to the same topic: gene regulation of cell death. The Fas receptor and its natural ligand (FasL) are transmembrane proteins that belong to the tumor necrosis factor family of receptors and protein ligands. Fas ligand is expressed by activated T cells that are cytotoxic. When Fas ligand is engaged, cells expressing Fas rapidly undergo apoptosis via activation of a specific intracellular signaling pathway. Dysfunction of the Fas system has recently been associated with disease states of the immune system where regulation of cell death is crucial. Mounting data indicate that Fas and FasL must be tightly regulated to prevent emergence of disease. Lymphoproliferative syndrome in mice and autoimmune lymphoproliferative and hyperesosinophilic syndromes in humans are now recognized to involve disordered Fas regulation:[3] hepatitis and Hashimoto's thyroiditis[1] are now added to the list. Note that thyroiditis involving immune cell loss related to activation of T lymphocytes is important in the development of hypothyroidism in the elderly.

An intriguing result of the Kondo studies is that modification of the FasL/Fas system after administration of a soluble form of Fas as well as the Fas null state in transgenic mice can limit otherwise lethal hepatic damage. Will it be possible in the future to target agents neutralizing FasL and Fas to specific tissues such as the liver or to organs where apoptosis is driven by the Fas cascade?

J.R. Shapiro, M.D.

References

1. Giordano C: Potential involvement of Fas and its ligand in the pathogenesis of Hashimoto's thyroiditis. *Science* 275:960–963, 1997.
2. French LE, Tschopp J: Thyroiditis and hepatitis: Fas on the road to disease. *Nature Med* 3:387–388, 1997.
3. Lenardo MJ: Fas and the art of lymphocyte maintenance. *J Exp Med* 183:721–724, 1996.

Genetics and Disease

Mutations in the Consensus Helicase Domains of the Werner Syndrome Gene

Yu C-E, Oshima J, Wijsman EM, et al (Veterans' Affairs Puget Sound Health Care System, Seattle; Univ of Washington, Seattle; Osaka Univ, Japan; et al)
Am J Hum Genet 60:330–341, 1997 5–48

Background.—A potential model of accelerated human aging is Werner syndrome, a rare autosomal recessive disorder. The features of accelerated aging include graying and loss of hair beginning in the second decade of life, sclerodoma-like skin changes, and voice alterations. Mutations in a gene, WRN, cause Werner syndrome. The gene encodes a predicted 1432–amino-acid protein with homology to RNA and DNA helicases. A previous study showed 4 Werner syndrome mutations in the 3' end of the gene. This mutation did not disrupt the helicase domain region of amino acids 569–859, but it resulted in predicted truncated protein products of 1060–1247 amino acids. The intron–exon structure of the gene was determined in patients with Werner syndrome, and they were also screened for mutations.

Methods.—Cosmid clones were isolated from a chromosome 8–specific cosmid library, and WRN-containing cosmids were identified from patients with Werner syndrome. The genomic structure of WRN was identified and mutation analysis was conducted.

Results.—With the coding sequences beginning the second exon, 35 exons were defined. The study identified 5 new Werner syndrome mutations, including a predicted truncated protein of 391 amino acids, a 1-base-pair deletion causing a frame shift, a mutation at a splice-junction site resulting in a predicted truncated protein of 760 amino acids; and 2 nonsense mutations at codons 369 and 889. Another deletion of more than 15 kb of genomic DNA included the exons 19–23, and the predicted protein was 1196 amino acids long. Four of these new mutations result in predicted protein products completely missing the helicase region or partially disrupting the helicase domain region.

Conclusions.—Werner syndrome is caused by mutations in the WRN gene. The presence of absence of the helicase domain in the protein does not influence the Werner syndrome phenotype, as evidenced by the location of the mutations, suggesting that Werner syndrome results from a complete loss of function of the WRN gene product.

► Werner syndrome is one of a group of extremely rare disorders that follow mendelian genetics and have features suggestive of premature aging, explaining why they have captured the collective imagination of the field of geriatric medicine. The molecular genetic basis of these diseases is being elucidated and elaborated. Patients with Werner syndrome prematurely appear old, with graying and hair loss beginning before adulthood. Diseases characteristic of aging show up early in adult life rather than in old age. The cause of death is cancer or cardiovascular disease, typically before age 50. Interestingly, fibroblasts cultured from young donors with Werner syndrome behave more like fibroblasts taken from older patients (i.e., they cease replication after only 10–20 doublings). The reduced replicative potential of fibroblasts, as well as the high rates of cancer, may be related genomic instability—which is also a part of the Werner syndrome phenotype, with elevated prevalence of chromosomal rearrangements and deletions. In 1996, the Werner syndrome gene, designated WRN, was identified by means of positional cloning. The WRN protein consists of 1,432 amino acids that contain a central domain with 7 motifs that are structural signatures of the proteins that constitute the DNA and RNA superfamily of helicases. In each case of Werner syndrome, some mutation was found in the gene, adding further evidence that this is the Werner syndrome gene. One mutation (designated 4) was found only among the Japanese; the authors present evidence that these patients have a common genetic founder (i.e., an ancestor in common who is responsible for providing the mutation to all the others in Japan who have this Werner syndrome mutation). The disease is autosomal recessive (i.e., both copies of the WRN gene had mutations). A large section of the WRN gene, covering more than 400 bases, is highly homologous to other helicases from a wide range of organisms—including bacteria, yeast, and *Caenorhabditis elegans*—and several human helicases. The function of a helicase is to help in the unwinding of DNA to allow portions of it to become exposed and thereby become involved in gene expression. The unwinding occurs with the concomitant hydrolysis of ATP. By analogy with the function of other helicases, the WRN protein could function in DNA repair, regulation of transcription, regulation of progression through the cell cycle, or any number of other potential functions involving DNA or RNA unwinding. Cockayne syndrome, another inherited disorder with features of premature aging, has been found to have mutations in a different helicase. Genes for other helicases have been implicated in other diseases, including xeroderma pigmentosum group B, Bloom syndrome, and the X-chromosome–linked α-thalassemia mental retardation syndrome.

J. Roth, M.D.

Substantial Genetic Influence on Cognitive Abilities in Twins 80 or More Years Old

McClearn GE, Johansson B, Berg S, et al (Pennsylvania State Univ, Univ Park; Univ of College of Health Sciences, Jönköping, Sweden; Karolinska Inst, Stockholm; et al)

Science 276:1560–1563, 1997 5–49

Background.—General and specific cognitive abilities have been shown to be similar in twins. Likewise, environmental influences throughout the life span can also affect these abilities. The effects of both hereditability and environment on general and specific cognitive abilities in elderly twins were studied.

Methods.—Twins over the age of 80 (median 82.3 years) with no cognitive, sensory, or motor impairments were selected from the Swedish Twin Registry. Ultimately 110 pairs of identical twins and 130 pairs of same-sex fraternal twins were tested. Subjects completed tests for verbal processing, spatial processing, speed of processing, and memory. General cognitive ability was determined based on the first principal component (PC) of the scores and a short form of the Wechsler Adult Intelligence Scale (WAIS). The environment in which the twin pair lived (shared or nonshared) was also documented.

Findings.—After adjustment for age and gender, factor analysis revealed that general cognitive ability accounted for 50% of the variance in test performance. Correlations from identical twins were significantly stronger

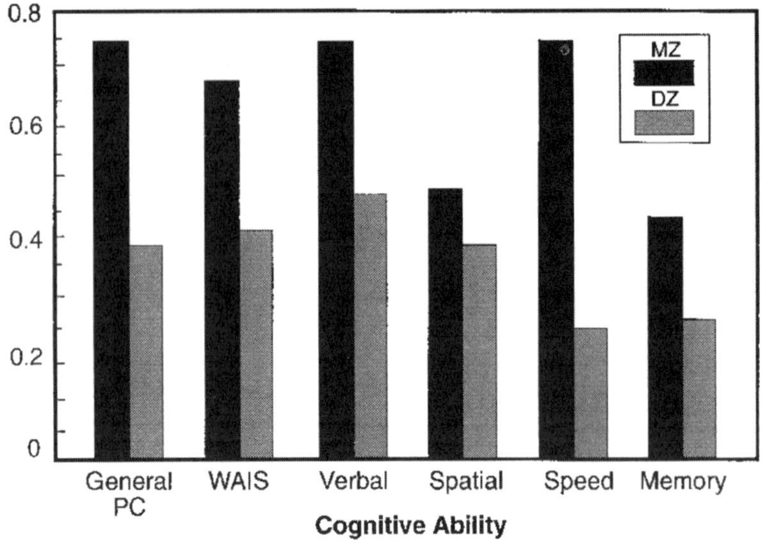

FIGURE 2.—Intraclass correlations for identical twins (MZ; *black bars*) and fraternal twins (DZ; *gray bars*) for general cognitive ability (PC and WAIS) and specific cognitive abilities. (Reprinted with permission from McClearn GE, Johansson B, Berg S, et al. Substantial genetic influence on cognitive abilities in twins 80 or more years old. *Science* 276:1560–1563. Copyright 1997, American Association for the Advancement of Science.)

than those from fraternal twins (Fig 2), reflecting a genetic influence. In fact, when best-fit models were constructed, dropping the genetic parameter significantly reduced the fit of the data, but dropping the shared environment parameter did not. Heritability (percentage of total phenotypic variance due to genetic variance) was 62% and 53% for the PC and WAIS measures of general cognitive ability, 55% for verbal ability, 32% for spatial ability, 62% for speed of processing, and 52% for memory (Fig 3). The shared environment parameter (i.e., that variance not due to heritability) accounted for 11% and 15% of the variance in the PC and WAIS measures of general cognitive ability, 20% for verbal ability, 13% for spatial ability, and 0% for speed of processing and memory.

Conclusions.—Genetic inheritance showed a significant influence on cognitive function in these older patients. Nonetheless, a large percentage (40%) of variance in cognitive abilities was due to environmental factors. These environmental factors are not related to a shared or unshared environment, indicating that idiosyncratic differences over the life span are important determinants of cognitive function.

▶ In this remarkable article, the authors show, using classical twin techniques (which takes advantage of natural cloning of individuals), the extraordinary hereditary influence on cognitive abilities that persists even over the age of 80. The details of the article were tough sledding for me, but the essence of the article is clear: the influence of genetics is strong and it persists well into old age. The other finding, equally surprising to me, was

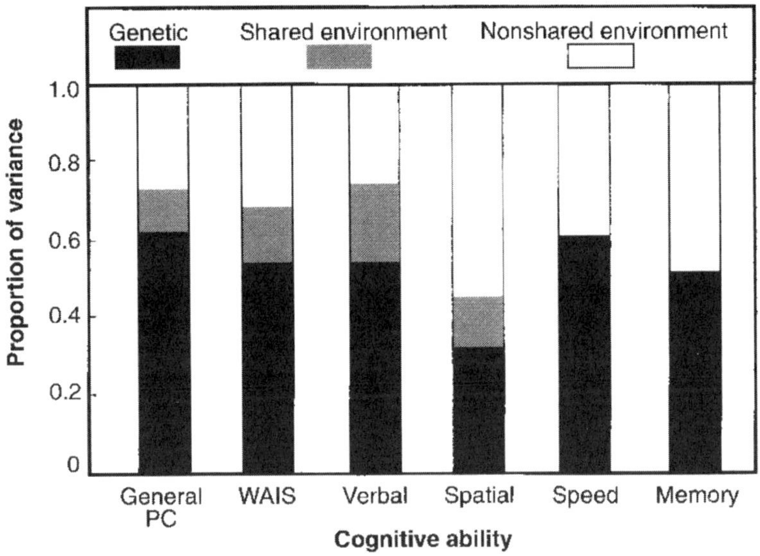

FIGURE 3.—Estimates of proportions of variance due to genetic influence (*black*), shared environment (*gray*), and nonshared environment (*white*), as derived from maximum likelihood, model-fitting twin analyses. For each measure, the full model fit well. Chi-squares with 3 degrees of freedom were 1.22 (p = 0.75) for PC general cognitive ability, 0.92 (p = 0.75) for WAIS general cognitive ability, 0.89 (p = 0.83) for verbal ability, 3.38 (p = 0.34) for spatial ability, 0.66 (p = 0.76) for speed of processing, and 2.8 (p = 0.42) for memory. Akaike fit indices also indicate that the full model fits well for each measure: −4.78, −5.08, −5.11, −2.62, −4.34, and −3.21, respectively. For each measure, the best-fitting model was one that only included genetic and nonshared environment parameters, with the following chi-squares with 4 degrees of freedom: 1.45, 1.72, 2.36, 3.70, 1.66, and 2.80, respectively. In other words, dropping the shared environment component of variance from the full model did not significantly reduce the fit of the model. In contrast, dropping the genetic parameter from the model significantly worsened the fit, with the following chi-squares with 4 degrees of freedom for the above measures: 9.64, 10.14, 12.74, 5.03, 12.30, and 7.54, respectively. (Reprinted with permission from McClearn GE, Johansson B, Berg S, et al: Substantial genetic influence on cognitive abilities in twins 80 or more years old. *Science* 276:1560–1563. Copright 1997, American Association for the Advancement of Science.)

the powerful effect of unshared environment (i.e., "idiosyncratic experience"). The accompanying editorial comment[1] puts this into the broader perspective of Drosophila, mouse, and the whole human genome. (Heritability of IQ[2] and an accompanying editorial[3] are worth examining as well.) We hope that this important area of science, which runs the risk of being contaminated by polemics, can be explored free of political and racial bias and rhetoric.

J. Roth, M.D.

References

1. Gottesman II: Twins: En route to QTLs for cognition (comment). *Science* 276:1522–1523, 1997.
2. Devlin B, Daniels M, Roeder K: The heritability of IQ (see comments). *Nature* 388:468–471, 1997.

3. McGue M: The democracy of the genes (editorial). *Nature* 388:417–418, 1997.

Notch3 **Mutations in CADASIL, a Hereditary Adult-Onset Condition Causing Stroke and Dementia**

Joutel A, Corpechot C, Ducros A, et al (Faculté de Médecine Necker-Enfants Malades, Paris; Hôpital St Antoine, Paris; Généthon, Evry, France; et al)
Nature 383:707–710, 1996 5–50

Background.—Cerebral autosomal dominant arteriopathy with subcortical infarcts and leukoencephalopathy (CADASIL) has been mapped to a mutant gene on chromosome 19. Also on human chromosome 19p13.1-13.2 is a cosmid that crosshybridizes with mouse *Notch3* deoxyribonucleic acid (DNA). Because *Notch* cosmids have been linked with another neurological condition (Alzheimer's disease), these investigators examined whether the *Notch3* pathway is involved in CADASIL.

Methods.—Mouse complementary DNA (cDNA) was used to isolate human *Notch3* cDNA from 58 patients with CADASIL and a 5,615-base pair string was constructed. Functional domains were identified, including 33 EGF domains, 3 Notch/Lin-12 repeats, and 3 Cdc10 ankyrin-like repeats. Then genomic DNA from controls and from patients with CADASIL was examined for gross rearrangements and point mutations in these domains.

Findings.—Although no gross rearrangement of DNA was found, at least 29 exons were identified from patients with CADASIL. Analysis of 14 of these exons for which flanking intron sequences were identified revealed 11 conformational variants. Nine of these mutations were found in distinct EGF-like domains and 1 was located within the *cdc-10* repeat domain (the eleventh mutation was found in both patients and controls). Sequencing revealed these aberrations were due to nucleotide substitutions, which resulted in a change in amino acid synthesis.

Conclusions.—The missense mutations identified in patients with CADASIL could severely disrupt *Notch3* protein synthesis. The exact relationship between *Notch3* mutations and the development of CADASIL is not known, but in *Drosophila*, mutations in Notch genes result in different phenotypic alterations depending on whether they are present in intracellular or extracellular domains. Notably, phenotypes did not differ between patients with mutations in EGF-like and Cdc-10 domains and those with mutations in distinct EGF domains. In summary, the Notch signalling pathway may play a role in the pathogenesis of CADASIL and other cerebrovascular diseases.

► Vascular dementia is the second leading cause of dementia after Alzheimer's disease. It may occur in a sporadic manner or in a familial pattern. Cerebral autosomal dominant arteriopathy with subcortical infarcts and leukoencephalopathy (CADASIL) is a recently described disease of small arteries mainly affecting the subcortical regions of the brain. It is an inherited disorder that has been the subject of genetic linkage studies in multiple families.[1] Starting during mid-adulthood, it involves recurrent ischemic attacks, either transient or permanent, resulting in multiple small, deep cerebral infarcts and leukoencephalopathy. CADASIL is a diffuse angiopathy of small cerebral arteries that has been demonstrated to include morphologic changes in vascular smooth muscle cells. Clinically, subjects experience attacks of migraine with aura, severe mood disorders, strokes, and eventually vascular dementia.[2]

Initial gene linkage studies localized the disorder to chromosome 19pl3.1.[3] Using positional cloning techniques based on localization to highly polymorphic microsatellite markers, this report describes mutations involving the *Notch3* gene which could be the defective protein in CADASIL patients. The *Notch1* gene has been implicated in adult T-cell leukemia. A remarkable fact is that the Notch gene family was initially described in *Drosophila* where it functions as a receptor which serves to transmit extracellular signals that play an essential role in specifying cell development. The ultimate question is how mutations in this gene affect vascular smooth muscle function in man.

J.R. Shapiro, M.D.

References

1. Chabriat H, Tournier-Lasserve E, Vahedi K, et al: Autosomal dominant migraine with MRI white matter abnormalities mapping to the CADASIL locus. *Neurology* 45:1086–1091, 1995.
2. Ragno M, Tournier-Lasserve E, Fiori MG, et al: An Italian kindred with cerebral autosomal dominant arteriopathy with subcortical infarcts and leukoencephalopathy (CADASIL). *Ann Neurol* 38:231–236, 1995.
3. Vérin M, Rolland Y, Landgraf F, et al: New phenotype of the cerebral autosomal dominant arteriopathy mapped to chromosome 19: Migraine as the prominent clinical feature. *J Neurol Neurosurg Psychiatry* 59:579–585, 1995.

6 Geriatric Nursing

Introduction

Providing science-based nursing care to older adults across a wide variety of settings continues to be a challenge for geriatric nurses. The literature is now developing rapidly, which will improve the scientific basis of nursing practice, and this year a variety of excellent papers have been selected to exemplify these advances. This chapter is divided into five subsections: (1) Decision-making and Patient Competence; (2) Caring for Residents with Dementia; (3) Patient and Family Education; (4) Cost-Effectiveness; and (5) Staff Training and Satisfaction.

A major theme in geriatric nursing literature this year was decision-making and patient competence. Four articles are included in this subsection to give readers a flavor of the discussion. Kelly-Powell (Abstract 6–1) provides a qualitative analysis of decision-making under potentially life-threatening conditions and Lander et al. (Abstract 6–2) discuss the effects of decisions, like involuntary relocation, on nursing home residents. End-of-life decisions continue to be discussed in the nursing literature because nurses have a major role in obtaining advance directions and in carrying them out, especially in long-term care settings. In this subsection Mezey and colleagues (Abstract 6–3) discuss the nurse's role in implementation of the Patient Self-Determination Act (PSDA). The final entry (Abstract 6–4) is an interesting study on nurses' views of appropriate medical care in nursing homes.

Providing compassionate, competent care to older adults who are unable to communicate their needs continues to be a challenge for geriatric nurses. At least one half of all residents of nursing homes, and many elderly cared for by family members at home, have some dementia that complicates the daily caregiving process and places them at risk of receiving poor care. An article by Algase et al. (Abstract 6–5)—redefining these behaviors from "disruptive" to "need-driven" and providing a framework for nursing interventions to reduce wandering, resistance to care, inappropriate sexual behavior, and verbal and physical aggression—leads off the second subsection. Other articles in this section (Abstracts 6–6 through 6–10) report strategies for making bathing more pleasurable, decreasing restraints, avoiding falls, assessing discomfort, and making tube feedings more nutritious.

In this era of technology, nurses have many options for obtaining good clinical outcomes through innovative patient and family education. This subsection (Abstracts 6–11 through 6–14) has articles discussing production of preoperative videotapes for at-home use, electronic monitoring of medication compliance, workshops for patients with urinary incontinence, and diabetic education for caregivers.

The cost of medical care, especially for the elderly, continues to be a hotly debated issue. Three articles in this section report on issues and approaches to improving cost-effective treatment of common problems: lack of up-to-date immunizations (Abstract 6–15), oral mucositis during cancer chemotherapy (Abstract 6–16), and acute stroke care and rehabilitation (Abstract 6–17). The final article (Abstract 6–18) demonstrates the cost-effectiveness of a comprehensive family caregiver program that decreases costs by delaying nursing home placement.

The final subsection of this chapter on geriatric nursing includes two articles (Abstracts 6–19 and 6–20) that discuss what is basic to the delivery of quality care in nursing facilities: a stable, knowledgeable staff. Their findings that Alzheimer's Special Care Units have greater staff satisfaction and less turnover than traditional units have implications for changes in educational and organizational policies in the entire nursing home industry.

Sharon K. Ostwald Ph.D., R.N., C.S.

Decision-making and Patient Competence

Personalizing Choices: Patients' Experiences With Making Treatment Decisions

Kelly-Powell ML (Edgewood College, Madison, Wis)
Res Nurs Health 20:219–227, 1997 6–1

Objective.—The variables involved in patients' choices of treatment for life-threatening illnesses have not been well studied. Results of a study of the decision-making experiences of patients making choices about treatment for a potentially life-threatening illness are presented.

Methods.—Interviews were conducted with 18 adults (9 women) being treated for heart disease ($n = 3$), cancer ($n = 5$), or renal failure ($n = 9$), including 1 who had terminated treatment for colon cancer. Interviews were repeated 1 month later with 15 patients, and a third interview was conducted with 4 patients. Interviewers' observations of patients' behavior, mannerisms, and physical appearance were included. Variables in the decision-making process were identified.

Results.—The core variable in the decision-making process was 'personalizing choices' and encompassed feelings of faith, trust, love, support, values, and beliefs. Interpretations of the past, including perceptions of family history, past personal experiences, and experiences of others also contributed to the decision-making process by providing a frame of reference. Patients' choices also involved sustaining normal lives and roles for themselves, protecting their psychic integrity, and preserving personal relationships. Patients selected options that allowed them to maintain hope and optimism for themselves or for their children. Most patients trusted their doctors. Although most refused to predict the course of their illnesses, they continued to feel they had made the right treatment decisions. Most patients were reconciled to the fact that they might die.

Conclusion.—Patients make treatment decisions in life-threatening situations based on personal values and beliefs and perceptions of self and family. Physician trust and attitudes of health care providers are important factors in choosing treatment options.

▶ The right of older patients to make decisions regarding their own lives—where they will live and what treatments they will permit—is sometimes called into question. However, the quality of one's life and the cost of health care hinge on those decisions. Little is known about how patients make treatment decisions. A better understanding of that process may enlighten the discussion of how to support patients in making difficult decisions and how to determine when they need assistance with those decisions. The author uses a grounded theory approach to describe decision-making under potentially life-threatening conditions. In another article, Willis[1] uses a longitudinal, quantitative approach to investigate the question of everyday cognitive competence. Willis concludes that for individuals with no known pathology, the decline in decision-making competence is very modest between the ages of 60 and 75. The rate of decline increases after the age of 75 and for individuals who are educationally disadvantaged. However, competence in making decisions is multidimensional, and nurses need to support the individual's right to make those decisions until proven incompetent.

S.K. Ostwald, Ph.D., R.N., C.S.

Reference

1. Willis SL: Everyday cognitive competence in elderly persons: Conceptual issues and empirical findings. *Gerontologist* 36:595–601, 1996.

Intrainstitutional Relocation: Effects on Residents' Behavior and Psychosocial Functioning

Lander SM, Brazill AL, Ladrigan PM (Univ of Rochester, NY; Monroe Community Hosp, Rochester, NY; Nazareth College of Rochester, NY)

J Gerontol Nurs 23:35–41, 1997 6–2

Objective.—The effect of relocation on the cognitively impaired elderly is not known because most studies have focused on elderly individuals who are able to make a cognitive appraisal of the process. Results of a prospective study comparing the effect of intrainstitutional relocation on the behavior and psychosocial functioning of nursing home residents with no psychological disorders versus those with cognitive, mood, and psychotic disorders are presented.

Methods.—Medical and nursing information and results of the Multidimensional Observation Scale for Elderly Subjects behavioral and psychosocial functioning assessment were obtained for 78 residents relocated intrainstitutionally 1 month before the move and at 1 and 3 months after the move. A comprehensive pre-move intervention involved patients; medical, psychiatric, and nursing staffs; families; departments; and construction, administration, and maintenance personnel 2 months before the move.

Results.—There was no correlation between relocation after 1 or 3 months and the number of emergency department or psychiatric visits, admissions, or consultations. There was a significant increase in the number of medical visits by 3 months after the move; a significant weight loss among those with a mood or psychiatric disorder from 1 month before to 1 month after the move; a nonsignificant increase in the number of falls 1 month after relocation, particularly in those residents who had been in the facility longer; and a significant difference in self-care and withdrawn behavior 3 months after the move in patients with a cognitive impairment. The mortality rate was unchanged from the previous year.

Conclusion.—Careful planning, premove interventions, and follow-up probably explain why residents involved in the relocation process did so well. The diet and weight of residents with mood and psychotic disorders should be monitored to avoid weight loss after relocation. Using family and volunteers to familiarize residents with their surroundings may decrease falls after relocation. Increasing staff and lighting during the first 2 weeks of a move and reinstituting normal routines quickly will help alleviate stress.

Clinical Significance.—A concerted premove effort to inform staff and elderly residents of, and involve them in, the relocation process can decrease the stress and resulting psychiatric and medical consequences of relocation.

► Although community-dwelling older persons change their residences only after much thought and significant preparations, residents in nursing homes may be moved with little warning at the discretion of the nursing facility. Not only are the vulnerable, frail elderly moved within nursing facilities, but also they may be moved to different facilities, especially following extended hospitalizations. Multilevel facilities are based on the fact that residents will be moved to higher levels of care, usually on different floors or in different buildings, rather than more intensive services being brought to them. This article is of interest because it documents prospectively some of the negative physical and psychological consequences of relocating residents during building renovation. The authors also suggest specific premove interventions to minimize relocation stress.

S.K. Ostwald, Ph.D., R.N., C.S.

Implementation of the Patient Self-Determination Act (PSDA) in Nursing Homes in New York City

Mezey M, Mitty E, Rappaport M, et al (New York Univ; RL Associates Inc, Princeton, NJ)

J Am Geriatr Soc 45:43–49, 1997 6–3

Objective.—Under the Patient Self Determination Act (PSDA), patients in a health care facility must be informed of their right to execute a living will or durable power of attorney for health care. The results of a New York City telephone survey developed to estimate how many residents made a directive are presented.

Methods.—Social workers in 109 (69%) nursing homes in New York City were surveyed by telephone regarding their knowledge of the following: the PSDA, information provided to residents about a living will and durable power of attorney, determination of a patient's capacity to make a responsible decision, perceptions of the effect of the PSDA, awareness of ethics committees, follow-up and documentation in the patient's medial record, and staff and community education.

Results.—Social workers were very familiar with the PSDA in 60% of nursing homes and unfamiliar with it in 20%. There were ethics committees in 47 nursing homes, with 74% having ongoing staff education. Of the 61% of homes offering community education, 87% provided information to family members, and 25% provided information to the community.

TABLE 3.—Size, Religious Affiliation, Ethics Committees, and Health Care Proxies Per Bed in Voluntary and Proprietary Nursing Homes in New York City (n = 100)

Characteristics	Voluntary (n = 44)	Proprietary (n = 56)	Significance
Size (mean ± SD)	325.12 (±98.84)	214.89 (±98.84)	$t(95) = -3.65$ $P < .001$
Proportion of patients with a health care proxy	0.1871 (±0.237)	0.1204 (±0.194)	$t(73) = 1.33$ $P = .188$
Religious affiliation			$\chi^2 = 7.3$, $df = 1$
% Yes (n = 45)	59	32	$P = .007$
% No (n = 55)	41	68	
Ethics Committee			$\chi^2 = 8.7$, $df = 1$
% Yes (n = 47)	63	34	$P = .003$
% No (n = 51)	37	66	
Always transfer terminally ill residents			$\chi^2 = 11.9$, $df = 1$
% Yes (n = 23)	10	33	$P = .001$
% No (n = 77)	90	67	
IVs in nursing home			$\chi^2 = 4.9$, $df = 1$
% Yes (n = 40)	52	30	$P < .03$
% No (n = 55)	48	70	
Honor verbal directives			$\chi^2 = 5.14$, $df = 1$
% Yes (n = 73)	82	68	$P < .03$
% No (n = 27)	18	32	

(Courtesy of Mezey M, Mitty E, Rappaport M, et al: Implementation of the patient self-determination act (PSDA) in nursing homes in New York City. *J Am Geriatr Soc* 45[1]:43–49, 1997.)

Individual patient PSDA counseling sessions were provided by 97% of the nursing homes surveyed. Reviews were conducted at least annually by 63% of the nursing homes surveyed. The patient's capacity to execute a directive was based on the physician's judgment alone in 39% of homes and on the physician's and social worker's judgment in 61%. Written procedures for determining capacity were available in only 35% of homes. In homes with an ethics committee, 45% had written procedures, compared with 26% of homes without an ethics committee. The percentage of residents with an advanced directive was more than 60% in 10% of homes, 21% to 60% in 47% of homes, less than 20% in 24% of homes, and no data were provided in 19% of homes. Voluntary homes were significantly more likely to honor the letter as well as the intent of the act (Table 3).

Conclusion.—Large, voluntary nursing homes are more likely to have ethics committees and to address PSDA issues with patients and staff.

Clinical Significance.—An effort needs to be made to help nursing homes implement the PSDA and address staff and patient education, determine patient capacity to make decisions, and establish an ethics committee, and ensure that patients' directives are reviewed and followed.

► Although all health care facilities are mandated by the Patient Self-Determination Act (1991) to inform patients of their right to execute an advance directive, the implementation of this act differs significantly from facility to facility. Generally, nursing homes have been more effective than hospitals in complying with this mandate. However, this process is complicated by the fact that a large proportion of patients admitted to nursing facilities have some degree of mental impairment. Researchers found that the majority of facilities did not have written policies for determining a resident's decision-making capacity. In a related retrospective cohort study in a different state, Bradley et al.[1] concluded that substantial numbers of nursing home residents may be excluded from participating in discussions because of difficulties in determining their capacity to discuss their treatment wishes. Because a fundamental intent of the PSDA is to give the individual control over his or her own medical decisions, gerontological professionals need to re-examine the process for providing information and determining decision-making capacity. Because nurses are most often charged with informing patients about advance directives, the readers are referred to a protocol by Mezey et al.[2] to assist them in this important role.

S.K. Ostwald, Ph.D., R.N., C.S.

References

1. Bradley E, Walker L, Blechner B, et al: Assessing capacity to participate in discussions of advance directives in nursing homes: Findings from a study of the Patient Self Determination Act. *J Am Geriatr Soc* 45:79–83, 1997.
2. Mezey M, Bottrell MM, Ramsey G, et al: Advance Directives Protocol: Nurses helping to protect patients' rights. *Geriatr Nurs* 17:204–210, 1996.

Medical Care in Old Age: What Do Nurses in Long-term Care Consider Appropriate?

Gillick MR, Mendes ML (Beth Israel Hosp, Boston; Harvard Med School, Boston; George Washington Univ, Washington, DC)

J Am Geriatr Soc 44:1322–1325, 1996 6–4

Background.—In discussions of advance directives, it is generally assumed that people's choices depend solely on personal preference, with little attention to their health status before acute illness. However, for elderly people preexisting health status may affect not only quality of life and preferences for care, but also the capacity to tolerate medical interventions. People may opt for progressively less vigorous treatments as they progress from good health to frailty. This hypothesis was tested in a study of nurses working in a long-term care facility who know about the various conditions affecting older people.

Methods.—The study included nurses working at a large long-term care facility with a mean resident age of 88. Of 145 eligible nurses, 102 completed the study questionnaire. Respondents completed a specific advance directive for themselves, indicating what care they would desire under various conditions: terminal illness, dementia with chronic illness, chronic illness while living in a nursing home, chronic illness while living in the community, and robust health while living in the community. The results were assessed in terms of refusal rate, that is, the mean number of interventions refused per respondent.

Results.—Under all 5 conditions combined, the overall refusal rate was 72%. Refusal rate was highest, 91%, for the terminal illness scenario. For the other conditions, refusal rate was 82% for dementia plus chronic illness, 69% for dementia while living in a nursing home, 71% for chronic illness while living at home, and 50% for robust health while living at home. Refusal rates in the different scenarios varied by the severity of the interventions (Table 1). Nurses who worked with more impaired patients tended to refuse more interventions.

Conclusions.—Nurses who are experienced in working with institutionalized elderly people express strong preferences for the types of medical interventions they would want to have in old age under varying health conditions. These health-care professionals indicate that they would refuse more interventions as their level of physical and cognitive impairment increased. Advance planning is needed to find out what treatments would be considered appropriate under varying circumstances, not just terminal illness, dementia, or coma.

▶ With increases in technology and concern over scarce resources, prolonging life has become increasing controversial. Previous research has shown that health-care professionals are impacted by providing care that they consider to be futile. In an earlier study by Solomon et al.,[1] approximately 50% of nurses claimed to have acted against their consciences in giving care to the terminally ill. Although the discussion of medical futility

TABLE 1.—Refusal Rates for Aggressive, Moderately Aggressive, and Minimally Aggressive Interventions

	Healthy Age 85 years	Chronically Ill Age 75 years	Demented in NH	Demented, Chronically Ill, in NH	Dying
Aggressive interventions					
CPR, Ventilator, Dialysis, Chemotherapy	76.8%	92.6%	91.3%	96.3%	98.5%
Moderately Aggressive interventions					
Major surgery, invasive tests, artificial nutrition, blood transfusion	50.6%	78.2%	79.0%	89.9%	97.0%
Minimally aggressive interventions					
Minor surgery, simple diagnostic tests, antibiotics	13.6%	31.6%	25.8%	50.7%	75.1%
P value	<.001	<.001	<.001	<.001	<.001

(Courtesy of Gillick MR, Mendes ML: Medical care in old age: What do nurses in long-term care consider appropriate? *J Am Geriatr Soc* 44[11]:1322–1325, 1996.)

has primarily occurred in the acute hospital setting, especially in intensive care units, nurses in long-term care facilities are faced daily with caring for residents with severe mental and physical disabilities. It is not a surprise to find that nurses working in long-term care favor limitations of treatment in old age, especially for those with severe physical and cognitive impairment. This finding does not suggest that individual nurses should limit care, but rather that discussions be expanded to include what constitutes appropriate care in a broad range of circumstances. It also suggests that long-term care facilities need to discuss the possibility of facility-wide futility policies, such as is occurring with increasing frequency in acute care settings.

S.K. Ostwald, Ph.D., R.N., C.S.

Reference

1. Solomon MZ, O'Donnell L, Jennings B, et al: Decisions near the end of life: Professional views on life-sustaining treatments. *Am J Pub Health* 83:14–23, 1993.

Caring for Residents with Dementia

Need-driven Dementia-compromised Behavior: An Alternative View of Disruptive Behavior

Algase DL, Beck C, Kolanowski A, et al (Univ of Michigan, Ann Arbor; Univ of Arkansas, Little Rock; Wilkes Univ, Wilkes Barre, Pa; et al)

Am J Alzheimer Dis 11:10–19, 1996 6–5

Objective.—Attempts to explain the disruptive behaviors of elderly demented patients have not been completely successful. These behaviors may arise from a need by the cognitively impaired individual to express needs. An investigation of background factors may explain these need-driven, dementia-compromised behaviors (NDB) (Fig 1).

Wandering, Vocalizations, and Aggression.—Wandering may reflect a loss of ability to find one's way, forgetting a destination or goal, walking toward something that attracts attention. The need to communicate may be impaired because of memory loss. Vocalization may express a need for sensory stimulation or to draw attention to discomfort. Aggression results from frustration, cortical damage, and need for assistance with activities of daily living.

Background Factors Affecting NDB.—Neurologic damage, regional CNS damage including poor parietal lobe functioning, reduction in the brain's ability to use or eliminate excess neurotransmitters, lessening ability to process information, and disturbed circadian distribution of locomotor and motor activity to satisfy personal needs.

Cognitive Factors.—Basic attention and memory skills may be impaired and result in resistive behavior. Perceptual and sensory skills impairment may lead to inability to identify what is seen, heard, and smelled. Inability to express one's needs with language may result in dysfunctional vocalizations.

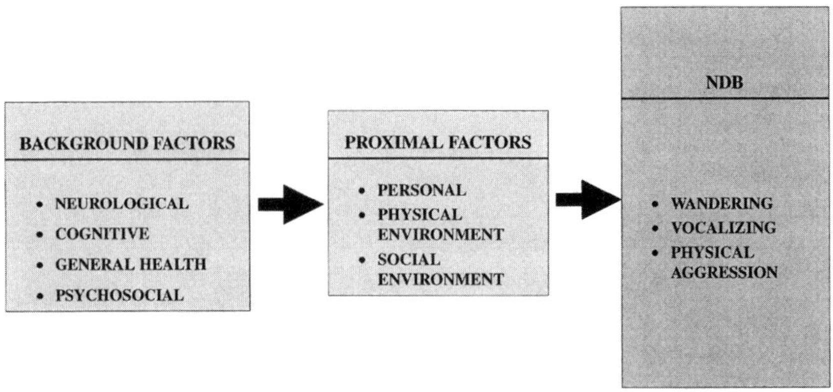

FIGURE 1.—Factors affecting NDB (Courtesy of Algase DL, Beck C, Kolanowski A, et al: Need-driven dementia-compromised behavior: An alternative view of disruptive behavior. *Am J Alzheimer Dis* 11:10–19, 1996).

Health Status.—Patients with more physical problems tend to exhibit more aggressive behaviors. The decline in functional behavior parallels the decline in cognitive function.

Psychosocial Factors.—Associations between demographic factors and behavior have not been demonstrated unequivocally. Personality change is associated with NDB. Wandering may be a stress-coping behavior. Aggression is more often found in patients with delusions or those with financial problems during their lives.

Personal Factors Affecting NDB.—Need states such as pain, fatigue, and hunger; an inability to perform because of caregiver or environmental constraints or decline in function performance; restrictions imposed by the physical environment; or a decline in social contacts may result in NDB.

Applications to Practice and Research.—Developing a conceptual framework that would integrate clinical findings and empirical data to predict behaviors on the basis of a pattern of cognitive impairments may result in improving communication with demented patients. Patients, for example, may respond better to gestures rather than conversation, may wander less if their social interactions are increased, may decrease vocalizations if provided with stimulation, and may stop or decrease aggressive behaviors if made to feel more secure or respected.

► A significant number of residents of long-term care facilities who have a diagnosis of dementia display behaviors that are labeled as "disruptive" by the staff. Algase and colleagues propose a framework for studying these behaviors that considers their purpose or meaning to the residents who display them. This framework appears to have the potential to organize some of the disparate research that currently exists on resident behaviors and, thereby, facilitate the development of new, more effective interventions. Additional help for the gerontologic nurse who is currently confronting the need to manage disruptive behaivors can be found in the November 1996 issue of the *Journal of Gerontological Nursing.* A series of 5 articles discuss the same disruptive behaviors (categorized using Kolanowski's 1995 formulation) that are addressed in the framework presented by Algase et al. These articles include detailed decision trees in which strategies for managing the behaviors are linked to the theoretically corresponding etiology.[1-5]

S.K. Ostwald, Ph.D., R.N., C.S.

References

1. Coltharp W Jr, Richie MF, Kaas MJ: Wandering. *J Gerontol Nurs* 22:5–10, 1996.
2. Potts HW, Richie MF, Kaas MJ: Resistance to care. *J Gerontol Nurs* 22:11–16, 1996.
3. Philo Sw, Richie MF, Kaas MJ: Inappropriate sexual behavior. *J Gerontol Nurs* 22:17–22, 1996.
4. White MK, Kaas MJ, Richie MF: Vocally disruptive behavior. *J Gerontol Nurs* 22:23–29, 1996.
5. Chou KR, Kaas MJ, Richie MF: Assaultive behavior in geriatric patients. *J Gerontol Nurs* 22:31–38, 1996.

Reducing Aggressive Behavior During Bathing Cognitively Impaired Nursing Home Residents

Hoeffer B, Rader J, McKenzie D, et al (Oregon Health Sciences Univ, Portland; Benedictine Inst for Long Term Care, Portland, Ore)

J Gerontol Nurs 23:16–23, 1997 6–6

Objective.—The physically aggressive behavior displayed by cognitively impaired nursing home residents during caregiving is a defensive response to a perceived threat. A pilot study was instituted to test interventions aimed at preventing or reducing aggressive behavior of cognitively impaired nursing home residents during bathing.

Methods.—Ten severely cognitively impaired, aggressive residents (8 women), age 86–98, housed at least 5 months in a 76-bed proprietary intermediate care facility, were bathed by 3 nursing assistants. A clinical nurse specialist (CNS) observed the bathing procedure and worked with each assistant for 3–8 baths to help the assistant change the psychosocial and physical environment by introducing flexibility into the schedule, modifying verbal and nonverbal approaches, evaluating the residents' behavioral cues, and developing an individualized bathing plan. Residents' behaviors and nursing assistants' ratings before and after interventions were recorded.

Results.—Scores for physical and verbal aggression and being upset declined significantly from preintervention to postintervention. Assistants found postintervention bathing to be significantly less frustrating, challenging, or frightening, and it was accomplished more quickly. Assistants' feelings toward residents were essentially unchanged.

Conclusion.—Changing the psychosocial and physical bathing environment of aggressive, cognitively impaired nursing home residents and individualizing the bathing plan significantly reduced aggressive behavior.

▶ It is well known that many of the aggressive behaviors displayed by cognitively impaired individuals occur while they are receiving personal care and that personal care, such as bathing, is usually assigned to the least prepared staff members—the nursing assistants. This article presents a compassionate approach to increasing the pleasure of nursing home residents with the bath, thus reducing aggressive behaviors during bathing and making the experience more positive for the nursing assistants. This study occurred in a teaching home where the clinical nurse specialist was available to teach, role model, and support new bathing behaviors. It is important that nursing assistants receive organizational support for making care more personalized and humane. The entire May 1997 issue of the *Journal of Gerontological Nursing* is devoted to bathing updates, which readers may wish to peruse. In particular, Miller[1] offers suggestions for improving the safety of residents and nursing staff on a dementia unit, and Skewes[2] discusses the use of a bag bath.

S.K. Ostwald, Ph.D., R.N., C.S.

References

1. Miller MF: Physically aggressive resident behavior during hygienic care. *J Gerontol Nurs* 23:24–39, 1997.
2. Skewes SM: Bathing: It's a tough job! *J Gerontol Nurs* 23:45–49, 1997.

A Clinical Trial to Reduce Restraints in Nursing Homes

Evans LK, Strumpf NE, Allen-Talyor SL, et al (Univ of Pennsylvania, Philadelphia)

J Am Geriatr Soc 45:675–681, 1997 6–7

Objective.—Approximately 300,000 nursing home residents spend part of every day in restraints, despite research indicating that restraints, can lead to poor physical and psychological functioning, complications, falls, or death. No randomized clinical trial of the effects of reducing restraints has been conducted. A prospective 12-month clinical trial was conducted in 3 nursing homes, which were randomly assigned to a restraint education (RE), restraint education-with-consultation (REC), or control (C) group.

Methods.—The 6-month RE program, taught by a gerontologic nurse specialist, consisted of ten 30- to 45-minute sessions on the effects of physical restraint, resident behaviors, fall risk, preventing interference with medical treatment, and coping with patient behaviors. The REC program used the RE program, supplemented by 12 hours a week of concurrent, unit-based consultation. The control sites received no instruction or consultation. The nursing homes had a total of 643 residents over the age of 60. Restraint use was evaluated at baseline and at 1 year.

Results.—There were 463 residents who remained in the study for 1 year. At baseline, the control group had a significantly higher prevalence of restraint use than the RE or REC groups did. The average, relative decline from baseline in the use of restraints was 11% for the control group, 23% for the RE group, and a significant 56% for the REC group. The decline was preserved for 6 months after the study. The difference between the REC and C groups was significant, and the difference between the REC and RE groups was almost significant. The differences remained significant at each time point, regardless of attrition or differences between groups at baseline. If restraint use decreased, REC residents were 25% to 40% less likely to be restrained than C or RE residents, respectively. At 12 months, vest restraint use had declined 41%, 77%, and 85% for the RE, REC, and control groups, respectively. There was no increase in staff hours per resident during this time, and fall rates declined significantly during the study period.

Conclusion.—A 6-month program of restraint education and consultation significantly reduced restraint use in nursing homes without increasing staff hours or fall rates.

▶ The use of restraints to control behavior of residents in nursing homes was identified as a major problem in the 1980s. During the ensuing 10 years, a consensus was reached within the long-term care community that restraints do more harm than good. However, the question remained of how to best move toward restraint-free facilities. Drs. Evans and Strumpf have been leaders in demonstrating the value of staff education and consultation in moving toward that goal. This report of a clinical trial demonstrates the success of using a master's-prepared gerontologic nurse to provide staff education and consistent on-site staff consultation.

S.K. Ostwald, Ph.D., R.N., C.S.

Case-Control Study of Exposure to Medication and the Risk of Injurious Falls Requiring Hospitalization Among Nursing Home Residents

Mustard CA, Mayer T (Univ of Manitoba, Winnipeg)

Am J Epidemiol 145:738–745, 1997 6–8

Objective.—Medications may be an important and modifiable risk factor for falls among the elderly population. However, reports disagree about the risk of falls associated with specific types of medications. Confounding by indication poses potential problems with validity in this line of research. A case-control study was performed to assess the association between medication use and falling risk among the elderly, with an emphasis on maximizing external validity and controlling for underlying medical condition.

Methods.—The study used insurance data on 1,560 initial injurious falls among 14,744 residents of nursing homes in the Canadian province of Manitoba. In each case, the injury was severe enough to require hospital

TABLE 2.—Odds Ratios of Injurious Falls Associated With Medication Use in the Previous 30 Days, by Medication Class, Manitoba, Canada, 1987–1992

Medication class	Medication prevalence (% of cases)	Series 1—Controls matched on age and sex (n = 1,486 matched pairs)		Series 2—Controls matched on age, sex, dependency level, and duration of residence (n = 1,486 matched pairs)		Series 3—Controls matched on age, sex, dependency level, duration of residence, and underlying disorder (n = 1,486 matched pairs)	
		OR	95% CI	OR	95% CI	OR	95% CI
Inotropic agents	8.2	0.76*	0.60–0.97	0.73†	0.57–0.94	0.69†	0.54–0.89
Calcium channel blocking agents	3.6	1.00	0.65–1.52	1.01	0.67–1.52	1.02	0.68–1.51
Beta blocking agents	2.6	1.03	0.64–1.67	0.97	0.62–1.52	1.04	0.64–1.63
Antihypertensive agents	5.6	1.01	0.73–1.38	1.05	0.76–1.45	0.91	0.68–1.26
Vasodilating agents	6.3	1.08	0.79–1.48	1.02	0.75–1.38	0.86	0.64–1.17
Other cardiovascular agents	0.7	0.89	0.37–2.04	1.12	0.47–2.67	0.64	0.29–1.40
Nonsteroidal antiinflammatory agents	17.5	1.17	0.97–1.41	0.95	0.79–1.15	1.11	0.92–1.33
Antidepressants	13.3	1.18	0.95–1.46	0.93	0.76–1.14	0.92	0.75–1.12
Antipsychotic agents	15.6	1.32†	1.08–1.62	1.51‡	1.23–1.85	1.31†	1.06–1.61
Anxiolytics/sedatives/hypnotics	14.5	1.59‡	1.27–1.98	1.28*	1.03–1.58	1.35†	1.09–1.68
Diuretics	20.2	0.97	0.82–1.16	1.05	0.89–1.29	0.97	0.82–1.15
Narcotic/opiod analgesic	16.7	1.34†	1.08–1.64	1.39†	1.13–1.70	1.18	0.96–1.45

*$P < 0.05$.
†$P < 0.01$.
‡$P < 0.001$.
Abbreviations: OR, odds ratio; *CI*, confidence interval.
(Courtesy of Mustard CA, Mayer T: Case-control study of exposure to medication and the risk of injurious falls requiring hospitalization among nursing home residents. *Am J Epidemiol* 145:738–745, 1997.)

admission for treatment. Pharmacy records were used to assess medication use. The study used 3 series of pair-matched single controls for each case, with increasingly stringent matching for age, sex, level of dependency, duration of residence, and chronic diseases.

Results.—On multivariate analysis, 4 classes of drugs were significantly related to risk of injurious falls in at least 1 case-control series: inotropic agents, antipsychotic agents, anxiolytics/sedatives/hypnotics, and narcotic/opioid analgesics (Table 2). In the most stringently controlled series, 2 medication classes significantly increased the risk of injurious falls if dispensed within the previous 30 days: antipsychotic agents, odds ratio 1.31, and anxiolytics/sedatives/hypnotics, odds ratio 1.35. Surprisingly, inotropic agents had a protective effect against falls, odds ratio 0.69. Confounding by indication did not seem to pose a significant threat to these inferences.

Conclusions.—Among nursing home residents, use of psychotropic medications is an independent risk factor for injurious falls. The data suggest that about 20% of the risk of injurious falls may be attributed to anxiolytic/sedative/hypnotic agents and antipsychotic agents. It may be possible to prevent some injurious falls in the nursing home through the use of nonpharmaceutical approaches to behavioral management.

▶ Many studies have identified risk factors for falls among the elderly. However, this study is particularly helpful in that it uses a large database of nursing home patients, carefully defines injurious falls, and has specific and accurate information on the use of medications at the time of the fall. Because the offending medications (antipsychotics and sedatives/hypnotics) are primarily used to control behavior, it is clear that nonpharmacologic strategies need to be strongly encouraged as the primary management tools for behavioral problems in frail elderly nursing home residents. Nursing staff need to be thoroughly educated in the use of behavioral analysis and understand the array of appropriate nursing interventions that can reduce the need for medications which increase residents' risk for injury.

S.K. Ostwald, Ph.D., R.N., C.S.

The Assessment of Discomfort in Elderly Confused Patients: A Preliminary Study

Miller J, Neelon V, Dalton J, et al (Univ of North Carolina, Chapel Hill)
J Neurosci Nurs 28:175–182, 1996 6–9

Introduction.—There are several possible causes of discomfort in hospitalized elderly patients, including chronic diseases, treatment-associated pain, and problems related to immobility. A reliable, clinically applicable tool is needed for effective management of discomfort in confused elderly patients. Several measures of discomfort were evaluated for use in evaluating nursing interventions to reduce or prevent discomfort in confused elderly hospital patients.

Methods.—Four different approaches were evaluated: questioning the patient about discomfort; using the discomfort thermometer, which used the concept of the visual analog scale; using the Discomfort Screen, a modification of a tool developed in a previous study of confused elderly patients; and using the Discomfort Scale for Patients with Dementia of the Alzheimer's Type (DS-DAT), a 9-item objective measure. Other instruments included the NEECHAM Confusion Scale and the Katz Index of ADL. Elderly hospitalized patients were evaluated each day for confusion and discomfort by all 4 instruments. All assessments were performed in the morning, when many procedures involving possible patient discomfort are done.

Results.—The analysis included 46 patients with an average age of 83. Twenty-seven percent could not provide complete information because of communication or cognitive deficits. The range of scores on the DS-DAT was similar in situations that were not likely to involve discomfort. However, the mean discomfort score was higher in situations involving likely discomfort. There were problems in administering the physical assessment subscale of the Discomfort Screen—certain items were grouped together, whereas others were not well defined. Thirteen percent of patients could not respond to questioning about discomfort. Patients with higher NEECHAM scores were better able to report comfort or discomfort. Even with cueing, nearly three fourths of patients could not use the discomfort thermometer. Overall, responses to the question of discomfort were significantly related to the discomfort score on the DS-DAT. Scores on the discomfort thermometer were not significantly related to the patients' observed discomfort.

Conclusions.—Patient self-report appears to be inadequate for the assessment of discomfort in confused elderly patients. The DS-DAT is a potentially useful observational measure. However, in its current form it is not practical for use in routine nursing care. Nurses caring for acutely confused elderly patients must be aware of the likelihood of patient discomfort and provide appropriate interventions.

► This study explores the clinical use, validity, and reliability of 4 different approaches to nursing assessment of discomfort in elderly confused patients. It is a welcome addition to the literature. Nurses who work with the confused elderly have long maintained that patient self-report, the most common practice for assessing pain, is inadequate in this cohort. The finding from this study, that current standards of practice that rely on patient self-report of discomfort are not an adequate means of assessing confused elderly patients, opens the door for further exploration of better ways to assess pain. Anticipating the likelihood of pain is the first step toward developing strategies that provide for comfort, and perhaps even decrease confusion, in elderly patients.

S.K. Ostwald, Ph.D., R.N., C.S.

The Effect of Dietary Fiber in Tube-fed Elderly Patients

Bass DJ, Forman LP, Abrams SE, et al (Harris Continued Care Hosp, Fort Worth, Tex; Appalachian State Univ, Boone, NC; East Tennessee State Univ, Johnson City; et al)

J Gerontol Nurs 22:37–44, 1996 6–10

Objective.—Elderly patients receiving nutrition through a feeding tube are frequently at risk because of complications resulting from prolonged diarrhea. Soluble fiber delays voiding, increases fluid and nutrient absorption, and maintains the bacterial content of the gut. Controlling diarrhea by using fiber-containing enteral feeding formulas is a promising new treatment.

Methods.—A retrospective review was conducted of records of 50 patients (21 females), age 28–83, who required tube feeding for a least 3 weeks. Feeding formulas were coded as fiber-containing or fiber-free (Table 2). The fiber formula contained a soy polysaccharide and had an osmolality of 300–350. Bowel movements and consistencies were recorded.

Results.—Patients receiving the FCF formula had significantly more liquid/loose stools than patients receiving the FFF diet (12.9 vs. 3.0) and significantly more formed stools (49.6 vs. 19.5). Age was not correlated with number or consistency of stools.

Conclusion.—Nurses, dieticians, and physicians need to cooperate in designing protocols that maximize the benefits to patients of tube feeding. Nurses in particular are interested in decreasing the incidence of diarrhea in patients on long-term enteral support. Careful attention should be paid to elimination patterns of these patients to improve their outcome and control the cost of care.

► Diarrhea is a common complication of enteral feedings that may lead to dehydration, electrolyte imbalance, skin breakdown, and pressure ulcers in patients in acute and long-term care settings. This retrospective study, documenting the effect of dietary fiber in decreasing diarrhea in tube-fed

TABLE 2.—Comparison of Groups That Did/Did Not Consume Fiber

	FCF* (+Fiber)	FFF† (No Fiber)	Statistical Significance
Number of patients	35	15	
Mean age (yrs)	66.4	70.3	
Mean serum albumin concentration (g/dL)	2.77	2.73	
Mean number of liquid/ loose stools over 21 days‡	3.0±0.78	12.9±3.49	$p<0.014$
Mean number of formed stools over 21 days‡	49.6±4.14	19.5±2.84	$p<0.001$

*FCF: fiber-containing formula.
†FFF: fiber-free formula.
‡mean±SEM.
(Courtesy of Bass DJ, Forman LP, Abrams SE, et al: The effect of dietary fiber in tube-fed elderly patients. *J Gerontol Nurs* 22[10]:37–44, 1996.)

patients in a continuing care facility, is an example of an inexpensive interdisciplinary study that can have a significant impact on the quality of life of patients in long-term care settings. Additional observational and experimental studies are needed to determine the best nutritional supplements and enteral feeding protocols to prevent common complications, like diarrhea, in these patients.

S.K. Ostwald, Ph.D., R.N., C.S.

Patient and Family Education

A Video Approach to Interactive Patient Education

Maller CE, Twitty VJ, Sauve A (Veterans Affairs Med Ctr, Albuquerque, NM)
J PeriAnesth Nurs 12:82–88, 1997 6–11

Introduction.—The focus of the Joint Commission on Accreditation of Healthcare Organizations (JCAHO) on patient education requires a new approach to preoperative teaching programs as outpatient surgery becomes more prevalent. Using videotapes for patient education has proven to be as effective as other presentation methods and more effective than written information alone. Patients have responded positively. Little study has been devoted to the cost, time, and collaboration involved in producing a video. Formation of an interdisciplinary team to focus on patients' preoperative concerns led to a collaborative effort to develop patient education videotapes.

Methods.—Involving consumers in all phases of production of the videotapes fulfilled the JCAHO directive to make patient education interactive. A quality improvement model was designed to include teaching objectives such as allaying anxiety and enlisting the cooperation and participation of patients and their families in the surgical experience. Attendance was taken at education classes to assess the effectiveness of the videotape. To improve attendance, a more patient-centered approach was developed to provide better preoperative instruction to patients and their families. Improvements identified by patients included earlier information about surgery. Videotapes could be viewed continuously and privately at home. Patient education delivered by videotape was more available, more accessible, and more consistent.

Results.—The videotape received positive reviews from consumers. The estimated cost of production is $1,000 per minute, or $14,000 for the 14-minute tape. The tape allowed perianesthesia care unit nurses to reach and instruct more patients. Patients meet on tape the medical staff that will be treating them in the hospital. Patients are given the option of attending a class, viewing the videotape at home, or reading printed materials.

Conclusion.—Patients approve highly of instructive preoperative videotapes that prepare them for surgery. Although the tapes are expensive to produce, they can be used again by other patients when they are returned.

▶ Shortened hospital stays and a dramatic increase in day surgery have posed challenges for nurses who are charged with providing interactive preoperative education to patients and their families. Last minute or inadequate patient education may have particularly negative consequences for older patients, who may need a slower paced delivery or repetition of important points. This article describes a process for working with consumers to produce personalized educational videotapes of common surgical procedures that can be viewed by patients in their homes before hospital admission. This also increases the likelihood that family members will receive the accurate information they need to provide optimal postoperative support. Video self-instruction kits also have proven effective for teaching older women the skills for performing breast self-examinations and for detecting lumps on the simulation model.[1] As society becomes more computer literate, the Internet will probably replace videotapes as the most accurate tool for providing education, freeing up time for nurses to address unique situations and specific questions.

S.K. Ostwald, Ph.D., R.N., C.S.

Reference

1. Wood RY: Breast self-examination proficiency in older women: Measuring the efficacy of video self-instruction kits. *Cancer Nurs* 19:429–435, 1996.

Assessing Medication Adherence by Pill Count and Electronic Monitoring in the African American Study of Kidney Disease and Hypertension (AASK) Pilot Study

Lee JY, for the AASK Pilot Study Investigators (Univ of Alabama, Birmingham; et al)

Am J Hypertens 9:719–725, 1996 6–12

Objective.—Accurate assessment of outcomes of clinical trials requires objective measures of medication adherence. Pill counts can be used but may be inaccurate and do not provide information on the interval between doses. Electronic monitors such as the Medication Event Monitoring System (MEMS) provide information on the date and time of bottle cap openings. There are few data about adherence to antihypertensive drug use among minority populations. Electronic monitoring and pill counts were used to assess medication adherence among patients in the African American Study of Kidney Disease and Hypertension (AASK) Pilot Study.

Methods.—The AASK Pilot Study included 94 African-American patients with hypertension and moderate impairment of renal function. They were randomized to 1 of 2 levels of blood pressure (mean arterial pressure at a low goal of 92 mm Hg or lower or the usual goal of 102 to 107 mm Hg) and to 1 of 3 antihypertensive drug regimens (a calcium channel blocker, an angiotensin converting enzyme inhibitor, or a β-blocker). For 91 patients, adherence was assessed by both MEMS recordings and pill counts. Adherence data were collected on a total of 313 regularly scheduled follow-up visits during an average follow-up of 5 months. As assessed

TABLE 4.—Proportion of Study Participants Who Achieved Goal Blood Pressure Medication

Pill Count	MEMS Adherent	MEMS Nonadherent	Total
Adherent	9/18 (50%)	5/32 (16%)	14/50 (28%)
Nonadherent	1/14 (17%)	3/17 (18%)	4/31 (13%)
Total	10/32 (31%)	8/49 (16%)	18/81 (22%)

(Reprinted by permission of Elsevier Science Inc. from Lee JY, for the AASK Pilot Study Investigators: Assessing Medication Adherence by Pill Count and Electronic Monitoring in the African American Study of Kidney Disease and Hypertension [AASK] Pilot Study. *Am J Hypertens* 9:719–725. Copyright 1996 by American Journal of Hypertension, Inc.)

by pill count, adherence was defined as acceptable if no more than 20% of the prescribed pills were returned to the clinic. By MEMS, adherence was deemed acceptable if the intervals between pill bottle openings were within 24 ± 6 hr. The effect of adherence on blood pressure control was analyzed.

Results.—Pill counts suggested that adherence was adequate for 68% of follow-up visits. However, the MEMS data showed noncompliance in 47% of these visits. Fifty percent of patients who were adherent by both pill count and MEMS throughout follow-up achieved their blood pressure goal. For patients who were nonadherent by either method, this figure dropped to 14% (Table 4).

Conclusions.—Electronic monitoring can aid in assessing compliance with antihypertensive medications. Providing MEMS data to patients and staff may offer a way of improving adherence. Some type of intervention is needed to promote medication adherence in African-American patients with hypertension.

▶ Patient adherence to medication schedules is a challenge, especially in those diseases, like hypertension, where patients experience few symptoms when they skip their medication doses. In this study, an electronic monitor that records the date and time the medication bottle was opened was added to the traditional pill counts to assess patterns of adherence. It provides a good example of how current technology can be used to provide information on adherence. Health professionals working with outpatients with chronic diseases should be encouraged to adopt this type of technology so they can provide more reliable feedback to patients and, thus, increase adherence to medication regimens and ultimately decrease complications from chronic diseases.

S.K. Ostwald, Ph.D., R.N., C.S.

Urinary Outcomes in Older Adults: Research and Clinical Perspectives

Palmer MH, Czarapata BJR, Wells TJ, et al (Natl Inst of Nursing Research, Baltimore, Md; Univ of Wisconsin, Madison)

Urol Nurs 17:2–9, 1997 6–13

Background.—Patient outcomes can be used clinically to measure treatment effectiveness and in research to identify groups of patients who could benefit from treatment and treatment modifications for various patient subgroups. A symposium at a recent Society of Urologic Nurses and Associates conference focused on urinary outcomes in older adults. The clinical and research uses of continence outcomes in long-term care and in the community are discussed.

Continence Outcomes in Long-term Care.—There are several types of interventions for long-term care residents with urinary incontinence. Habit training seeks to identify the voiding pattern and to keep that person dry with assistance. Decreased incontinence, rather than a normal micturition pattern, is the expected outcome. Prompted voiding aims to increase dryness and increase patient requests to use the toilet. The goals of scheduled checks and changes are to prevent infection and skin breakdown, enhance quality of life, and promote patient and staff satisfaction. Bladder training may be indicated for cooperative residents with the potential to achieve a normal micturition pattern.

In behavior modification interventions, compliance is essential to positive outcomes. Experience with these types of interventions in the long-term care setting has identified some factors important to achieving positive outcomes. The facility's administration must be supportive of the treatment program. This may range from tolerating the program to full support, including mandatory counseling for employees who do not comply with the program. Nursing staff support is also essential, including the nursing administration, continuing education personnel, and aide staff.

Continence Outcomes in Community Care.—The key principles for continence interventions in the community are to be clear about the treatment and to make no assumptions. In research, particularly for behavioral interventions, it is essential to define the treatment and its rationale exactly. It should not be assumed that the patient understands the directions in a certain way, that the patient is performing the treatment as instructed, and that the targeted behavior or physiology is being affected. It is important to test the patient's understanding of instructions and to determine the target of the treatment in the mechanism of urine control. The next step is wetting outcome measurement. There is no universally accepted measure for this outcome; options include the patient's opinion of wetting outcomes, patient diaries, and pad tests. Instruments for measuring the consequences of wetting include the Incontinence Impact Questionnaire and the Coping with Incontinence Scale. Outcome measurement is increasingly required for regulatory purposes. Having a common language about outcomes will facilitate communications among patients, clinicians, and researchers.

Genitourinary conditions are among the most frequently encountered diagnoses in home health care, and urinary incontinence is the most common of these. The psychological, physical, social, and financial consequences of this problem demand a consistent and systematic approach. There is no standard technique for evaluating the cause or severity of urinary incontinence, or for suggesting actions for further evaluation and treatment. There are few data on the treatment of patients with "intractable" urinary incontinence—these are usually impaired, frail elderly people who cannot respond to behavioral interventions. Measures to maintain social continence are a primary part of nursing care. They are widely used in homebound patients, often with the goal of management rather than cure. Still, knowledge of how to use these interventions, their complications, and the relevant patient outcomes may be lacking. The complex nature of urinary incontinence will increase the need, use, and cost of nursing care for homebound elderly patients. Nursing research must emphasize assessment of the outcomes of basic nursing interventions for this patient population.

Discussion.—The research and clinical implications of urinary outcomes in the elderly are discussed. Clinicians and researchers must work together to identify outcomes that better reflect incontinence interventions in terms of cost, quality, and effectiveness.

► Incontinence is a major problem for older adults. It has negative social consequences which can trigger institutionalization among frail older persons who live at home and can lead to medical complications, including infections and skin breakdown, for incontinent individuals regardless of their setting. This article presents four experts' perspectives on research issues and interventions that produce positive outcomes for older adults with urinary incontinence. The authors provide specific recommendations for measurement instruments which may help standardize the research into urinary outcomes. This article serves as a good update for nurses who work in community and long-term care settings and a call to test the effectiveness of nursing interventions with these patients. Readers also may wish to refer to two additional articles in the same issue that describe specific educational programs for urinary incontinence. Gallo and Sasso describe a pelvic floor stimulation pyramid of patient education that can be implemented in a busy clinical setting.[1] Gerard describes a 2-hour group education class that covered anatomy and physiology and treatment options, including behavior modification and pelvic muscle exercise.[2]

S.K. Ostwald, Ph.D., R.N., C.S.

References

1. Gallo M, Sasso K: Key components of patient education for pelvic floor stimulation in the treatment of urinary incontinence. *Urol Nurs* 17:10–16, 1997.
2. Gerard L: Group learning behavior modification and exercise for women with urinary incontinence. *Urol Nurs* 17:17–22, 1997.

The Care of Older Persons With Diabetes Mellitus: Families and Primary Care Physicians

Silliman RA, Bhatti S, Khan A, et al (Boston Univ; New England Med Ctr, Boston)

J Am Geriatr Soc 44:1314–1321, 1996 6–14

Purpose.—Studies have shown that family members are important care providers for frail elderly people. However, there are few data on the role they play in helping elderly patients with chronic diseases. Type II diabetes is a chronic disease of old age in which patients must actively cooperate in management for a prolonged period of time. The extent to which family members help older persons with diabetes manage their disease was examined.

Methods.—The longitudinal study included 357 family members of patients age 70 or older who were participating in the Patient Outcomes Research Team Study of type II diabetes. The current report presents the sample's responses to baseline questionnaires. The dependent variables analyzed were the extent to which family members assisted in diabetes-related care and in diabetes-related medical encounters.

Results.—Seventy-six percent of the family members were women, most often the wives of diabetic patients. Their mean age was 66. Depending on which aspect of diabetes care they were questioned about, 22% to 50% of family members reported helping the patient with diabetes care. Thirty-six percent were regular participants in the patient's medical encounters. In a multiple linear regression model, factors affecting family assistance with diabetes-related care included the patient's physical function, the family member's relationship to the patient, assistance with basic activities of daily living, and understanding of disease management issues. Factors affecting family members' participation in medical encounters included patient age and function, assistance with instrumental activities of daily living, and assistance with diabetes-related care.

Conclusions.—Many older patients with diabetes receive help in managing their disease from family members. In addition, one third of the family members studied participate in the patient's medical encounters. Patients with functional disability are more likely to receive help from their family members. Older patients with diabetes and other chronic diseases and their involved family members need education about care issues and support for their roles in managing the disease.

▶ Although literature is abundant on the role of family caregivers in caring for the frail elderly, especially patients with dementia, less is known about the family's role in the management of chronic diseases such as diabetes. This study adds to the body of literature, making it clear that regardless of the disease process, elderly spouses and adult children are involved in the care of elderly family members who are functionally disabled. It is important for health-care professionals to recognize this and to provide education and support and treat them as partners in the management of chronic diseases in the frail elderly.

S.K. Ostwald, Ph.D., R.N., C.S.

Cost-Effectiveness

A Pilot Study for the Development of a Hospital-based Immunization Program

Scarbrough ML, Landis SE (Mission–St Joseph's Health System, Asheville, NC; Mountain Area Education Ctr, Asheville, NC)
Clin Nurse Spec 11:70–75, 1997 6–15

Objective.—Immunization is one of the most effective, cost-effective, and underused methods of disease prevention. Results of a pilot study of a hospital-based immunization program for adults are presented.

Methods.—Baseline data gathered on 2 adult medical–surgical floors of the hospital showed a need for the following vaccinations: 44.9% of the 215 patients surveyed needed tetanus and diphtheria (Td) toxoids; 57.1% needed pneumococcal polysaccharide; 51.9% needed influenza virus; and 1.4% needed measles-mumps-rubella (MMR). The baseline rate of immunization before initiation of the immunization program was 2.6%. Two protocols were developed for administration of adult vaccines before discharge, and the staff was trained in their implementation. Three nursing units used a family nurse practitioner (FNP)-managed strategy, wherein

TABLE 2.—Immunization Rates in Intervention Study by Immunization Strategy

Characteristics	MD-managed (*N* = 821) *N* (%)	FNP-managed (*N* = 431) *N* (%)	*p* value
Patient vaccine status assessed	375* (46.0)	431	
No vaccine needed	78 (9.5)	180 (42.0)	
Vaccine needed†			
Any	272 (33.0)	201 (46.0)	
Td	228 (27.8)	140 (32.5)	
Pneumovax	123 (15.0)	135 (31.3)	
Rubella	12 (1.5)	3 (0.7)	
Measles	11 (1.3)	2 (0.46)	
Patients receiving vaccine (of those who needed vaccine)‡			
Any	10 (3.7)	69 (34.0)	<0.001
Td	7 (3.1)	42 (29.5)	<0.001
Pneumovax	5 (4.1)	43 (31.8)	<0.001
Rubella	0 (0)	1 (33.3)	
Measles	0 (0)	1 (50.0)	

*Incomplete assessments were frequent.
†Patients could need more than 1 vaccine.
‡Patients could receive more than 1 vaccine.
Abbreviations: MD, physician; *FNP*, family nurse practitioner; *Td*, tetanus-diphtheria.
(Courtesy of Scarbrough ML, Landis SE: A pilot study for the development of a hospital-based immunization program. *Clin Nurse Spec* 11[2]:70–75, 1997.)

the FNP reviewed charts, interviewed patients, and ordered the necessary vaccines. Three nursing units used an MD-managed protocol, which involved integrating immunization history and patient and staff education into the daily activities of doctors and nurses. Outcome was defined as administration of vaccines. Rates of vaccination were statistically compared after 3 months for both strategies.

Results.—Ten of 821 MD-managed patients received vaccines and 69 of 431 FNP-managed patients received vaccines (Table 2). The FNP-managed patients were significantly older than those in the MD-managed group. They also were more likely to be male, on Medicare, and have any of the following conditions: chronic heart disease, chronic obstructive pulmonary disease, or diabetes. However, they were less likely to have cancer than MD-managed patients.

Conclusion.—A hospital-based immunization program for adults before discharge is a cost-effective way to promote vaccination. Progressive vaccination and education programs should be encouraged.

▶ Although much attention has been devoted to the importance of immunizations for young children, the issue of adult immunization has been largely ignored. Most adults are unaware of their own immunization status, and the majority of adults over 70 have never received the initial series for tetanus and diphtheria (Td). This article reports an innovative, cost-effective way to promote immunizations by vaccinating patients before their discharge from the hospital. Although this approach will not be appropriate or acceptable for all patients, it still provides a useful adjunct to the current practice of outpatient immunizations, which misses the majority of the adult population.

S.K. Ostwald, Ph.D., R.N., C.S.

Randomized Clinical Trial of Chlorhexidine Versus Placebo for Prevention of Oral Mucositis in Patients Receiving Chemotherapy

Dodd MJ, Larson PL, Dibble SL, et al (Univ of California, San Francisco; Univ of Philadelphia, Pa)

Oncol Nurs Forum 23:921–927, 1996 6–16

Objective.—Patients receiving chemotherapy for cancer frequently have oral mucositis, a dose-limiting side effect. The effectiveness of a nurse-initiated systematic oral hygiene teaching program combined with the use of mouthwashes in preventing incidence, delaying onset, and reducing severity of chemotherapy-induced mucositis was tested.

Methods.—The nurse-initiated PRO-SELF:Mouth Aware (PSMA) program, a randomized, double-blind, placebo-controlled, clinical trial, provided either chlorhexidine or sterile water as mouthwash to 222 patients (68% female), average age 56.66 years. They were undergoing chemotherapy at 23 outpatient sites. Colon or breast cancer patients followed a daily mouth care regimen for 3 chemotherapy cycles. The Oral Assessment

Guide was used to evaluate oral health, and incidence, onset, and severity of mucositis were reported.

Results.—Eighty-nine patients (40%) did not complete the study, due mostly to the discontinuation of chemotherapy (n = 25), a dislike for the taste of the mouthwash (n = 12), or death (n = 14). There were no significant differences in the incidence, days to onset, or severity of chemotherapy-induced mucositis between the two mouthwash groups. The estimated incidence of chemotherapy-induced mucositis of 44% was reduced to 26%. Patients using chlorhexidine, at $20 per pint, did not demonstrate a significant effect in preventing mucositis when compared to those using sterile water as a mouthwash. Therefore, the same reduction in mucositis could be achieved using sterile water at a tremendous cost savings when multiplied by the 400,000 patients per year who develop oral cavity complications.

Conclusion.—This study suggests that the use of a systematic oral hygiene program may reduce the indicidence of chemotherapy-induced mucositis. When combined with sterile water mouthwashes, this represents a cost-effective treatment for prevention of mucositis in the outpatient setting. Research is now testing the effectiveness of the mouthwashes without the accompanying PSMA program.

Nursing Implications.—Nurses can offer patients the knowledge and skills they need to perform twice daily systematic assessements and oral care hygiene. Nurses should encourage their patients to use water as a mouth rinse to help reduce costs.

▶ Geriatric nurses can expect to encounter increasing numbers of older persons who are receiving chemotherapy. This article reports on a multisite, randomized clinical trial testing the effectiveness of a nurse-initiated oral hygiene protocol for patients receiving chemotherapy. The findings suggest that a sterile water mouthwash will prevent mucositis as well as a more expensive medicated mouthwash, thereby providing data that can save millions of health care dollars each year. It provides an award-winning example of clinical nursing research that can increase patient comfort and contain costs.

S.K. Ostwald, Ph.D., R.N., C.S.

Acute Stroke Care and Rehabilitation: An Analysis of the Direct Cost and Its Clinical and Social Determinants

Jørgensen HS, Nakayama H, Raaschou HO, et al (Bispebjerg Hosp, Copenhagen)

Stroke 28:1138–1141, 1997 6–17

Objective.—The costs of treating stroke patients have a significant impact on health care economics. Because most of the direct costs of treatment are incurred during hospitalization, the factors that contribute to

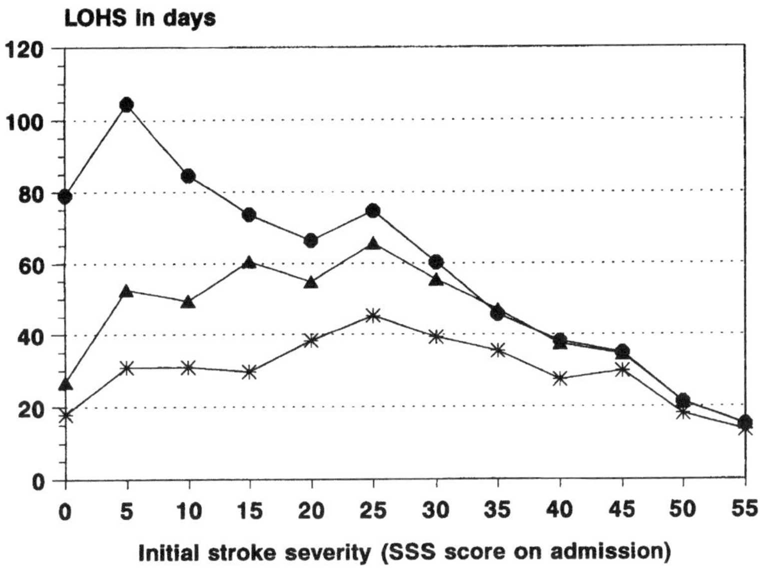

FIGURE.—Mean LOHS as a function of initial stroke severity as measured by the Scandinavian Stroke Scale score on admission. Shown are actual LOHS (▲), actual LOHS in survivors (●), and adjusted LOHS, actual LOHS minus time spent for nonmedical reasons (*). (Courtesy of Jørgensen HS, Nakayama H, Raaschou HO, et al: Acute stroke care and rehabilitation: An analysis of the direct cost and its clinical and social determinants. *Stroke* 28:1138–1141, 1997. Reproduced with permission of *Stroke*. Copyright 1997, American Heart Association.)

length of hospital stay (LOHS) were evaluated in an attempt to study more cost-effective treatment.

Methods.—Between September 1991 and October 1993, 1,197 consecutive stroke patients were enrolled in the Copenhagen Stroke Study. All patients received acute care and rehabilitation in the 63-bed stroke unit of Bispebjerg Hospital. Patients were discharged to go home or to a nursing home after rehabilitation and were evaluated clinically at 6 months. Total LOHS was recorded.

Results.—There were 250 deaths in the hospital. A total of 177 patients were discharged to nursing homes, and 770 were sent to their own homes. Mean LOHS was 37.4 days, with 27% of those days spent waiting for a place in a nursing home after rehabilitation. This adjusted LOHS (27.1 days) was used in subsequent calculations. Length of hospital stay was influenced by stroke severity, marital status, and death. When LOHS was stratified according to stroke severity, increasing stroke severity increased LOHS until a Scandinavian Stroke Scale score of 25 was reached. Then, the LOHS decreased as a result of increased mortality (Figure). Survival increased LOHS significantly by an average of 33.5 days.

Conclusion.—Treatment of stroke patients in a dedicated stroke unit takes 4 weeks on average and costs $12,150 per patient in Denmark. The only medical factor that significantly influences LOHS is stroke severity.

Reducing the cost of treating stroke involves reducing the severity of the initial stroke and speeding the rate of recovery.

▶ Stroke is the third leading cause of mortality and chronic disability in older persons in the United States and thus is a major health care cost. This interesting study from Copenhagen calculates the direct cost of acute stroke care based on the length of hospital stay. Surprisingly, comorbidity did not increase the hospital rehabilitation time. Although the severity of a stroke was the most important predictor, almost one third of the overall stay (10.3 days) was the result of factors related to posthospital care. The study supports the need for nurses and social workers to be involved in the care plan early in the hospitalization so that discharge planning issues can be addressed and resolved in a timely and appropriate manner. In our environment of cost-containment, too often patients are discharged with little advance planning and little education of family caregivers who assume most of the responsibility for home care.

S.K. Ostwald, Ph.D., R.N., C.S.

A Family Intervention to Delay Nursing Home Placement of Patients With Alzheimer Disease: A Randomized Controlled Trial

Mittelman MS, Ferris SH, Shulman E, et al (New York Univ; Columbia Univ, NY; New York State Psychiatric Inst)

JAMA 267:1725–1731, 1996 6–18

Objective.—Because the rate of deterioration of patients with Alzheimer's disease (AD) varies, caregiving can be a long-term commitment. Caregivers who want to delay placement of a loved one in a nursing home for as long as possible need a lot of support and assistance. Psychosocial intervention to prevent or postpone nursing home placement was provided in a randomized, controlled 3½-year study.

Methods.—In an outpatient clinic in New York City, 206 spouses of AD patients living at home and having at least 1 relative living in the area, were randomized to a control or treatment group. The treatment group received 2 individual and 4 family counseling sessions lasting 1–3 hours each. The sessions were provided within the first 4 months of enrollment and dealt with the following: task-oriented, problem-solving, and behavioral management techniques; family communication; and improvement of emotional and instrumental support of the primary caregiver. At the end of the 4-month period, caregivers were required to join a support group. Continuous counseling was made available to caregivers to deal with crises and with the changing nature and severity of the illness. The control group received no structured counseling but was offered the services usually provided to caregivers of AD patients. Time to institutionalization was the outcome measure.

Results.—Time to placement was 329 days longer for the intervention group than it was for the control group. Female caregivers were more likely to place their spouses in a nursing home than male caregivers were. Patients with lower incomes were more likely to be placed in nursing homes than were patients with higher incomes. Patients with more severe dementia were more likely to be placed in nursing homes. Patient age increased the risk of placement by 32% for every 10 years of patient age. An increase in caregiver symptoms of depression and reaction to the patient's behavior increased the risk of placement. After adjusting for caregiver sex, patient age, and patient income, caregivers in the intervention group were only 66% as likely as control group caregivers to place their spouses in a nursing home. The effect of intervention was most apparent for spouses who were mildly or moderately demented.

Conclusion.—Caregiver intervention programs can significantly delay nursing home placement of AD patients, particularly in the early or middle stages of the disease.

▶ It is well recognized that caregiving takes a physical and emotional toll on family members who are providing care at home. This excellent article takes a different approach to the issue by using life table methods with multiple time-dependent covariates to evaluate the effectiveness of a comprehensive intervention program that combines individual and family counseling with education and support group participation. Of particular interest are factors such as family income and gender that influenced the family's placement decisions. The issue of the degree to which the caregiver's enmeshment with the patient contributes to caregiver burnout and the decision to institutionalize the patient deserves additional attention and has implications for all health professionals caring for the frail elderly at home.

S.K. Ostwald, Ph.D., R.N., C.S.

Staff Training and Satisfaction

Staff Training and Turnover in Alzheimer Special Care Units: Comparisons With Non-Special Care Units

Grant LA, Kane RA, Potthoff SJ, et al (Univ of Minnesota, Minneapolis)

Geriatr Nurs 17:278–282, 1996 6–19

Objective.—Although staff in Alzheimer special care units (SCUs) require special training, there is little information on the availability of dementia-specific training programs. The specialized training in dementia care and turnover among licensed nurses and nursing assistants was evaluated for 124 Minnesota nursing homes.

Methods.—Personal interviews were conducted with education supervisory nurses and education coordinators in 400 nursing units. Intensity of dementia training was measured by training methods, training content, and staff categories trained. The index for training content was the total number of content areas included in training programs for each unit. The measure for staff categories trained were yes–no scores indicating whether housekeeping, food services, activity, and social services were included.

TABLE 1.—Comparison of SCUs and Non-SCUs on Selected Measures

	SCUs (n = 64)	Non-SCUs (n = 321)	Non-SCUs in SCU facility (n = 182)	Non-SCUs in non-SCU facility (n = 139)
Mean score on training methods (SD)	19.6 (5.8)	16.2 (6.9)	17.7 (6.1)	14.2* (7.4)
Percentage of units using training method:				
1. Licensed nursing staff attend outside workshops or seminars on dementia care	95.2	87.6	88.1	87.0
2. Films or videos are used by aides to learn about dementia care	98.4	89.4†	95.1	82.0
3. Outside consultants are used to give talks about dementia care during in-service training	90.6	84.4	90.7	76.3*
4. Reading materials about dementia care (e.g., newsletters or articles) are given to staff	93.8	81.6†	84.1	78.4
5. Films or videos are used by nurses to learn about dementia care	98.4	87.5‡	95.1	77.7*
6. A training manual about dementia care is used by licensed nursing staff	53.2	31.0*	41.2	18.0*
7. A training manual about dementia care is used by aides	46.8	27.5‡	37.3	15.1*
8. One or more in-house experts on behavior management work with staff on this unit to deal with difficult behaviors	98.4	89.3†	98.9	77.0*
9. In-house staff gives talks about dementia care during in-service training sessions	95.3	86.3†	94.0	76.3*
10. Role playing techniques are used to train aides about caring for residents with dementia	70.3	65.7	68.7	61.9
11. An orientation program about dementia care is provided to new staff coming onto the unit	78.1	69.8	73.6	64.7
Mean score on training content (SD)	7.8 (2.2)	7.2 (2.5)	7.5 (2.2)	6.8‡ (2.9)
Percentage of units offering training by content area:				
1. Information regarding dementia care	98.4	91.0†	95.1	85.6‡
2. Management of difficult behaviors	92.2	88.8	92.3	84.2†

3. Dealing with family or friends of residents with dementia	71.9	63.6	66.5	59.7
4. Mental health in elders	60.9	56.1	60.4	50.4
5. Normal effects of aging	90.6	90.3	91.8	88.3
6. Physical, cognitive, and behavioral changes associated with Alzheimer's disease/dementia	93.8	87.8	91.2	83.2†
7. Communication skills with dementia residents	95.3	87.9	92.9	81.3‡
8. Family support techniques for families of cognitively impaired residents	45.3	38.0	34.1	43.2*
9. Community resources for family/friends of cognitively impaired residents	54.7	34.9‡	42.9	24.5*
10. Death and dying	81.3	85.0	87.9	81.3
Mean score on staff categories trained (SD)				
Percentage of units offering training by staff category:	3.1 (1.2)	3.0 (1.4)	3.0 (1.3)	3.0 (1.5)
1. Housekeeping staff	77.4	72.6	71.4	74.1
2. Activities staff	92.2	84.1	90.1	76.3*
3. Social service staff	89.1	93.5	89.0	76.3‡
4. Food services staff	54.7	59.5	50.5	71.2*
Mean score on staff stability (SD)	7.9 (1.1)	7.5* (1.3)	7.6 (1.2)	7.2‡ (1.4)
Mean nursing assistant turnover (SD)	0.14 (0.20)	0.18 (0.23)	0.16 (0.17)	0.20 (0.30)
Mean licensed nurse turnover (SD)	0.08 (0.12)	0.10 (0.15)	0.09 (0.14)	0.11 (0.16)

*$P < 0.001$.
†$P < 0.05$.
‡$P < 0.05$.
Abbreviation: SD, standard deviation.
(Courtesy of Grant LA, Kane RA, Potthoff SJ, et al: Staff training and turnover in Alzheimer special care units: Comparisons with non-special care units. *Geriatr Nurs* 17:278–282, 1996.)

Staff stability was assessed based on consistency in nursing staff assignment and staffing patterns across shifts, units, and days.

Results.—Overall turnover rate among nurse assistants and licensed nurses was 17.0% and 9.4%, respectively. When SCU and non-SCU scores were compared, there were no significant differences (Table 1). Training methods varied considerably with low nursing assistant turnover, rural location, less staff stability, high licensed nurse turnover, high prevalence of dementia, and SCU facility predicting more diversity in training methods. Turnover rates among nurses was positively correlated with turnover rates among nursing assistants. Turnover among licensed nurses was especially high when turnover among nursing assistants was high. Low turnover for nursing assistants was predicted by low turnover among licensed nurses, more diversity in training methods, fewer units in the facility, and nonprofit ownership.

Conclusion.—Low turnover appears to be the result of training that increases the knowledge and skills needed to do the job and the presence of an SCU that decreases job stress by better management of problematic behaviors of patients. More diverse training methods can lower turnover and decrease staff stability, especially when a high proportion of residents have dementia.

Perceptions of Job Satisfaction in a Long Term Care Facility: A Comparison Between a Dedicated Alzheimer's Unit and Non-Alzheimer's Units

Hays AM, Dowling-Williams T (Regis College, Weston, Mass)

Am J Alzheimer's Dis 12:35–39, 1997 6–20

Objective.—It is understood that special care units (SCUs) provide advantages for patient care, but little is known about the job satisfaction of the SCU staff. The job satisfaction of nursing staff who work on SCUs and the staff who care for Alzheimer's patients in traditional skilled nursing care units were compared.

Methods.—Professional, paraprofessional, and temporary or agency nursing staff in a 332-bed skilled nursing care facility completed the Index of Work Satisfaction Tool (IWT) addressing areas of remuneration and benefits, autonomy, task requirements, organizational policies, formal and informal social and professional interaction, and professional status. Surveys were analyzed using univariate and bivariate statistical methods.

Results.—Of the 235 questionnaires distributed, only 61 could be evaluated. Approximately 75% of questionnaires were completed by staff working in general nursing home units, and 25% were completed by staff working on a SCU. Of the 61 respondents, 67% were paraprofessionals, 33% were professionals, 33% were age 17–28 years, and 33% were older than 40. Using a Z Matrix with weighting coefficients to rank the variables, pay and autonomy ranked the highest, and interaction and organizational policies ranked the lowest. Special care unit staff ranked profes-

TABLE 4.—Comparison of Job Satisfaction Components Between Alzheimer's Unit Staff and Non-Alzheimer's Unit Staff (N = 61)

	Alzheimer's unit staff N = 15	**Non-Alzheimer's unit staff N = 46**
Interaction		
Mean	5.28	4.70
SD	0.69	1.11
t = −1.92 p = 0.06		
Professional Status* Mean		
SD	5.95	5.41
t = −1.28 p = 0.03	0.77	0.85
Organizational Policy*		
Mean	3.95	3.11
SD	0.98	1.24
t = −2.47 p = 0.02		
Autonomy		
Mean	4.75	3.95
SD	1.11	1.45
t = −1.94 p = 0.06		
Tasks		
Mean	3.46	2.99
SD	1.00	1.15
t = −1.39 p = 0.17		
Pay		
Mean	3.61	3.06
SD	1.10	1.57
t = −1.27 p = 0.21		
Total IWS*		
Mean	13.92	11.97
SD	1.97	2.42
t = −2.83 p = 0.006		

*Significant variables.

(Courtesy of Hays AM, Dowling-Williams T: Perceptions of job satisfaction in a long term care facility: A comparison between a dedicated Alzheimer's unit and non-Alzheimer's units. *Am J Alzheimer's Dis* 12:35–39, 1997.)

sional status, interaction, organizational policies, and autonomy as the most important factors influencing job satisfaction. The mean scores of Alzheimer's unit staff were significantly higher than those of non-Alzheimer's unit staff on professional status, organizational policy, and total IWST (Table 4).

Conclusion.—Job satisfaction scores for SCU staff were significantly higher than they were for staff in non-Alzheimer's units. Study results argue for additional research into determinants of job satisfaction for nursing staff in long-term care, development of recruiting and retainment programs, importance of professional status, interaction, and organizational policies for SCU staff.

► As turnover rates in nursing homes soar and recruitment becomes more difficult, the nursing home's ability to guarantee consistent high quality care is compromised. Previous research has suggested that organizational policies and perceived autonomy are related to job satisfaction and that job satisfaction is related to lower turnover rates. The two studies summarized here (Abstracts 6–19 and 6–20) compare the staff satisfaction and turnover rates between Alzheimer Special Care Units (SCU) and Non-Special Care Units. While the authors use different methodologies in different geographical regions of the country, they find greater satisfaction and lower turnover rates in SCUs. Both articles have important implications for organizational policies and staff education. Readers may also wish to consult the article by Mistretta and Kee for further discussion of organizational and educational strategies that may improve staff job satisfaction and resident care in SCUs.[1]

S.K. Ostwald, Ph.D., R.N., C.S.

Reference

1. Mistretta EF, Kee CC: Caring for Alzheimer's residents in dedicated units: Developing and using expertise. *J Gerontol Nurs* 23:41–49, 1997.

Subject Index

A

B

D

E

F

G

H

J

K

L

N

O

Q

R

S

T

U

V

Author Index

A

B

C

D

E

F

G

H

I

J

K

L

M

N

O

P

R